The Innovation and Evolution of Medical Devices

S. Abbas Shobeiri
Editor

The Innovation and Evolution of Medical Devices

Vaginal Mesh Kits

Springer

Editor
S. Abbas Shobeiri
INOVA Health System
Falls Church, VA
USA

ISBN 978-3-030-07298-8 ISBN 978-3-319-97073-8 (eBook)
https://doi.org/10.1007/978-3-319-97073-8

Softcover re-print of the Hardcover 1st edition 2019

This Springer imprint is published by the registered company Springer Nature Switzerland AG
The registered company address is: Gewerbestrasse 11, 6330 Cham, Switzerland

On behalf of my contributing authors, we would like to dedicate this work to patients and those who share their journeys with them.
This book is our attempt to understand and appreciate the perspective of each entity involved in the production and utilization of a medical device. We pledge to continue our journey together to improve the process to achieve the creation of zero harm medical devices.
To my trainees, I can teach you things. But the important thing, the only important thing, how to listen, how to see things through the patients' eyes, how to feel their sorrows, how to have unconditional empathy and compassion, should have started at home long before you met me. Be humble and always practice evidence-based innovation that places patients' well-being first and foremost.
Lastly, this book is dedicated to my family, the most and the only important thing.

Preface

In the distant past, when there were no antibiotics and surgeons were mere glorified barbers, trials and chronic catastrophes were part of a surgeon's existence. It was not unusual for a gynecological surgeon to perform 30 vaginal fistula procedures and to have all fail. From today's ethical point of view, we look at past experimentations on patients and marvel at how barbaric they were only 100 or 200 years ago. While preoccupied with surgical success in the absence of antibiotics and anesthesia, these surgeons increased patients' suffering. James Marion Sims—whose statue was recently taken down from New York City's Central Park, whose disgrace caused the American Urogynecologic Society to retire the annual lectureship in his name, and who was every gynecologists' hero—experimented on slave women "given" to him by their owners at Sims' expense to find a cure for vesicovaginal fistula. In his day what Sims did was perhaps noble and heroic. There were no medical standards, laws or regulations to motivate Sims to behave otherwise. Just as the concept of consent was different in Sims' time and now, future generations will look at us in amazement at how we failed on multiple levels by allowing what they would view as practical experimentation with medical devices that lacked appropriate design or adequate scientific evidence for their use. The experimentations with medical devices today is much different than the experimentations that surgeons performed 200 years ago. While the motivation of the surgeon has always been to simply cure disease, the motivation of a medical device innovation process is much more complicated and culminates in a modern corporation's fiduciary responsibility to the shareholders. The experimentations still go wrong despite many advances over the past 200 years, advances such as more refined ethical standards, evidence-based medicine, regulatory processes from the US Food and Drug Administration, and local hospital peer review and safety initiatives.

Although in this book we use vaginal mesh kits as a case study of a nearly failed gynecological product, the failed medical device corollaries can be found in any organ system from cardiac stent to orthopedic hardware. This book aims to understand the process of medical device approval and to examine why years after a product is approved, the device is withdrawn from the market for either lack of efficacy or for causing harm to the patients. The bar for approving medical devices is being raised everyday constantly moving. With recent loosening of some regulatory processes in an attempt to bring lucrative manufacturing jobs to the United States, patients and the health care system in general may pay a hefty toll in exchange. Once a medical device has hit the market, investors are anxious to reap the benefits, and there is simply no incentive to perform efficacy trials. The product is sold to as many and as quickly as possible before the device is inevitably withdrawn from the market and litigation ensues.

In the face of financially driven medical innovation and loosening federal and local regulations, there remains evidence-based medicine, taught in medical schools, as the only hope for patient safety. Although medical societies have taken some leadership to demand hard data by creating registries and sponsoring randomized controlled trials to protect their patients, the fee-for-service system rewards physicians who use the devices the most. While double-blind studies such as those performed for drugs may be seen as difficult for medical devices, it is imperative for us to change the way we approve and oversee medical devices if we are to achieve zero harm to our patients. Furthermore, the current system rewards the quantity of procedures performed, not the quality of patient outcomes. We need more robust monitoring and demand for improved outcomes data by the insurers.

Historically, medical devices were produced by the industry and "consumed" by the surgeons and hospitals. The medical device industry has had a better price-to-earnings ratio with 23–25% operating margin compared to other major stock market indices. The current changes in technology and the development of new disruptive frontiers have resulted in the breakup of well-entrenched industries, value chains, and value-creating strategies. Technological advances have made the metamorphosis of commercial models possible, favoring centralized purchasing, contracting, and call points.

This book discusses the disruptive forces that will determine the medical device industry's direction in the near future. Although it is estimated that market forces will greatly decrease the value generated by each dollar for the research and development of new medical devices, the forecast depends on shifting from a fee-for-service to a value-based healthcare model. This book discusses medical device innovation, the regulatory process, and the ethics of medical device marketing in detail and adds the largely lost patient perspective. The book emphasizes the fact that the sectors that produce, approve, and utilize medical devices operate with a silo mentality and not necessarily in the patients' best interest. The system should change such that innovators, industry, regulators, physicians, patients, and hospitals communicate in a way that improves patient outcome and eliminates suffering by utilizing evidence-based medicine principles while enhancing the product life cycle and go-to-market strategies that are in the interest of the investors.

Falls Church, VA, USA S. Abbas Shobeiri

Contents

Contributors

Pakeeza A. Alam Section of Female Pelvic Medicine and Reconstructive Surgery, MedStar Washington Hospital Center, Departments of Obstetrics/Gynecology and Urology, Georgetown University School of Medicine, Washington, DC, USA

Jonia Alshiek, MD, MSc Department of Obstetrics and Gynecology, Gynecologic Subspecialties, Inova Women's Hospital, Virginia Commonwealth University, Falls Church, VA, USA

Tel Aviv Sourasky Medical Center, Sackler Faculty of Medicine, Tel Aviv University, Tel Aviv, Israel

Elizabeth T. Brown, MD, MPH Department of Urology, MedStar Georgetown University Hospital, Washington, DC, USA

Laura Chang-Kit, MD Department of Urology, Albany Medical Center, Albany, NY, USA

Roberta N. Clarke, MBA, DBA Health Care Management Program, Questrom School of Business, Emeritus Boston University, Boston, MA, USA

Roger R. Dmochowski, MD, MMHC Department of Urology, Vanderbilt Medical Center, Nashville, TN, USA

Tanaz Ferzandi, MD, MBA, MA Division of Urogynecology and Pelvic Reconstructive Surgery, Department of Obstetrics and Gynecology, Tufts Medical Center, Boston, MA, USA

Farzeen Firoozi, MD Center for Female Pelvic Medicine & Reconstructive Surgery, The Arthur Smith Institute for Urology, Northwell Health, Lake Success, NY, USA

Zucker/Northwell School of Medicine of Hofstra University, Hempstead, NY, USA

Howard B. Goldman, MD Glickman Urological and Kidney Institute, Cleveland Clinic, Cleveland, OH, USA

Cheryl B. Iglesia, MD Section of Female Pelvic Medicine and Reconstructive Surgery, MedStar Washington Hospital Center, Departments of Obstetrics/Gynecology and Urology, Georgetown University School of Medicine, Washington, DC, USA

Melissa R. Kaufman, MD, PhD Department of Urology, Vanderbilt Medical Center, Nashville, TN, USA

Katrina Knight, PhD Department of Medicine, School of Medicine, University of Pittsburgh, Pittsburgh, PA, USA

Neeraj Kohli, MD, MBA Boston Urogynecology, Newton-Wellesley Hospital/ Brigham and Women's Hospital, Wellesley, MA, USA

Department of Obstetrics and Gynecology, Harvard Medical School, Boston, MA, USA

Rui Liang, MD, MSc Department of Obstetrics, Gynecology and Reproductive Sciences, University of Pittsburgh, Pittsburgh, PA, USA

Vincent R. Lucente, MD Department of Obstetrics and Gynecology, St Luke's University Health Network, Bethlehem, PA, USA

Pamela Moalli, MD, PhD Division of Urogynecology and Pelvic Reconstructive Surgery, Department of Obstetrics, Gynecology and Reproductive Sciences, Magee-Womens Hospital of UPMC, Magee-Womens Research Institute, University of Pittsburgh, Pittsburgh, PA, USA

Miles Murphy, MD, MSPH The Institute for Female Pelvic Medicine and Reconstructive Surgery, North Wales, PA, USA

Sherrie J. Palm Association for Pelvic Organ Prolapse Support, Mukwonago, WI, USA

Bruce Patsner, MD, JD Department of Obstetrics and Gynecology, Virginia Commonwealth University School of Medicine, Richmond, VA, USA

Quality and Patient Safety, Inova Fairfax Women's Hospital, Falls Church, VA, USA

Department of Obstetrics and Gynecology, Inova Fairfax Women's Hospital, Falls Church, VA, USA

Ghazaleh Rostaminia, MD, MSc Female Pelvic Medicine and Reconstructive Surgery NorthShore University Health System/University of Chicago, Skokie, IL, USA

S. Abbas Shobeiri, MD, MBA, FACS, FACOG, CMPE INOVA Health System, Falls Church, VA, USA

Michael Ting, MD Division of Minimally Invasive Gynecologic Surgery, Department of Obstetrics and Gynecology, St Luke's University Health Network, Bethlehem, PA, USA

Chapter 1
Introduction: Why a Case Study of Vaginal Mesh Kits?

S. Abbas Shobeiri

A vaginal mesh kit representative walked into my clinic and declared that I was a "thought leader," and, as such, he wanted me to use his vaginal mesh kit product because, once I had done a certain number, I could lecture on the subject and go around and proctor others how to do it. As a brand-new assistant professor of obstetrics and gynecology, I did not think of myself as a thought leader, and, since he did not know anything about me, I was not sure what brought him to the conclusion that I was a thought leader. When people compliment you in ways that are disingenuous, it is wise not to accept their compliment and instead wonder what their motives are. This was the first time that I was seeing a vaginal mesh kit. I held it and inspected it. I politely asked for safety data, and he said that it has been used successfully in Europe and that a major publication on its use will be coming soon. Plus, he said not to worry: the device is approved by the US Food and Drug Administration (FDA). I was not familiar with the FDA 510(K) process, which allows a premarket submission made to FDA to demonstrate that the device to be marketed is at least as safe and effective—that is, substantially equivalent—to a legally marketed device (21 CFR §807.92[a][3]) that is not subject to premarket approval. I did not understand much about the FDA process back then and again politely asked for the FDA studies that led to the approval of the device. As physicians, we are used to double-blind, randomized studies that drug companies are expected to perform before marketing their drugs, and I expected a similar publication for the vaginal mesh kit sitting on the desk in front of me. The representative stated that the mesh had been used for hernia repairs for years, and the trocars were similar to those used in tension-free vaginal tape devices (Fig. 1.1). As such

S. A. Shobeiri
INOVA Health System, Falls Church, VA, USA
e-mail: Abbas.shobeiri@inova.org

S. A. Shobeiri (ed.), *The Innovation and Evolution of Medical Devices*,
https://doi.org/10.1007/978-3-319-97073-8_1

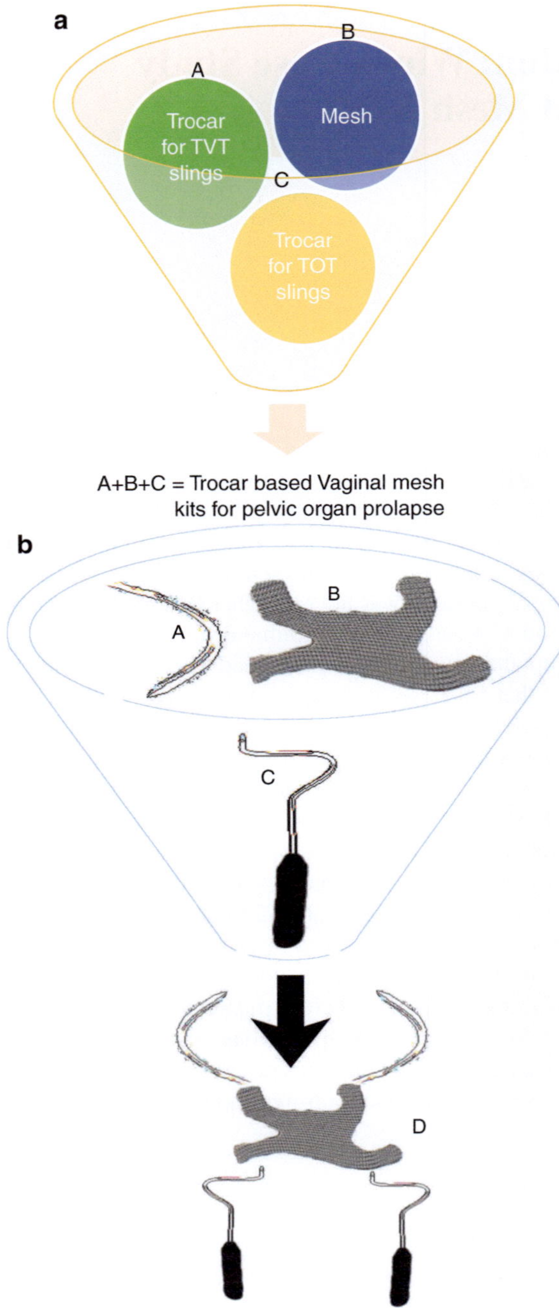

Fig. 1.1 The genesis of various vaginal mesh kits via the FDA 510 K process. Three already approved devices, **A**, tension-free vaginal tape (TVT) trocar, **B**, mesh, and **C**, trans-obturator tape (TOT) trocar, were put together to create a new untested device, **D**, the vaginal mesh kit. (**a**) Schematic of the conceptual process. (**b**) Schematic assembly of these products into new products. By minor changes to the trocars and mesh, different companies rushed to benefit from this new market. (© Shobeiri)

no randomized trials were necessary, and the device was approved based on existing safety data.

I found his response very curious and confusing. I stated that as a member of an academic institution, we would be happy to use the device in research setting. Otherwise, we will wait for the publication before using the device. He asked me to please use it once just to see how it feels. I said it felt OK in my hands, but I could not use it without evidence. I said again that we will be happy to use it in a clinical research setting if the company is willing to fund the research. He countered again that the device is FDA-approved and does not require further investigations. I asked a series of questions: What is the incidence of bladder injury? What was the incidence of rectal injury? Was the device associated with other adverse outcomes such as pain? What would happen to the mesh in my patient's body in 10, 20, or 50 years? Would the mesh shrink like the abdominal meshes? Would it not become contaminated in the course of introduction through the vagina? The representative was rather irritated and left, stating that there was no reason I should not use the device, that it was absolutely safe, and that I was doing a disservice to my patients.

Thinking back, I am proud of that moment and the moments like that when I remembered evidence-based medicine from my medical student days and did not fall prey to pressure tactics by various industry representatives who either threatened to take my business to the competition or tried to wine and dine me. I may not have been a "thought leader," but I was an assistant professor of anatomy, and my thesis was on pelvic floor muscles and neuroanatomy. The vagina is not like abdominal hernias. It is not static. It is more like the human mouth. It is a functional organ that is associated with ordinary activities such as urination, defecation, and sexual intercourse that we take for granted except when they don't work any longer and women become miserable.

Pelvic floor dysfunction patients are some of the most grateful patients on the planet. The surgeon reconstructs the anatomy, returning function to the appreciative patient. To my astonishment, the vaginal mesh kit representative who had come to my office went on to market his device to the community obstetrician/gynecologists and urologists by telling them that a "thought leader" (me!) had held the device and said it felt good. In the years to come, some companies did fund limited "multicenter" studies, during which our site performed a limited number of cases. We later discovered that these studies were never meant to be submitted to peer review for possible publication but were meant to introduce the devices to high-value hospitals and surgeons. None of the studies we participated in were published. Generally, once the quota of five or ten study cases were completed, the representative would ask if the surgeon wanted to continue using the vaginal mesh kit. Very quickly, I observed first hand adverse effects that were alarming. Recurrent prolapse, pain, pudendal neuralgia, recurrent bladder infections, and voiding and defecatory dysfunction to name a few.

When I told the representatives that my personal experience was contrary to what they were reporting from Europe, they did not have any advice. In patients with recurrent prolapse, they would give advice like "Place another kit in the same compartment." In patients with pain, they would say, "Let's wait and see." I invariably removed such symptomatic mesh quickly and performed old-fashioned repairs. To this day I lose sleep about my patients who were asymptomatic but are walking around with vaginal mesh kits like ticking time bombs, their bodies incorporating mesh that can erode into their rectum or bladder and extrude into vagina. My solace is that I performed only a few number of these cases.

As time passed it seemed there were more and more companies entering the market with variations on the theme of the vaginal mesh kit (see Fig 1.1b) [1]. They each had different needles, mesh, and route for introduction. I started seeing other occasional vaginal mesh complications. I recommended that my partner write a case report. Three months later, I recommended to another partner to write a case series because now we had more cases. The reports started pouring from all across the country. A few years later, we looked at the referral patterns of vaginal mesh complications and realized the patients were not referred to us by their surgeon [1]. The surgeons did not know what to do and the patients would find us via word of mouth.

By early 2010, a major portion of our patient volume seemed to be taking care of vaginal mesh kit complications. I wondered what compelled other physicians to perform vaginal mesh kit procedures. Why were they not directly referring the patients with complications to us? What was I to do with the horrendous complications no other surgeon had ever seen before? Why weren't the companies concerned enough to sound the alarm? What was the role of the government in this? Were these complications just limited to my geographic locale because the surgeons were so bad?

It turned out that it was not the surgeons who were bad. The vaginal mesh kit was undergoing contraction and freezing the function of the bladder or rectum. The mesh arms were irritating the major nerve going to the pelvis. To use an analogy, the vagina is a functional organ similar to the human mouth. It would be inconceivable for an oral surgeon to place mesh in the mouth or place mesh next to the trigeminal nerve that supplies the whole face. If they did, the risks would be pain, migraines, nerve paralysis or irritation, inability to eat or drink, and a life of constant misery. No one would consent to such an oral procedure, so why did the vaginal mesh kit industry make such a device? Why did so many doctors implant the vaginal mesh kits? And how did so many women consent to the procedure? The "medical device Swiss cheese systematic failure" to protect patients was becoming rapidly evident as the reports of complications were made public (Fig. 1.2). In many ways the failure of mesh kits represented a perfect storm where failure occurred at multiple levels concurrently (Fig. 1.3):

Level I: Failure of innovation, ideation, and industry (Fig. 1.4)
Level II: Failure of regulation (FDA)
Level III: Failure of medical school education, evidence-based medicine, professional societies, and postgraduate education (Fig. 1.5)
Level IV: Failure of local regulations—hospital credentialing of the product, physician peer review, patient consenting, and education (Fig. 1.6)

The complications were being reported from all across the United States. Many of my surgeon colleagues whom I respected and believed did not report any complications arising from their own vaginal mesh kit placements, but they did report

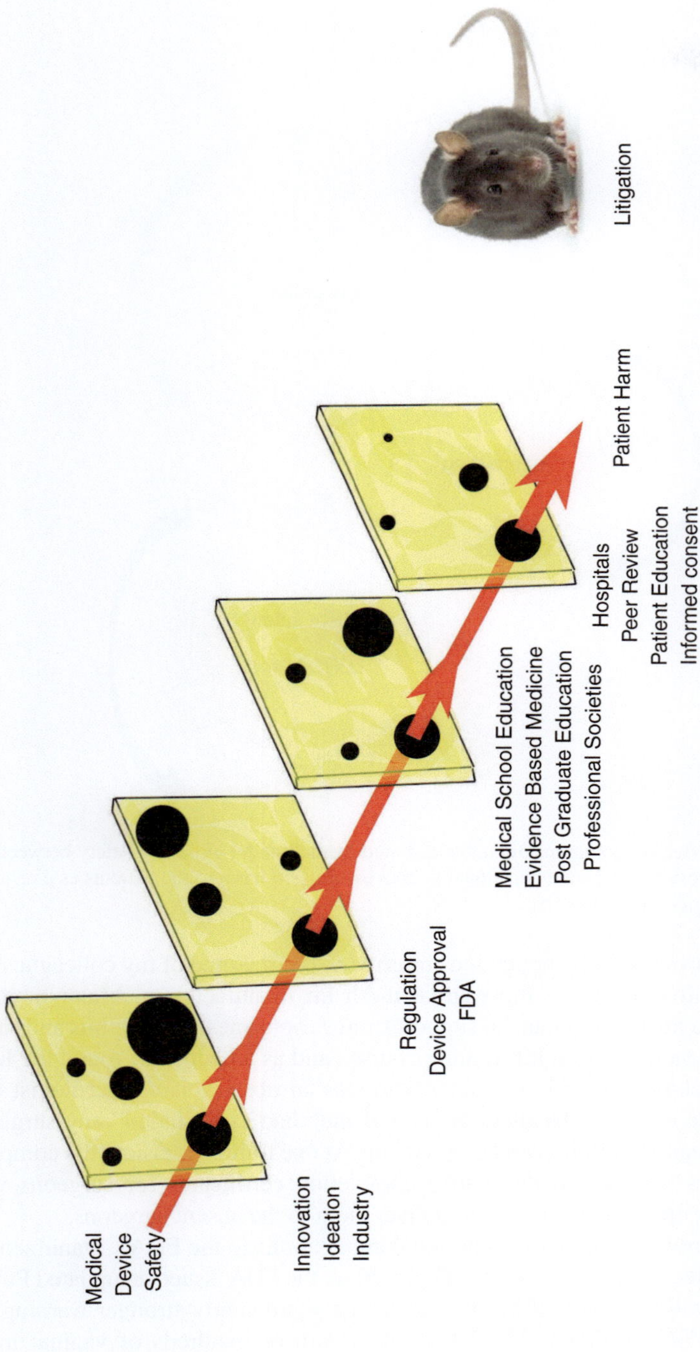

Fig. 1.2 Schematic of the medical device failure Swiss cheese theory. The layered human processes that are meant to create security are like slices of cheese with holes. When the holes in each process line up just perfectly, a medical device hazard passes through all layers of defenses and causes patient harm. Ideally, weaknesses in one process is stopped by additional layers of security, and patient harm is not materialized. (© Shobeiri)

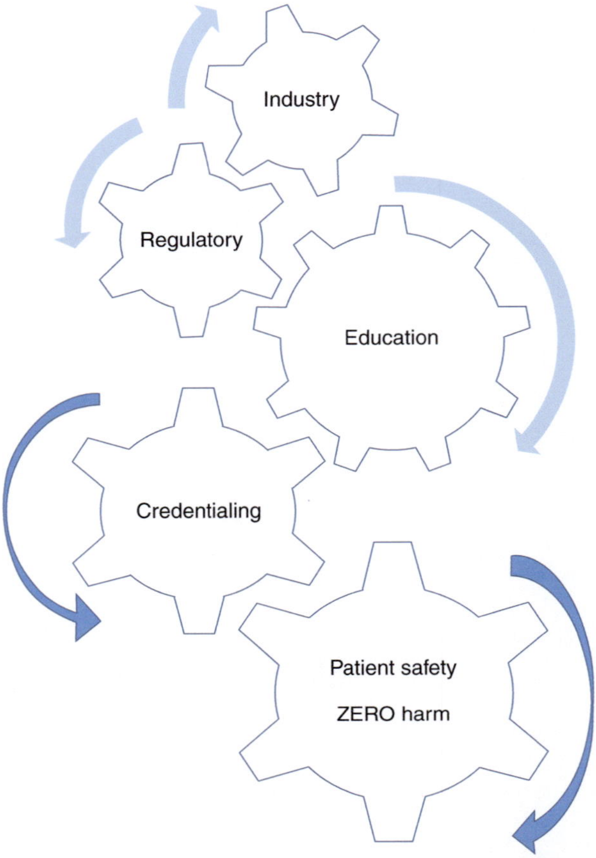

Fig. 1.3 Only effective communication and a shared mental model of patient safety between the industry, regulatory bodies, and educational system assure *zero* harm to the patients as a result of new medical devices. (© Shobeiri)

having seen horrendous complications referred to them. Some of my colleagues felt comfortable advertising for the vaginal mesh kit manufacturers. Major national meetings were flush with financial support from various mesh kit exhibits and funding. I went to vaginal mesh kit training courses and as an educator found the level of training lacking. I asked the trainer who was an obstetrician/gynecologist colleague and the company business director if they had ever "failed" any surgeons during their years of training, and they said no. At one training session, the company representatives were given the course completion certificates for surgeons who failed to show up so they could hand deliver them to the absent surgeons.

With the growing number of reported complications to the FDA's Manufacturer and User Device Experience (MAUDE) database, the FDA issued an updated Public Health Notification in July 2011 and included a significantly stronger warning for transvaginal POP mesh kits [2]. I had taken care of hundreds of vaginal mesh

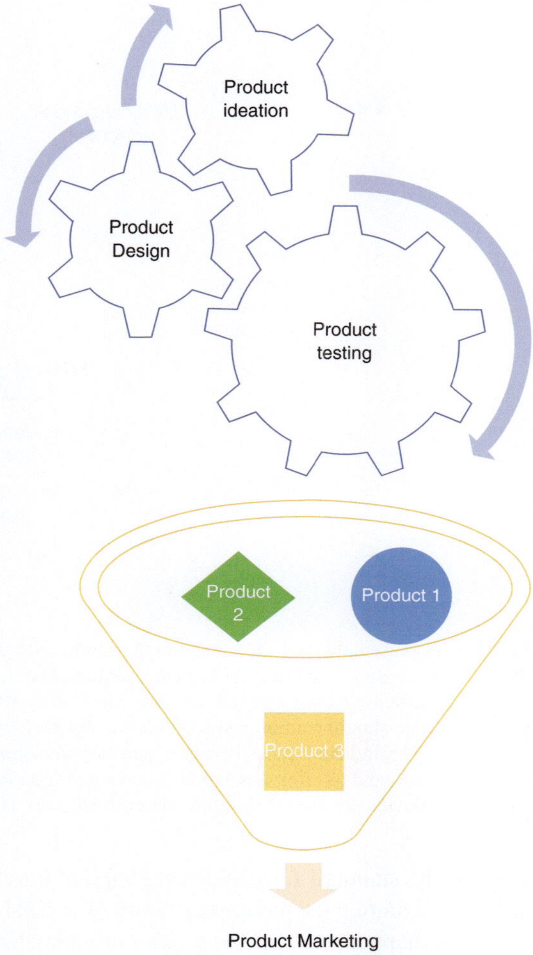

Fig. 1.4 Schematic of the innovation and ideation process that leads to marketing of new products. Each product can have unintended consequences if it is not tested in its intended environment. The term product testing in the setting of medical devices is broad and generally has been taken as biomechanical testing. Medical devices should undergo rigorous long-term, double-blind randomized trials to demonstrate safety and efficacy. (© Shobeiri)

complications before the FDA warning from MAUDE database came out. Neither I nor any of my other partners had reported cases to MAUDE because we were simply ignorant of the process. If it were true that not all surgeons and hospitals were reporting vaginal mesh kit complications, I knew the magnitude of the problem was much larger than the mere 1000 cases in FDA MAUDE database. I wondered about the ethics of marketing medical devices that were untested and how such an occurrence could have been allowed. I knew I was witness to multiple levels of systematic failure: the failure of medical education, of industry, and of government oversight, and the patients suffered because of it (see Fig. 1.2).

In an effort to see what was happening to the vaginal mesh kits, we drove innovation using ultrasound to better localize and treat vaginal mesh kit complications. It was shown that ultrasound was superior for diagnosing vaginal mesh complications [3]. We presented our findings at various meetings, and 3D pelvic floor ultrasound

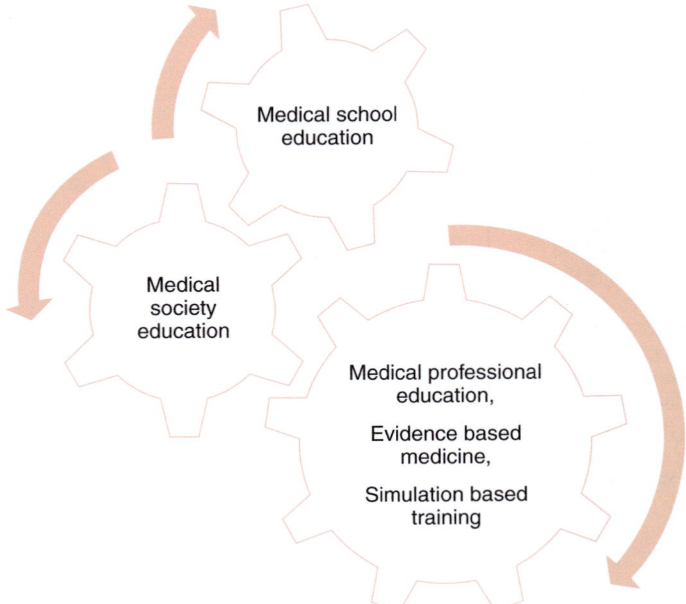

Fig. 1.5 Representation of the educational system with parts working together. It is imperative that evidence-based evaluation skills and the critical thinking that are taught in medical schools are carried to medical practice and reinforced by the CMEs offered by the medical societies. A physician in practice should continuously ask for the highest level of evidence before using a new medical device. The industry should partner with the societies to perform the necessary safety and efficacy studies and to offer simulation-based training to the membership after the safety and efficacy of the device are proven through randomized trials. (© Shobeiri)

became the standard for visualizing vaginal mesh [3]. The ultrasound was invaluable in elucidating the pathophysiology of vaginal mesh complications and in showing what happens to the mesh after implantation [4]. Surgically, some patients improved after mesh removal, while others had major nerve injuries and scarring that were not curable [4]. We all tried to understand what was happening, and some of us felt we could not be content with half the truth. The missing half of the truth was that only industry knew the total number of vaginal mesh kits sold, and our half of the truth was that we could extract how many vaginal mesh kit complications had occurred. To this date the denominator of how many vaginal mesh kits were sold has not been released by the industry; thus the prevalence of vaginal mesh kit complications can only be estimated. The only available estimate is from FDA for 2010. FDA market data from manufacturers indicated that in 2010 approximately 300,000 women underwent surgical procedures in the United States for POP. According to the FDA, approximately one-third (100,000) of POP surgeries used mesh, and of those, three-fourths (75,000) utilized vaginal mesh. The mean rate of vaginal mesh complications from the literature is 14.5% [2]. Combining these data, it can be estimated that 10,875 patients had complications due to vaginal mesh procedures for

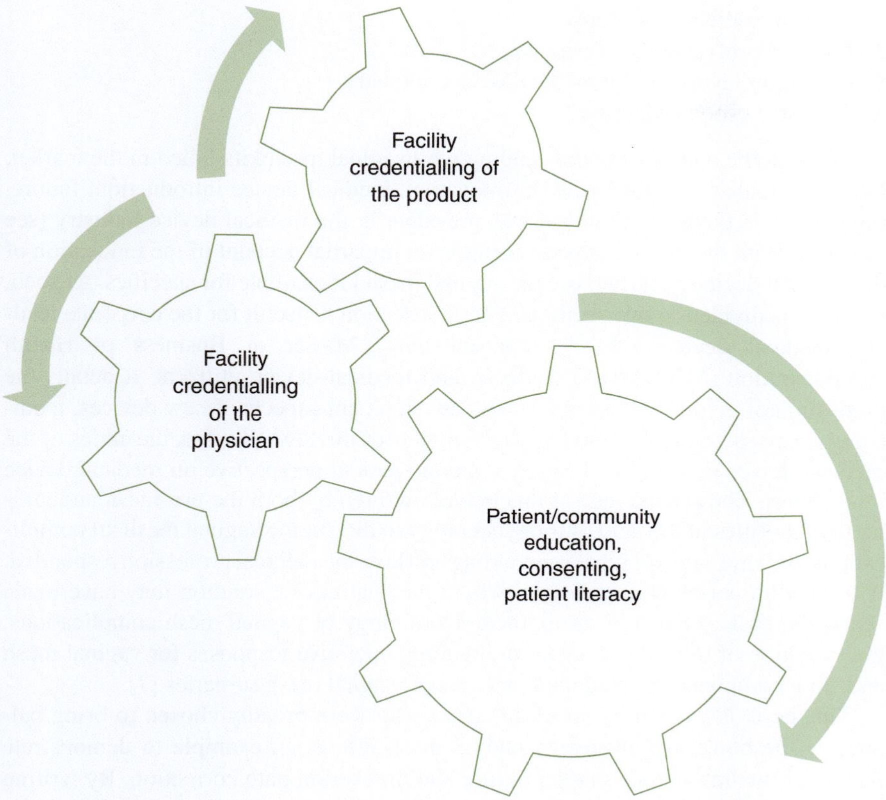

Fig. 1.6 Schematic of last safety mechanisms. The hospitals should not utilize a device that has not been proven efficacious and safe in patients through randomized trials. The physicians should undergo independent education and evaluation separate from the industry to assure evaluation integrity. The patients should be offered up-to-date and comprehensive counseling on the risks, benefits, and alternatives to the new medical device being utilized. The physician should recount honestly how many times they have performed a particular procedure and what their personal outcome has been in their cohort. (© Shobeiri)

POP in 2010 alone [5]. Almost 11,000 patient harms per year should have been enough to sound the alarm in any other industry. Multiplying this number of harms by all the years that the vaginal mesh kits were sold underscores the enormity of the problem and begs for solutions so that such a grave failure does not happen again.

In May 2014, the FDA proposed to reclassify surgical mesh for transvaginal POP repair from class II devices to class III, thus requiring increased safety and efficacy data for mesh kits prior to FDA approval [6]. This reclassification was based on the tentative determination that the previously used mechanism of approval was not sufficient to provide reasonable assurance of safety and effectiveness for this device.

The product failure was followed by:

1. Governmental regulatory response

2. Medical societies' response
3. Medical professionals' response
4. Litigation involving the medical device industry
5. Industry response/defense

Through the course of understanding why vaginal mesh kits failed in the market, I came to realize that the cycle of innovation, medical device introduction, failure, litigation, and device withdrawal was prevalent in the medical device industry (see Fig. 1.2). With this book I hope to compile an impartial account of the innovation of the medical device cycle and use the vaginal mesh kit example for specifics. As such, the book is divided in two sections. The first section is useful for the corporate leaders, medical device industry representatives, Master of Business or Health Administration (MBA/MHA) students, and medical device utilizers. It details the innovation of medical devices, business development aspects of new devices, medicolegal aspects of medical devices and a review of the FDA process, the ethics of the medical device industry, and finally a unique patient perspective on medical device innovations. The second half of this book is written by both the pro-mesh and anti-mesh authorities in the field of urogynecology to dissect the vaginal mesh kit complications as a case study of what went wrong and how the medical profession responded. It starts with pertinent anatomy on why a medical device solution may have made sense, the basic science of mesh, the epidemiology of vaginal mesh complications, the evolution of ultrasound for mesh imaging, operative responses for vaginal mesh and sling complications, and the outcomes of vaginal mesh surgeries [7].

This book is written by various experts who were broadly chosen to bring balance to the book. We are using vaginal mesh kits as an example to demonstrate phases of medical device market failure and innovation path correction. By writing this book, I hope to create a resource for the medical industry representatives, corporate and hospital leaders, surgeons, medical students, and MBA or MHA students and to confer enhanced understanding of the medical device innovation and marketing process by addressing the concepts from all perspectives. In the long run, I hope that my efforts will eliminate the patient safety hazards created by unsafe and poorly tested medical devices that may be marketed in the future.

References

1. Rostaminia G, Shobeiri SA, Quiroz LH, Nihira MA. Referral pattern for vaginal mesh and graft complications to the University of Oklahoma Pelvic and Bladder Health Clinic. J Okla State Med Assoc. 2012;105(9):356–8.
2. Murphy M, Holzberg A, Raalte HV, Kohli N, Goldman HB, Lucente V, Pelvic Surgeons Network. Time to rethink: an evidence-based response from pelvic surgeons to the FDA Safety Communication: "UPDATE on Serious Complications Associated with Transvaginal Placement of Surgical Mesh for Pelvic Organ Prolapse". Int Urogynecol J. 2012;23(1):5–9.
3. Manonai J, Rostaminia G, Denson L, Shobeiri SA. Clinical and ultrasonographic study of patients presenting with transvaginal mesh complications. Neurourol Urodyn. 2016;35(3):407–11.

4. Javadian P, Quiroz LH, Shobeiri SA. In vivo ultrasound characteristics of vaginal mesh kit complications. Female Pelvic Med Reconstr Surg. 2017;23(2):162–7.
5. Javadian P, Shobeiri SA. The disability impact and associated cost per disability in women who underwent surgical revision of transvaginal mesh kits for prolapse repair. Female Pelvic Med Reconstr Surg. 2017. https://doi.org/10.1097/SPV.0000000000000489. [Epub ahead of print].
6. U.S. Food and Drug Administration. Reclassification of urogynecologic surgical mesh instrumentation. Executive Summary. Gastro-entrology-Urology Medical Devices Advisory Committee Panel. 26 Feb 2016.
7. Paul M, Littman D, Patrick J, Culligan M. The rapid evolution of vaginal mesh delivery systems for the correction of pelvic organ prolapse, Part I: clinical data. Female Patient. 2009;34:32–8.

Chapter 2
The Innovation of Medical Devices

S. Abbas Shobeiri

Introduction

Innovation in medical device industry doesn't require inventing something completely new. From an entrepreneurship perspective, it may involve applying the already available idea or product in a new setting or in a new "innovative" manner. In such an environment, (1) swift release of new medical devices and services backed with (2) scientific support of key opinion leaders, followed by (3) robust clinical education of practitioners in the field, with (4) clear communication of problems and flaws to the designers while (5) building and protecting brand equity and value, forms the five pillars of successful medical device launch.

From patients' point of view, they want a safe and effective procedure that will allow them to return to their normal activity quickly. From the operator/surgeons' point of view, they yearn for a device that is safe and efficient for the patient, that accomplishes the task quickly, and that is tied to fair compensation for their time and effort. Society looks for medical devices that decrease the cost to the society by either simplifying the existing procedures or by creating new solutions to old or unsolvable problems. As such, innovation may be significantly influenced by the patients, the care providers, the doctors, the payers, the policymaking groups, and the manufacturers or suppliers who can all effect real-world healthcare decision-making.

Once a device is ready to be released to the market, then the company has to tackle the country-specific regulatory requirements which are in place to protect the patient safety and guarantee the efficiency of the local markets. This is a fundamental

S. A. Shobeiri
INOVA Health System, Falls Church, VA, USA
e-mail: Abbas.shobeiri@inova.org

S. A. Shobeiri (ed.), *The Innovation and Evolution of Medical Devices*,
https://doi.org/10.1007/978-3-319-97073-8_2

bottleneck in time and cost for any medical device or biomaterial-based therapy [1]. Forces behind medical and specifically device innovation, the methods of disruptive innovations, the patenting process, and the marketing and economic considerations along with general regulatory considerations will be the focus of this chapter.

Factors That Determine Success or Failure of Medical Devices

In their paper on avoiding pitfalls on the road from original idea to certified product, Wieringa et al. state that "innovation in medical technology is a critical chain of events, ideally leading to an improved situation for patient and staff as well as a profit for the supplier of the innovation. Many innovative ideas are not successful in practice" [2]. This may be frequently because of lack of the following elements [3]:

- Relevance: Is the product needed in the market?
- Validity: Is the device based on sound technical principles?
- Reliability: Does the device function as intended?
- Ease of use: Is the device designed such that to reach maximum number of users?
- Robustness: Is the device designed such that it can withstand usage in the field?
- Compatibility: Is the device designed to withstand local factors such as heat, dust, fluids, and the other devices?
- Foolproof: Has the device been analyzed for improper handling to prevent use not according to intended purposes?
- Compliance: Has the device been designed in compliance with local regulatory affairs, pricing policies, and reimbursement criteria of health insurance organizations?

Ultimately, the majority of promising innovations are not effective in practice. Distinctive factors that govern the success of new medical devices are described in Table 2.1 [3]. In the case of pelvic organ prolapse, it takes a specialist at least 15 years of combined schooling and training to be able to perform the complex procedures that are done either vaginally or laparoscopically. The vaginal mesh industry tried to disrupt this process by creating easy to perform vaginal mesh prolapse surgeries that could be done by the vast army of general obstetrician/gynecologists and urologists, some of whom had never performed such procedures and were acutely unfamiliar with the anatomy.

Vaginal mesh kits constituted a "converging technology" that crossed borders between already established medical devices. Converging technologies may combine medical devices, pharmaceutical products, or human tissues. The medical products may be from the same or different categories [4]. Such convergent technologies may be both more acceptable to the users and more adaptable to a niche in the marketplace. However, such technologies are generally not viewed as breakthrough technologies. Bringing different technology silos with different processes together to create a convergent product requires communication. Members of a multidisciplinary team may simply lack the language to communicate with each

Table 2.1 Factors determining success or failure of medical devices [3] as applied to vaginal mesh kits

Factors determining success or failure of medical devices	Vaginal mesh kits
Relevance	The issue of pelvic organ prolapse is highly relevant to society because it is prevalent and bothersome to women. The vaginal mesh kits were designed to solve a real-life problem
Validity	The vaginal mesh kits were not validated as a single product. The initial studies performed in France used existing mesh and trocar material and did not take into account the basic properties of the mesh and whether or not it could be used in the vagina. This is an example of how sloppy validation of manufacturing processes, technical principles, and software issues can be very costly in the long run. Many vaginal mesh kit manufacturers went out of business. The validation process goes beyond device design. The instruction for use (IFU) package inserts in vaginal mesh kits failed to alert the physicians of the device dangers
Reliability	It seems that the engineers who put the vaginal mesh kits together had minimal or zero knowledge of the environment for which the product was intended. The mesh arms were placed next to the neurovascular structures that created short- and long-term pain and management dilemmas. The placement of the vaginal mesh kits were easy but came at the cost of disregard for relevant anatomy. The reliability of the vaginal mesh kits were shown to be "off" in various anatomical studies. The kits could not be placed in the same place reliably. The only "alarm" for incorrect device placement was the patient symptoms of pain, recurrent prolapse, or erosions and extrusions
Ease of use	The manufacturers stressed ease of use, as their customers were mostly inexperienced physicians. The devices were single-use disposable products. The training of physicians generally included a dinner outing followed by a quick cadaver lab/didactics and award of a training certificate. To our knowledge, no physician has ever "failed" a vaginal mesh training course. The physicians would return to their home institutions with a certificate of training that rendered the hospitals powerless, and they had no choice but to award the physicians the requested vaginal mesh kit surgery privileges
Robustness	There was almost no basic science testing of vaginal mesh kits as to how they would respond and perform in the intended vaginal environment. Mesh was originally intended for the *abdominal* wall, and groin hernia surgeries implanted deeply so as to minimize the exposure risk
Compatibility	There were never any robust studies before vaginal mesh was introduced to the market. To this day surgeons are seeing delayed reactions and unanticipated problems unique to the vaginal environment. Investigations of incidents would have shown that in many cases seemingly unimportant details such as mesh fiber diameter, weave, and anchoring method can cause huge effects. Changing from one mesh weave to another that may not withstand the forces will have huge differences in device function. The vaginal mesh needs to be tested in the human body for long periods of time to determine unforeseen problems

(continued)

Table 2.1 (continued)

Factors determining success or failure of medical devices	Vaginal mesh kits
Foolproof	"Foolproofness" of a device depends not only on appropriate device design but also on the education of the users. For a device to be foolproof, it requires intensive and meticulous education of the end user in regard to appropriate placement and anatomical knowledge
Compliance	Manufacturers in the United States traditionally seek the US Food and Drug Administration (FDA) 510(k) premarket approval process, by which a new device demonstrated to be "substantially equivalent" to a previously legally marketed device can be "cleared" by the FDA for marketing with some controls, but without the need for clinical trials. The industry rushed the products to the market. The R&D costs for vaginal mesh kits were minimal, as the manufacturers chose the 510(k) process

other. There is usually a lack of methodical feedback among the end users, buyers, inventers, and manufacturers of equipment [5].

After a device manufacturer bridges the divide between an idea and a certified product, the clinical introduction stage will prove if and how the projected innovation performs in widespread use in the harsh clinical environment. In developing medical devices, a thorough knowledge of human factors is perhaps more important than the technological know-how and expertise.

The Forces Behind Disruptive Device Innovation

Medical device innovations are socially relevant. Disruptive innovations are market-driven because of [6]:

- *Increasing demand for healthcare services*. Demographic changes such as aging, immigration, and increased or decreased births change the overall healthcare needs.
- *Increasing demand for higher efficiency*. While the numbers of procedures and patients have been increasing, the number of physicians delivering services has remained relatively constant. Primary care physicians see more patients and the surgeons do more procedures in the same amount of time.
- *Increasing empowerment of the patient*. Healthcare consumers are more educated. The libraries of the world are now at the fingertips of any individual with a cell phone. The chances are that the patient has consulted "Dr. Google" before reaching out to a provider for the problem. Most often, the patients go beyond that and present to the provider with a requested solution.

- *Increase in the effect of market forces*. The healthcare landscape is ever changing with new regulations, new payment models, and healthcare delivery models. A device choice may entirely depend on quality, safety, and innovative use of available resources.

Companies with mature and productive market positions may benefit from improvements of existing products rather than truly new disruptive innovations that disturb their own markets, challenge their recognized position, and at times render their hard-earned production facilities without utility [3]. Frequently, "market-driven" research will find industry-funded "curiosity-driven" innovation more risky. This mindset of maintaining a company's dominance in certain categories and not paying attention to the alternatives leaves the door open to the competition creating new markets (seeking the "blue ocean" [7]) for their products. Alternatively, companies with market dominance may purchase and buy out the emerging technologies to maintain status quo.

A blend of curiosity-driven and market-driven inventions creates a balanced portfolio for a company [8]. Medical innovation flourishes in the watershed of clinical (physicians and nurses) and academic (scientists, engineers, and human factors experts) confluences. Curiosity-driven, high-risk products are often developed with support from government grants or angel investors who are willing to sustain high risk.

Innovations That Disrupt the Market

Christensen et al. argue that disruptive innovations are generally simpler products that are all the customers really need [9]. Good examples of these are the Toyota Corolla, which couldn't even climb hills upon its introduction into the US market. Detroit carmakers did not take this threat seriously, but this simple car appealed to a large segment of the population and improved each year to create a niche market. Another example are the complicated disk operating system (DOS) computers. The customers were eager to use the computers, but they were difficult to use. The introduction of Apple computers overcame this barrier. Disruptive innovations are generally simpler, more convenient, and less costly offerings initially designed to appeal to the low end of the market. Figure 2.1 illustrates this dynamic [9]. The *top Green arrow* depicts the speed of technological sustaining innovations, the enhancements an industry creates as it introduces new and more progressive products to serve the more sophisticated customers at the high end of the market. The shaded area is the degree of improvement the market can absorb over a specified time period [9]. The *bottom red arrow* depicts the innovations that appeal to the lowest end of the market and over time become more sophisticated to appeal to the middle and the high end of the market. Because the sustaining innovations nearly always outperform even the dimensions of the most demanding customers, and because the existing market leaders want to meet and exceed the demands of the most demanding customers, there is a window of opportunity to introduce lower- or higher-performance products.

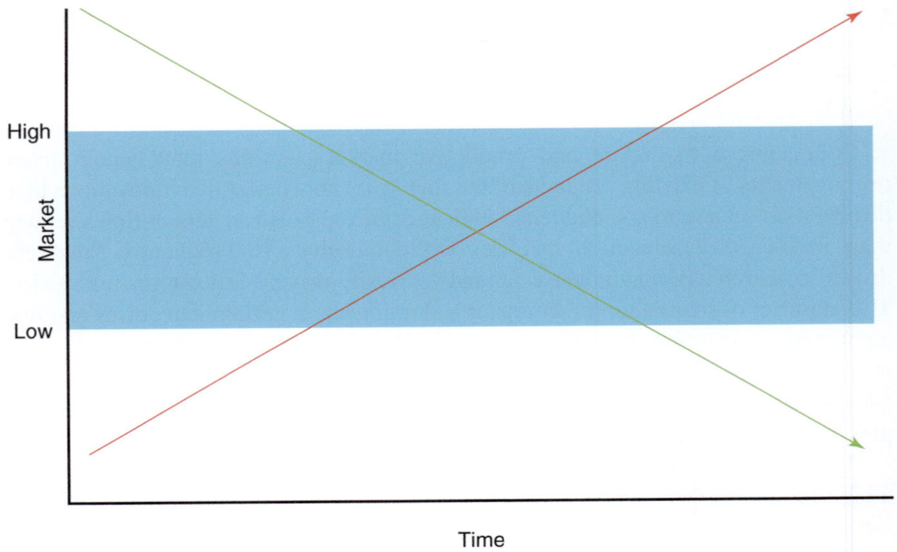

Fig. 2.1 The progress of disruptive innovation. (© Shobeiri)

If one views the performance of a physician as a product that is time dependent, it generally takes 13 years of higher education for a general surgeon to be board-eligible or in other words to have minimum performance criteria. A surgeon with 20 years of experience generally outperforms a younger colleague. The exception to this is when a new surgeon boosts their performance with new technology. For example, while cardiothoracic surgery was the standard for many years, invasive cardiologists took the major part of this market by utilizing technologically superior stents that did not require major surgeries performed by cardiothoracic surgeons.

Similarly, major healthcare institutions such as medical schools, general hospitals, specialist physician groups, and research organizations have overdelivered on the level of care actually required to keep the vast majority of patients healthy. But at the same time industry creates demands in the areas previously untapped. While our medical education system has churned out specialists and subspecialists with extraordinary capabilities, new markets, such as erectile dysfunction in men and demand for zero postoperative pain, have overburdened the system. In developing world countries, most conditions that afflict patients are emergencies and relatively straightforward disorders such as diabetes and hypertension whose diagnoses and treatments most often do not even require physician expertise. In the United States, the high number of patients asking for newer and more advanced surgical treatments, coupled with miserable reimbursement to the primary care physicians, has left the door open for mid-level providers such as nurse practitioners and physician assistants to serve the primary care markets, while the primary care physicians have been fleeing these markets in search of more profitable business models [9].

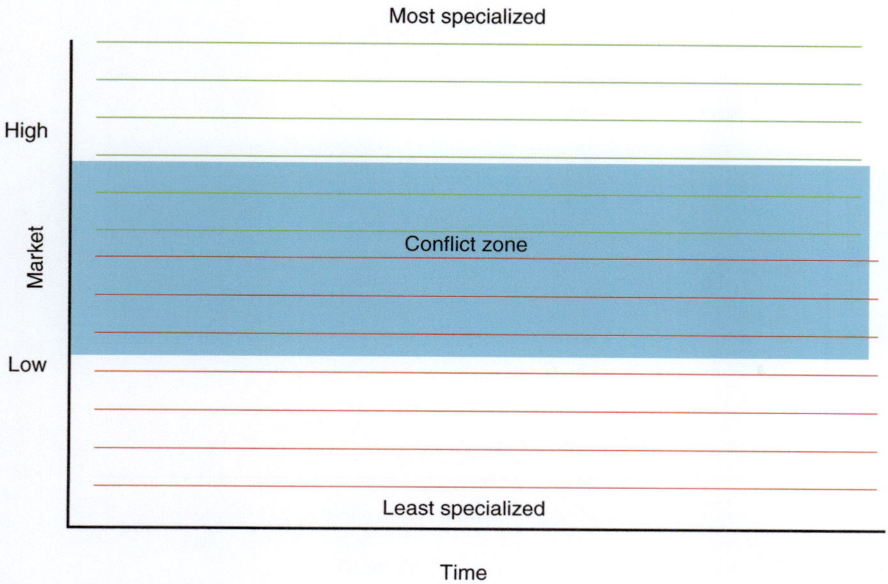

Fig. 2.2 Disruptions of healthcare professions. (© Shobeiri)

Similarly, in the medical device industry, the industry may profit from a larger population of less skilled people to perform in a more convenient, less expensive way tasks that previously were only performed by more expensive specialists in centralized and inconvenient locations [9]. The industry actively searches for the "blue ocean" opportunities to create solutions from the least to most complex solutions that can be addressed by self-care and telemedicine to highly specialized care offered only at major hospital settings. By simplifying the procedures such that they can be done in the office setting in a more convenient and cost-effective way, physicians can provide new innovative disruptive technologies. Figures 2.2 and 2.3 suggest how disruptive innovations might transform healthcare markets [9].

In many ways the vaginal mesh companies attempted to disrupt the practice of urogynecologists as the highly trained professionals that provided highly specialized care. Pelvic organ prolapse surgeries were traditionally performed by highly trained and skilled individuals who were mostly fellowship trained in urogynecology/female pelvic medicine and reconstructive surgery (FPMRS). Vaginal mesh kit manufacturers sought to recruit these specialists as the "thought leaders," with the intention of marketing the device to the larger community of general obstetrician/gynecologists and urologists. The majority of these physicians had never done vaginal reconstructive surgeries before being approached by the vaginal mesh kit salesmen. One of the strategies commonly employed to entice the academic physician was to offer them the opportunity to participate in multicenter studies. Each center was asked to recruit five to ten patients, and after the enrollment was complete, they would be asked to continue using the device clinically while waiting for the results

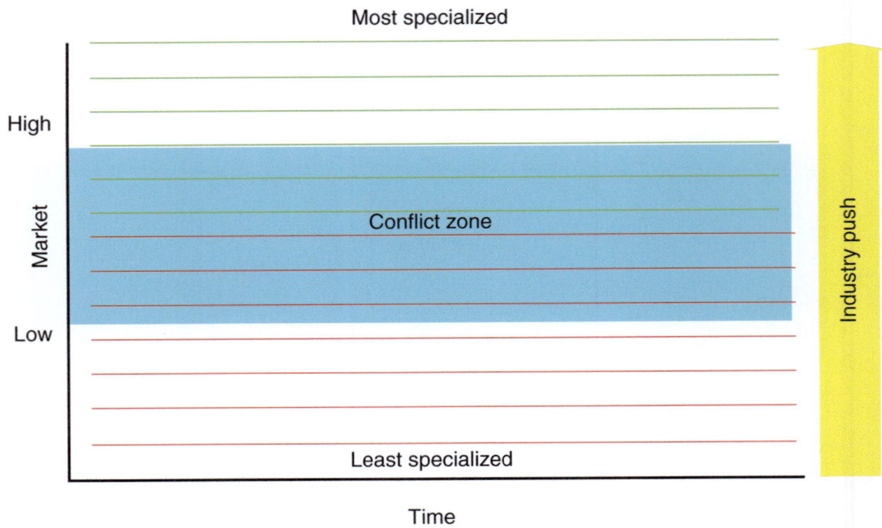

Fig. 2.3 Disruptions of healthcare institutions. (© Shobeiri)

of the study to be published. Most of these studies were never published. Meanwhile, even if the academic surgeon did not continue to use the device clinically, their names would be used in the community as the "thought leader" who has used or endorsed the device.

Additionally, with the industry focus on creating procedures that were easily done as simple outpatient procedures, with cheaper devices and equipment, the expense of performing pelvic organ prolapse surgeries would be less since surgeries would shift from the teaching hospitals to outpatient surgery centers.

Innovations of medical devices continuously transform pockets of the healthcare system and bring about higher quality, greater convenience, and lower cost [9]. After the introduction of the tension-free vaginal tape (TVT) system, the TVT-Secure TM (Gynecare, Ethicon, Somerville, NJ, USA) was introduced as a procedure that aimed appeal to a larger number of surgeons. The traditional sling procedure that used patients' own tissue was associated with a high complication rate and was dreaded both by the physicians and the patients. Not many of these surgeries were done, while a large number of women suffered from urinary incontinence. By utilizing a less expensive and effective technology, urogynecologists were now able to treat urinary incontinence in a less costly and more efficient manner. When care is multifaceted, costly, and troublesome to obtain, many afflictions simply go untreated.

Because the innovation of medical devices, although socially necessary, is entirely economically driven, and because of multiple medicolegal debacles involving past medical devices in addition to seemingly reputable studies that were designed to show the value of a product and were later discredited, seasoned physicians are understandably not early adapters of the new entrepreneurs' technology. Novice physicians, on the other hand, may be early adapters, using the new technology as a marketing tool to gain market share. Such physicians invariably become entangled in lawsuits involving untested products and learn to become more hesitant and cautious over time. There is a push in medical schools to teach students and residents to use evidence-based medicine that improves marketing and practice bottom line. Also, there is more recently an emphasis in medical schools to teach students how a product is patented and brought to the market.

The Patenting Process

The patent owner, in principle, has the exclusive right to prevent or stop others from commercially exploiting the patented invention. Patent protection dictates that the invention cannot be commercially made, distributed, imported, used, or sold by others without the patent owner's consent. The patent process generally occurs early on at the concept and design stage [10]. Patents are territorial rights, and exclusive rights are applicable only in the region or the country in which a patent has been granted and filed, in accordance with the law of that region or country [11].

- Rationale for patents
  - Publicly revealing how something works in exchange for a limited monopoly
  - New patents build on prior patents, enhancing technological innovation
- Requirements
  - New (not publicly known, published)
  - Inventive (nonobvious)
  - Useful (practical for any use)
- Right to exclude
  - Typically, 20 years from date of filing
  - Rights may be sold, licensed, etc.
  - Bayh-Dole Act (1980)—US P.L. 96-517
    - Allows universities/hospitals to commercialize inventions derived from federal funds
    - Must share royalties with the inventor
    - Government maintains "march-in" rights

(Figs. 2.4 [12], 2.5 [11], 2.6 [11], 2.7 [13], and 2.8 [10]), (Table 2.2) [11]

The Economic Perspective

In the case of vaginal mesh kits, physicians and patients did not have enough data to assess the efficacy of the new mesh kits advertised to them by the new mesh kit producers or multinational conglomerates that were the major medical equipment manufacturers. Hospitals constantly look for ways to trim medical expenditure. The

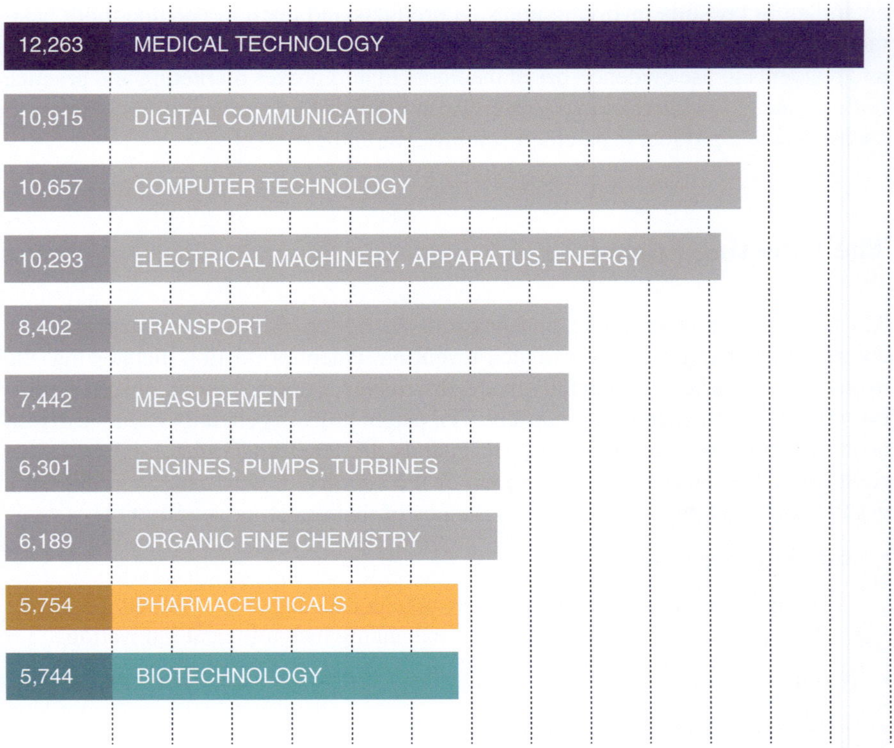

Fig. 2.4 Top ten technical fields in patent applications. Number of patent applications filed with European Patent Office (EPO), 2016 (EPO, MedTech Europe calculations. Medical technology as defined by World Intellectual Property Organization (based on the World Intellectual Property Organization IPC-Technology concordance as revised in August 2014). European countries refer to EU + Norway, Switzerland. Patents are attributed by the country of residence of the applicant.) (From MedTech Europe [12], with permission)

number one expense for hospitals is labor followed by supply chain management. What has been done traditionally by specialists, if simplified, can be done by generalists, and what was done by physicians in general, if simplified, can be now done by the nurses and so on. Yet, this constant down-marketing has not decreased the US gross domestic product (GDP) expenditure on healthcare. The savings from such equipment and personnel innovations does not necessarily translate to better care for the patients. It has resulted in more top-heavy hospital management, healthier instrument manufacturer stocks, and flat physician salaries, but it has not resulted in less healthcare spending.

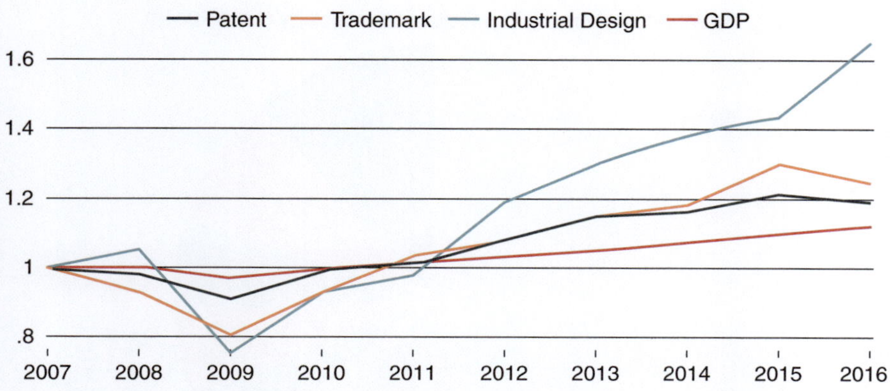

Fig. 2.5 Internet protocol (IP) filings and economic growth (set first available year to 1) in the United States 2007–1016 (From World Intellectual Property Organization (WIPO) [11], with permission)

The Valley of Death for Medical Device Development

In the research and development (R&D) process, between the stage in which the government predominantly invests (fundamental research) and the stage in which industry predominantly invests (commercialization of reliably profitable products)) lies technology's "valley of death" (Fig. 2.9) [14, 15]. That's the gap where private investment markets fail to finance the research needed to support the so-called "platform" technologies. This investment failure occurs because generic technologies are either expensive or risky or both for industry to develop the product on its own. Ironically, it is these platform technologies that are the seed corn for new devices and products and, in many cases, entire new market categories [15, 16].

Prior to becoming commercially available in the market, a medical device must first achieve a set of standards and comply with regulations designated by its class. Class I, II, or III device classification is based on risk of the device and the level of control needed to insure efficacy and safety [1] (Fig. 2.10) [17].

Low-risk devices are designated Class I and are subjected to general controls only. Conversely, most implants are considered high-risk Class III and are subject to the most complete and stringent standards. They are granted a preliminary investigational device exemption (IDE) to use the device in a US Food and Drug Administration (FDA)-regulated clinical trial in order to assemble required safety and efficacy data needed to justify safe introduction to markets [1].

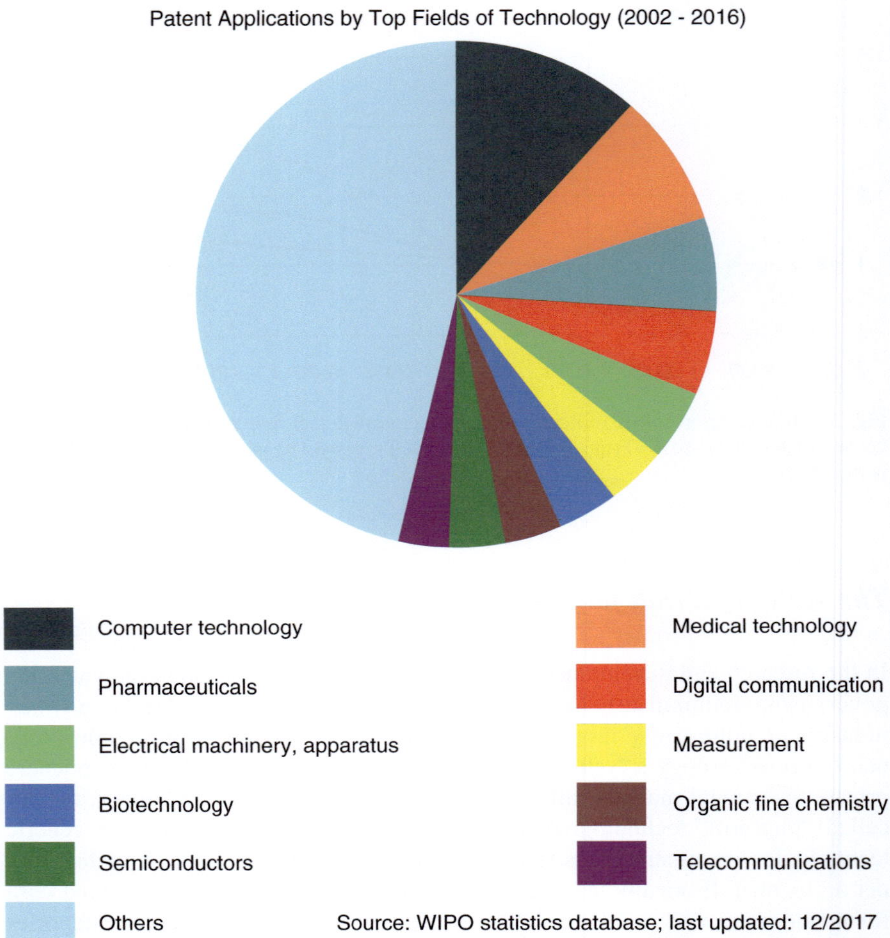

Fig. 2.6 Patent applications by top fields in technology in the United States (2002–2016) (From World Intellectual Property Organization (WIPO) [11], with permission)

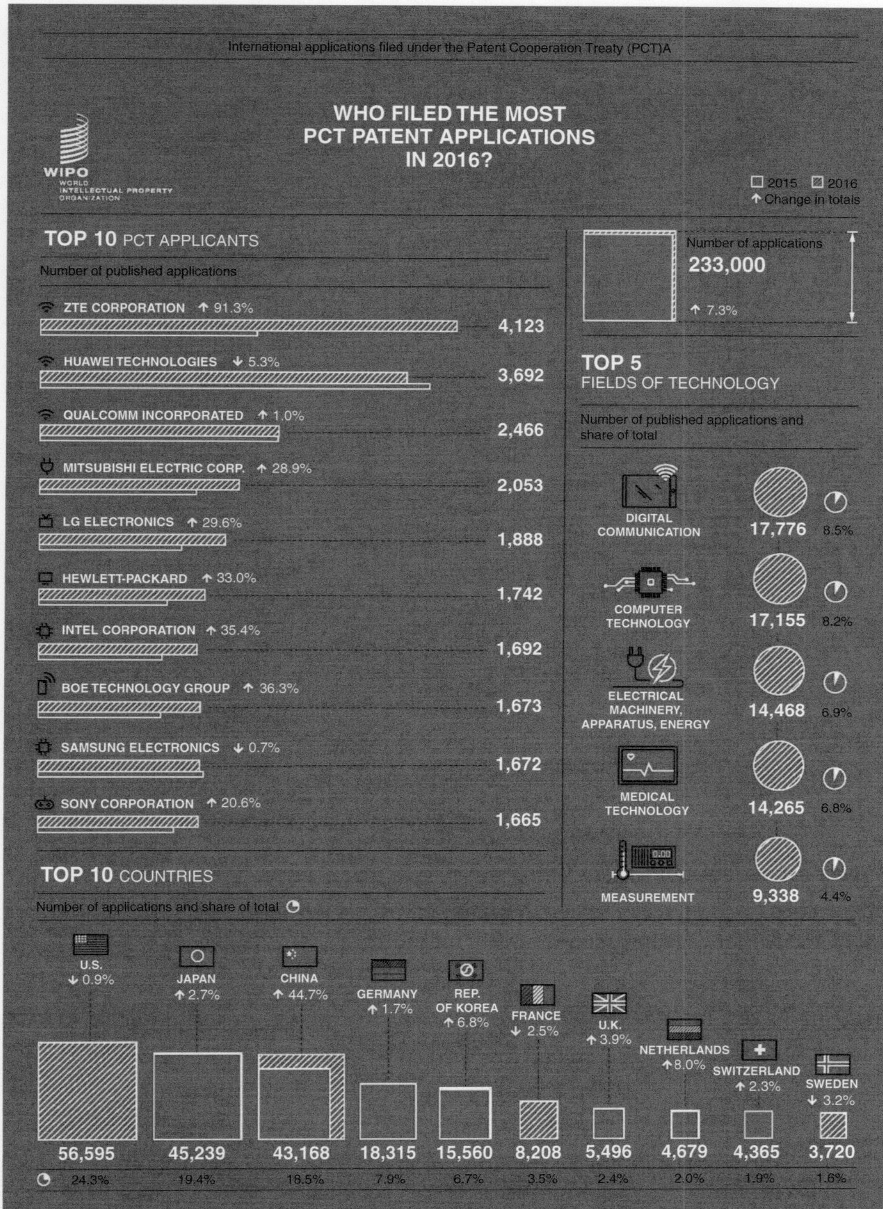

Fig. 2.7 International applications filed under the Patent Cooperation Treaty (PCT) 2016 (From World Intellectual Property Organization (WIPO) [13] with permission)

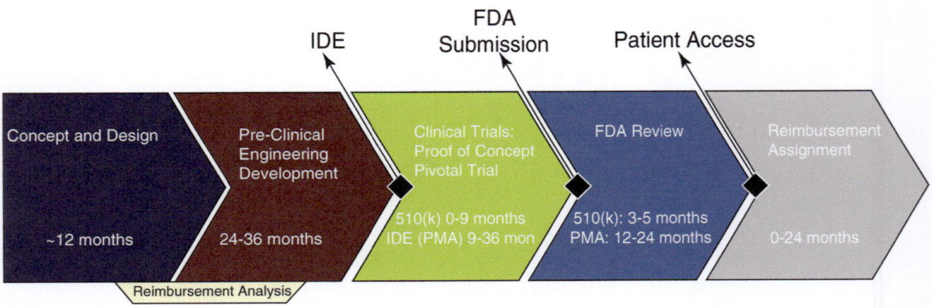

Fig. 2.8 US Food and Drug Administration (FDA) medical device regulatory approval process

Table 2.2 Patent Cooperation Treaty (PCT) top patent applicants in the United States (Publication year = 2016)

Applicant	Publication	Rank
Qualcomm Incorporated	2446	3
Hewlett-Packard Development Company, LP	1742	6
Intel Corporation	1692	7
Microsoft Technology Licensing, LLC	1528	12
Halliburton Energy Services, Inc.	1097	19
3M Innovative Properties Company	653	27
Procter & Gamble Company	624	28
Google Inc.	584	30
Apple Inc.	450	33
General Electric Company	434	35

From World Intellectual Property Organization (WIPO) [11], with permission

Investigation of R&D from Biomaterials Laboratory to the Preclinical Facilities

There are many organizations that adhere to a set of standards and a framework within which studies are planned, performed, monitored, recorded, reported, and archived. The International Organization for Standardization (ISO), the Good Laboratory Practice (GLP), and the Association for Assessment and Accreditation of Laboratory Animal Care International (AAALAC), a private, nonprofit organization that promotes the humane treatment of animals in science, through voluntary accreditation and assessment programs accredit the R&D processes and facilities when their standards are met. The group that is brought together to conduct the R&D are both academic and development-oriented members who investigate early on and before the start of large investment:

- If the medical device is really novel
- The nature of the current patent need for the device internationally

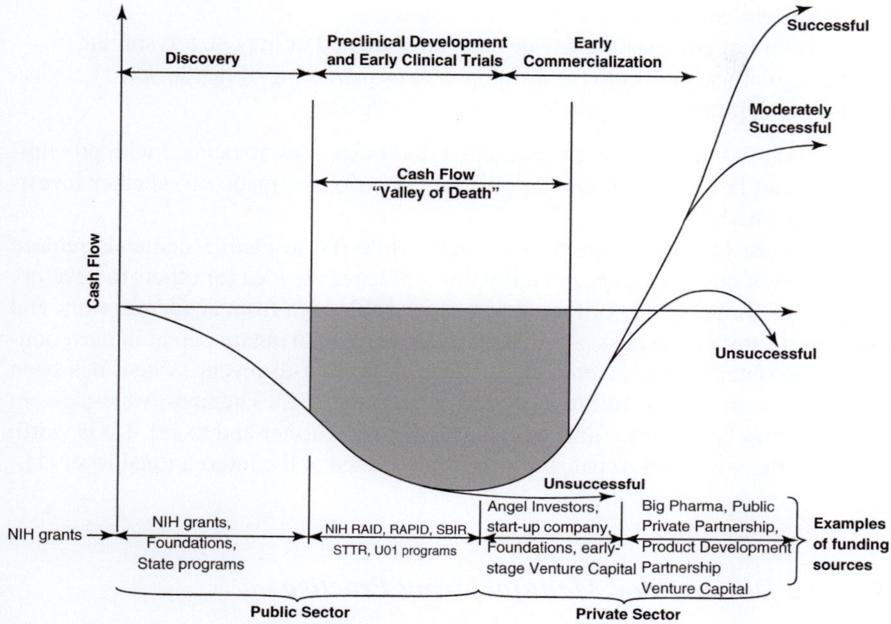

Fig. 2.9 Cash flow "valley of death" diagram. The cash flow "valley of death" as a function of development stage (time) with typical funding sources at various stages (Adapted from Murphy et al. [14]). *RAID* Rapid Access to Intervention Development, *SBIR* Small Business Innovative Research, *RAPID* Rapid Access to Preventive Intervention Development, *STTR* Small Business Technology Transfer (From Steinmetz and Spack [15], with permission)

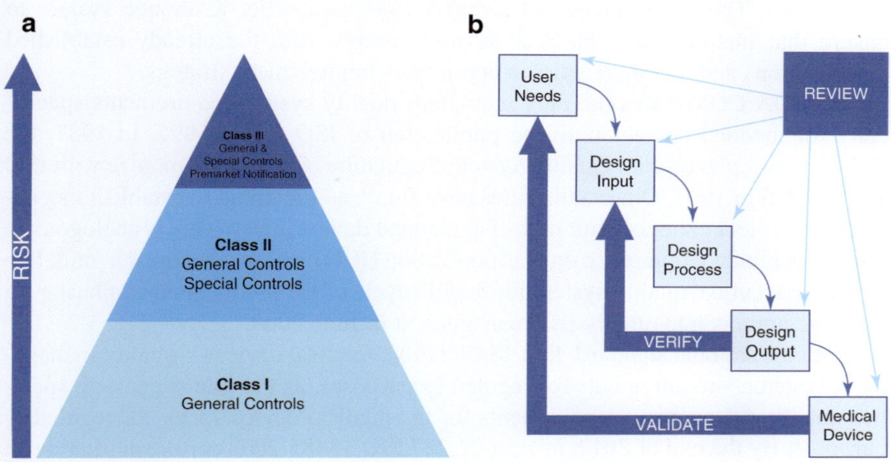

Fig. 2.10 Classification of medical devices and the design control process for device design. (**a**) Classification of medical devices is based on the degree of risk to the patient. Greater risk necessitates a greater degree of regulatory control for device market approval. (**b**) The design control model is suggested by the US Food and Drug Administration (FDA) for medical device development. Adapted from FDA, "Design Control Guidance for Medical Device Manufacturers," Guidance for Industry and Food and Drug Administration Staff, 11 Mar 1997 (From Morrison et al. [17], with permission)

- The current competing devices on the market
- The nature of any existing devices that are patented or may be too similar
- The regulatory hurdles to the development or marketing of the device
- The development and marketing costs of the device

Based on this knowledge, the estimated R&D expenses associated with preclinical work can be evaluated, and an objective decision be made on whether investment is worthwhile [1].

A problem for developers may be that, while the academic demands require publication of one's findings, in reality this will leave the idea for others to develop. As such it is important to differentiate a marketable idea from academic work and to obtain a patent as soon as possible. An alternative is to obtain patent in one country first to obtain a 1-year protection because the first-to-invent system has been substituted with the first-to-file-a patent system since 2013. The first-to-file-a patent system allows the inventor time to evaluate the idea further and to see if it is worth obtaining the next level of patent protection afforded at the international level [1].

Medical Device Good Manufacturing Practice

The FDA was the first to mandate medical device quality system requirements to ensure the safety and effectiveness of medical devices. The FDA issued a ruling, prescribing CGMP (current good manufacturing practice) requirements for medical devices, which required establishing a method of documentation and record keeping to investigate problems regarding quality and patient injuries associated with medical devices. The government and industry use this quality assurance system to ensure that manufactured medical devices comply with the already established specifications and that there exists a continuous improvement strategy.

The FDA CGMP was the only regulatory quality system requirements specifically for medical devices until the publication of ISO 13485:1996. In 1987, the CGMP was replaced with Quality System Regulation (QSR) to harmonize with ISO 13485:1996 in 1997. Other authorities have followed this trend to establish mechanisms to protect patients from high-risk medical device injury. This is analogous to the International Conference on Harmonization (ICH) which developed a guideline on pharmaceutical quality system for the life cycle of the product and emphasized a cohesive approach to quality risk management in June 2008.

The international standard, ISO 13485:2003, medical devices—quality management systems—requirements for regulatory purposes, as the title suggested, specifies quality management requirements for the medical device sector for regulatory purposes. By the end of 2012, at least 22,237 ISO 13485:2003 certificates had been issued in 97 countries and economies. The 2012 total represents an increase of 2388 (+12%) over 2011. The top three countries for the total of certificates were Germany, the United States, and Italy, and the top three in growth since the 2011 survey were Italy, Germany, and the United States [18].

Post-market surveillance programs instituted by medical device companies are vital to capturing unforeseen hazards as well as proper device performance. When a medical device fails expectation and regulations once in widespread use, a worldwide recall might cost a manufacturer at least 50 million dollars, not counting the loss of future income. The direct litigation costs are formidable, and indirect litigation costs such as loss of reputation and loss of market share can drive the products out of the market. In calculating the profitability of a medical device, the manufacturers often include the cost of future litigation as a cost of doing business. Because the bigger manufacturers generally choose to avoid the development of newer products with the high regulatory or liability risks, this leaves the market open for small- and medium-sized companies (SMEs) to navigate the innovation process and regulatory processes (e.g., 510[k], premarket approval [PMA], combination product) toward market approval, but also if the innovation fails, it will be easier for an SME to dissolve. The customer and the constantly changing regulatory environment represent both innovation challenges and opportunities for SME medical device companies because the larger companies are more resistant to expose themselves to risk [1]. Conversely, an SME can conveniently go bankrupt if the burden of litigation is too severe as demonstrated by vaginal mesh companies such as American Medical Systems. Many larger companies are not interested in purchasing a proof of concept. The SMEs use alternative funding concepts, technology transfer, and licensing methods to move scientific medical device innovation through an increasingly challenging and uncertain regulatory environment. The successful SME product launchers are subsequently taken over by the larger companies as their competitive threat becomes evident. Therefore a marketable device is the incentive for a successful SME to be absorbed by a larger company for many times their initial investment, either to be dismantled or incorporated into the product line of the larger company. Of all the ideas in all the world, in all the countries, and in all the companies, only a tiny fraction become products. Generally, in the pharma/biotech industry, only one-tenth of technology projects become a product that make it to the clinical trial stage [1], and very few become a best seller.

The innovative landscape in medical devices consists mainly of SMEs. In Europe, for example, 95% of the 25,000 medical technology companies are SMEs, which employ less than 50 people (small- and micro-sized companies) (Fig. 2.11) [12, 19]. The early stage innovations that are primarily financed at an SME level focus on a single product with high liability risk [20]. In this environment the quality aspects are at a low standard combined with high manufacturing optimization. The cost of goods sold (COGS) is high, which makes the initial SME devices expensive. The successful disruptive technology/product, easier-to-use innovations may be adapted by the large companies to make products through an already established reliable and cost-effective manufacturing method. These devices and products may be additionally upgraded by the acquired technology, by developing line extensions and second-generation incremental inventions [1].

In regard to medical device litigation, the US Supreme Court, after reviewing a case against Medtronics, ruled that medical device manufacturers may not be litigated under state laws by patients alleging harm from an FDA-approved medical

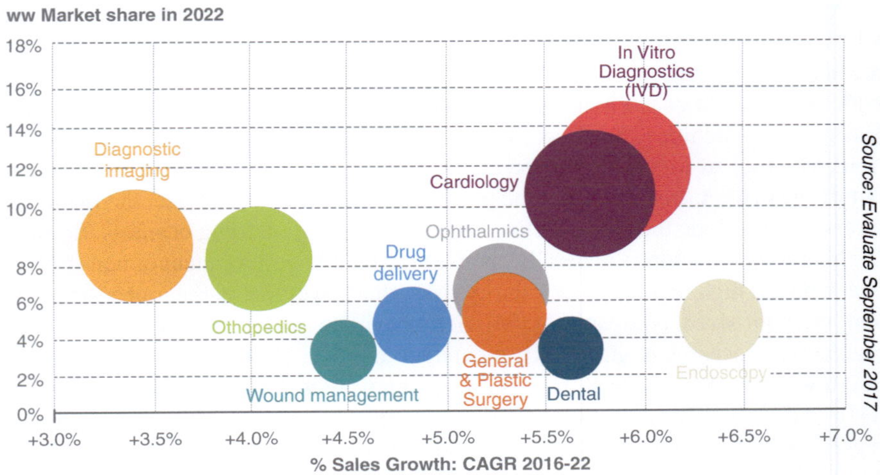

Fig. 2.11 World medical technology market by area and sales growth, 2014–2020. Worldwide market share in 2020. Medical technology offers solutions for many disease areas. On a worldwide perspective, in vitro diagnostics are the largest sector followed by cardiology and diagnostic imaging [19]. *CAGR* compound annual growth rate (From MedTech Europe [12], with permission)

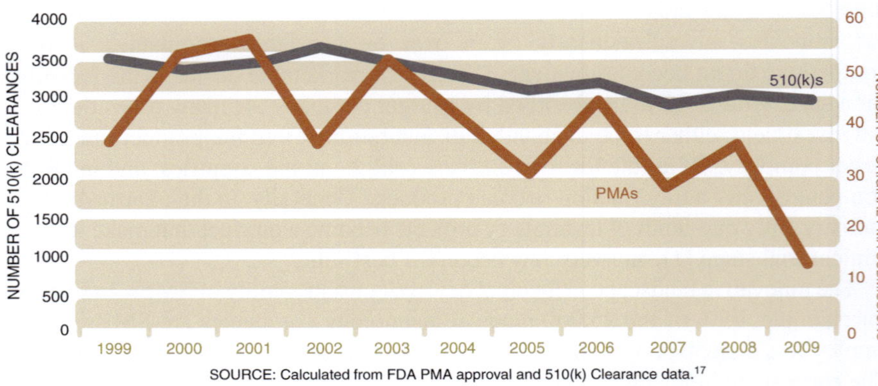

Fig. 2.12 Progressive declines in 510(k) and PMA submissions to the FDA between 1999 and 2009. Calculated from FDA data available at http://www.accessdata.fda.gov/scripts/cdrh/cfdocs/cfPMN/pmn.cfm and http://www.accessdata.fda.gov/scripts/cdrh/cfdocs/cfPMA/pma.cfm (22 Oct 2010). It was not possible to calculate the percentage change in clearances/approvals from year to year because data regarding the total number of 510(k) and PMA submissions are not made publicly available by the FDA (From Makower et al. [21], with permission)

device. But when a medical device has catastrophic failure, such as vaginal mesh kits, the legal actions are inevitable. Because of the FDA response and change in regulations and closing of the 510 K loophole, there has been a steady decline in both 510(k) and PMA submissions to the FDA (Fig. 2.12) [21, 22].

What Is the Large Medical Device Company Perspective in Regard to Collaboration or Innovation for Early Stage Medical Device Development?

By the virtue of the need to solve unique problems, medical device innovation can blend anatomy, biochemistry, physics, pharmacology, computation, and manufacturing technology to create solutions to previously unaddressed or poorly addressed problems. Just like a bridge exposed to hostile elements, implantable devices need to function in the human body and to sustain countless stresses. The manufacturing process integrates logistics, inventory control, tracking, reducing counterfeiting, and compliance with regulatory requirements.

In the United States, a major hurdle to device approval are clinical trials. The trials are performed at significant cost; therefore advance laboratory testing and preclinical evaluation reduce the risk of failure. Mimicking the disease process in the laboratory setting better predicts the device behavior in real life. Not only can the device fail in a clinical trial, but a poorly designed clinical trial can also fail the device due to poorly defined clinically relevant outcomes and/or quantifiable evaluation, unclear intermediate endpoints, or vague criteria for patient inclusion into the study [1].

The Reimbursement Challenge

A medical device development pro forma should take into account insurance policies for reimbursement for the device and the service provided. Even under the best circumstances, the prices and reimbursement are not as predicted. According to Advanced Medical Technology Association (AdvaMed), a US medical device trade association, the average price paid for medical devices has decreased in the United States. For example, drug-eluted stents decreased by 34% from 2007 to 2011. While the price decrease of medical devices may be partially explained by the reimbursement pressure, in reality a new successful device should expect competition closing in. The medical device has finite time to become profitable, to improve, and to dominate the market (Fig. 2.13) [23]. A successful device that provides a robust solution should reduce cost by developing value-for-money propositions for the payer to achieve acceptance. The current economic pressures dictate the need to do more with less.

Expanding Portfolio Challenge

Because of the advance of technology and new needs posed by a changing and aging population, the medical device industry has more opportunities in areas previously unavailable such as personalized, integrative, complementary, or regenerative

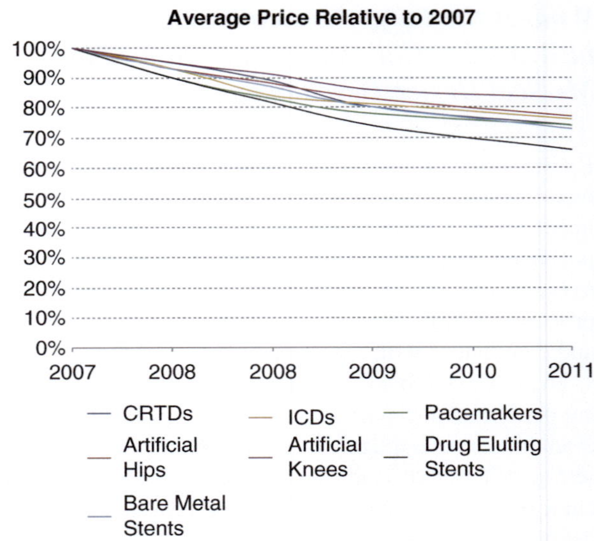

Fig. 2.13 Percent change in reported average real prices by medical device category 2007–2011. In real 2011 dollars (adjusted by medical care consumer price index [CPI]). Average price data provided by Millennium Research Group, Inc. (©2012 Millennium Research Group, Inc. [now Decision Resources Group] All rights reserved. Reproduction, distribution, transmission, or publication is prohibited. Reprinted with permission) (From Long et al. [23], with permission of Decision Resources Group)

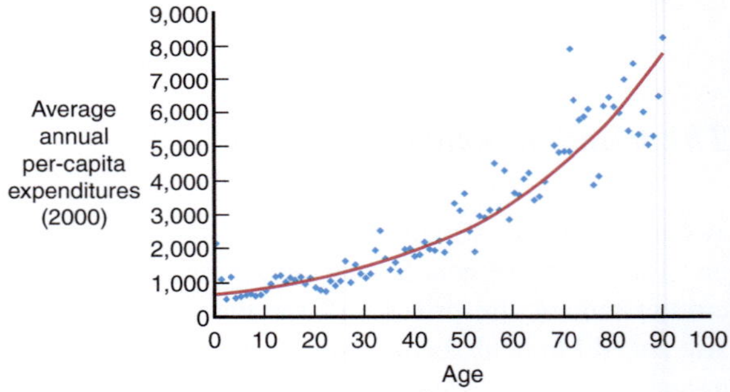

Fig. 2.14 Age is a powerful predictor of healthcare cost. Annual per capita expenditures in the United States by age (2000) (Goldman and McGlynn [24], with permission. Data from the Agency for Healthcare Research and Quality, 2000)

medicine, advanced therapy medical products, 3D printers, new biomaterials, and the Internet of things. The same fields create new challenges, as a product that previously could have a 20-year life span might quickly become obsolete because of new solutions previously unimaginable. For example, 3D printer technology allows new designs using materials with new and unique functionalities, which may result in personalized biomaterials solutions for the specific patient requirements.

Currently 27.4% of Medicare expenditures are used in the last years of life by a small portion of beneficiaries. Particularly in the United States, expenditure in healthcare increases sharply after the age of 60 (Fig. 2.14) [24]. If products are designed to last into these expensive years, overall healthcare spending will be reduced. New technologies can alert us to when body systems malfunction, enabling us to treat patients before expensive organ failure.

Cost-Effectiveness Research

The inventor and the manufacturing company cannot determine if their product benefits the society as a whole. Comparative effectiveness research (CER), which is a broad term encompassing many concepts, is used loosely as a key tool to lower costs and improve patient outcomes by policymakers. CER compares population outcomes, risks, and benefits when two or more therapies or devices are used. Policymakers, who are entities with access to large data banks, set goals for payers, physicians, and patients. This data in CER is used to make clinical and healthcare choices. The decision-makers use data dashboards that display relative risks and benefits of therapies to reduce what they view as unnecessary care, to direct resources to increase the use of effective therapies, and to lower overall costs. Like all data, the potential for CER to do good for the society depends on how the data is gathered, generated, or revised. For valid data to be created and used appropriately, it requires patients, medical practitioners, and the medical device industry to come together as multiple stakeholders. To show the benefit of a medical device or therapeutics, when is the optimal time to gather the data? The efficacies of many therapeutics increase with time. For example, Fig. 2.15 [22, 25–30] demonstrates the effect of changing the follow-up length on the number required to treat to save one life with implantable cardiac devices. The length of follow-up is of vital importance. In the case of vaginal mesh kits, if implanted in a 50-year-old patient, how do you obtain an informed consent from a patient about the risks of mesh erosion or extrusion 10–40 years down the road? All the available data so far go back only 10 years in the setting of badly designed retrospective trials. To perform long prospective trials, the medical device companies can incur high costs. For SMEs this is time that they do not have because investors will be seeking some return on investment in a specified period. Patients who need the technology want a safe and effective device quickly [22]. The needs of patients, physicians, and industry are conflicting, and the priority is created based on the data fed into the CER.

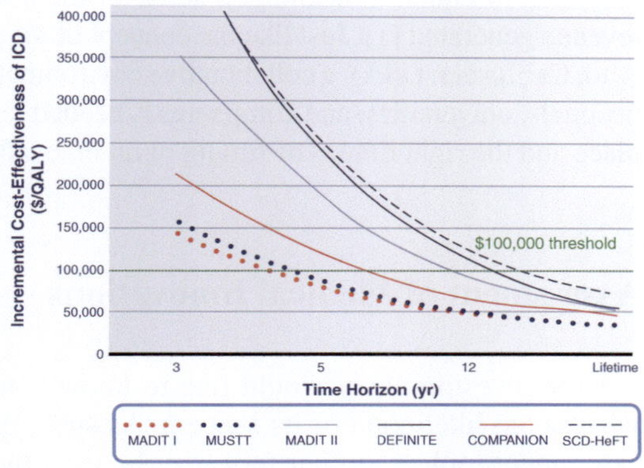

Fig. 2.15 Cost-effectiveness of implantable cardiac device (ICD) versus control over lifetime in 2005 US dollars (From Sharma et al. [22], with permission) [25–30]

From the medical device perspective, there is also the time required for the device to evolve through feedback and continuous improvement. Continuous improvement and evolution of the technology, procedure techniques, and physician skills influence clinical data endpoints to be considered in the setting of a CER [22]. In the example of vaginal mesh kits, it would have been important to place the device in the hands of highly trained competent surgeons to enhance and facilitate this evolutionary process by receiving reliable feedback to enhance the products. But as stated above, when an innovation is financially successful, the competition closes in, and the vaginal mesh kit manufacturers not only placed the devices in the hands of poorly trained physicians to harvest financial benefits, but also the feedback mechanism was lacking. To make matters worse, injured patients were hesitant to discuss in public issues concerning the damage caused by the devices.

Innovation Clusters

The commercial success of a medical device is not exclusively technology driven. It requires presenting cost-effective solutions to the market, ease of use for customers (e.g., doctors), robust clinical evidence, regulatory compliance, and effective marketing [1]. Commercial translation of a medical device can also be very expensive. Because larger companies may not invest in newer technologies, growing trends are the SME incubators located in major clinical settings and universities, with collaborative agreements that involve larger companies' investments and joint ventures. Universities and the health systems create incubators where the early stage companies are funded and sometimes have a physical presence on campus (e.g., INOVA Personalized Health Accelarator, Falls Church, Virginia, USA). Once an innovative idea is identified, the patent and intellectual property issues and the execution of business agreements (nondisclosure, collaborative research, material transfer) need to be instituted to obtain a meaningful sense of the costs and realistic expectations of the revenue generated [1]. Just like the concept of the global design company IDEO (Palo Alto, California, USA), a collaborative environment comprised of inventors, investors, hospitals, universities, and companies is needed to make the magic happen in the right place and the right time. The timing of an innovation is crucial to a successful launch.

Assessment of Medical Innovations

For the investors, they would like to know if a medical device will succeed and what is the likelihood of its success. As such, there are many models in use as an assessment tool. A similar tool may be used by the payers, as they would like to know the likelihood of adverse events and how much the device will cost. The health technology assessment (HTA) discipline was initiated about 30 years ago to evaluate how development, diffusion, and use of health technology impact the economic, social, medical, and ethical aspects of the environment in which it is introduced. In the era of CER and evidence-based medicine, the HTA is now in wide use to determine which health technologies might provide value for money [31]. Such models have proven to be complex and only as good as the data entered into them. For example, the cost-effectiveness assessment of diagnostic rather than treatment tools can be difficult, since they don't directly treat disease parameters but do influence mortality [3].

An interesting recurrent scenario for medical devices is that while the financial analysis for an SME may indicate that a device is not cost-effective to develop from healthcare perspective, the SMEs are not in the business of deciding if a technology is cost-effective from a societal perspective. For example, a donor laparoscopic nephrectomy is much more cost-effective from a societal perspective than from a healthcare perspective [3]. While it is common sense that CER and HTA should be concerned with the societal perspective, in countries such as the United States with free market healthcare, the decisions about appropriateness of devices and technologies are made in silos. Patient advocacy organizations, hospital associations, industry, and the other healthcare sectors lobby for their own financial benefit, which is not necessarily society's benefit. The more centralized societies such as those in Europe have a two-perspective approach for medical technology assessment. They calculate cost-effectiveness ratios for both the healthcare perspective and the common societal perspective [32].

Utilizing HTA should not be a one time exercise but rather part of continued improvement process as the data parameters entered into the models are constantly changing. Once a technology or medical device is employed, periodic assessments based on original assumptions used for modeling should be used. If the outcome of interest was used in the model, these need to be assessed. For example, many slings have been withdrawn from the market because they did not meet the efficacy endpoint. If there is a substantial negative variance from anticipated outcome, consideration should be given to forsaking the technology in favor of the assessment model [2].

While the HTA brings benefit to the patient, once this is proven, the healthcare worker aspects of the device need to be maximized. Minimally invasive surgery brought significant benefit to the patient, but the physicians were plagued with backache problems. The robotic technology addressed the healthcare worker issues [33–35]. To minimize the injury to healthcare workers, there is a constant evolution and adaptation from invasive to less invasive and even noninvasive procedures to replace traditionally open surgical procedures. Various new techniques are continuing to evolve and transform even the minimally invasive procedures. With decreased surgical invasiveness, instead of general anesthesia, minimal anesthesia could be used for minimally invasive urinary incontinence sling procedures. In the cancer treatment where resection was the norm, consideration is now given to imaging-guided radiofrequency ablation, microwave therapy, cryoablation, lasers and interstitial laser therapy, focused ultrasonography, and focused radiation with the same or better outcomes at much less cost [35]. The operating room of the future is a never achieved goal because the technology is constantly improving. The limitation to catching up with the ever-improving technology is understanding the human factors that dictate the performance of the surgical teams [36]. When technologies are overengineered for human performance, they create inefficiency as is seen with adaptation difficulties of the electronic medical records and telemedicine. The failure to reach technological potential stems from failure in human factor engineering [3]. Creating technologies that are not subservient to human limitations is an accident waiting to happen.

The Importance of Clear, Concise, and Closed-Loop Communication About Medical Device Adverse Events

Meager education of the users, poor implementation of a product, and the lack of a feedback loop mechanism form serious and commonly observed pitfalls in the road to successful evolution of an innovation. Human lack of acceptance of feedback and reluctance to acknowledge an incorrect choice should not be part of an objective assessment mechanism. For this reason, the inventors and investors should be separated from the assessment mechanism [3]. In the United States, there is a general perception by physicians and patients that a medical device is proven safe before it is marketed. What fuels the medicolegal industry is a cycle of products that are rushed to the market and withdrawn only after their complications become evident too late due to poor feedback loop mechanism.

Innovations in medical devices do not automatically translate in medical practice advances [37]. Positive technology impact in medicine requires human factor engineering to augment the skills of the healthcare team rather than seek the providers entirely with technology [38]. With human factor engineering, it is important to recognize that the nursing profession is crucial in the acceptance, application, and routine use of medical technological devices [3]. Medical devices can help physicians and their teams to be more efficient. Just like automobiles that have undergone continuous improvement, medical devices require several reiterations via technological improvement, which is only possible by an efficient feedback loop. The input of the whole team is a crucial component for such improvements. Ideally, medical sales representatives in the operating room should close the loop between the developers and users, but because of the incentive mechanisms in place, most representatives are most concerned with the sales of their items [3].

In this phase of innovation, many vaginal mesh companies under economic pressure did not form the communication loop. They marketed their products widely to a large number of novice users to demonstrate profitability. As a large number of problems occurred in the field, this did not translate to better product design. Although we have stated that good communication between physicians and industry is important, one method traditionally used by industry representatives was to wine and dine the physicians to create a report. This created a bias and conflicts of interest because of the close involvement of the physician and the industry. The Physician Payments Sunshine Act was created to increase transparency around the financial relationships between the physicians, the teaching hospitals, and the device manufacturers [39].

Investigating Incidents and Their Contributing Factors

While medical device-related adverse events can be divided into "device" or "operator" failure, this categorization is an oversimplification of an often difficult diagnostic issue. An objective structured approach is advocated. Understanding the functionality of the medical device in its clinical context assists with in-depth investigation of the causes. Generally such investigation should include a multidisciplinary team or committee at the hospitals tasked with purchasing medical devices. Medical device utilization involves devices, physicians, nurses, patients, scrub techs, and supporting infrastructure. Investigating the details of "medical device," "healthcare operator," or "infrastructure" failures enables a deep dive to uncover the actual reasons rather than simply crediting the failure to a device vs. user fault paradigm. The investigation should be performed in a safe and reassuring manner for the staff and instead focus on improving processes and recognizing patterns. The team can use Shepherd's global patterns of causes (Table 2.3) [40, 41].

Table 2.3 Shepherd's classification of medical device incidents

Device	Operator	Facility	Environment	Patient
(i) Human factors design	(i) Education/ training	(i) Human factors design	(i) Internal to hospital	(i) Active: patient action affected the outcome
(ii) Parts/circuit design: unexpected failure	(ii) "Use" error	(ii) Parts/circuits designs: unexpected failure	(ii) External to hospital	(ii) Passive: patient's condition affected the outcome
(iii) Deterioration: predictable failure that requires preventative maintenance (e.g., battery)	(iii) Diverted attention	(iii) Deterioration: predictable deterioration that requires preventative maintenance		
(iv) Maintainer error	(iv) Criminal intent	(iv) Maintainer error		

From Amoore [40], with permission. Data from AACE Health Technology Foundation, Clinical Alarm Task Force [41]

The general evaluation of medical device failures falls under *five failure types or groups*:

1. *Equipment*. The number of medical devices that may have the same function, the availability of equipment and its service readiness, and the requirements for maintenance and repair aspects should be evaluated [3]. Does the facility have many items of equipment for the same function with different operability? An example of this is stocking different trocars for laparoscopy procedures. Each may have different resistance during abdominal entry, which may increase the risk of viscus injury.

   One scheme for characterizing devices (https://www.mddionline.com/addressing-problem-medical-device-misuse) includes the following categories:

   - Normal use (the device is used as intended by the manufacturer)
   - Common use (the device is used consistent with the established standards of care)
   - Misuse subject to mitigation (the device is used in ways that a thorough human factor analysis reveals as predictable given the user population, the task, and the use environment)
   - Misuse not subject to mitigation (the device is used in ways not predicted by human factor analysis)
   - Abuse (the device is used in ways intended to cause damage and personal harm).

2. *Operator*. Analysis of possible device error should include evaluation of improper handling. This aspect of evaluation may be difficult, which is why medical devices should be used on a trial basis to evaluate human factors to predict improper handling that can occur during normally intended use or during reasonably foreseeable off-label use. It would be perhaps impossible for the manufacturer to predict how a medical device may be used in a not reasonably foreseeable off-label use [3]. Another scheme for characterizing product uses by the operator include:

   - Correct use (the device is used as intended by the manufacturer)
   - Use error (the device is used in a well-intentioned but incorrect manner)
   - Abnormal use (the operator is deliberately acting in omission or commission intended to produce adverse results)
   - (https://www.mddionline.com/addressing-problem-medical-device-misuse)

Examples of use not according to intended purpose(s) can be the repetitive usage of a disposable vaginal mesh trocar, which is not hygienic and raises the risk of infection, or opening a vaginal mesh kit and substituting the mesh to be used. At one of the international meetings, a video was presented on laparoscopic application of a vaginal mesh kit. Watching the video, it was hard to distinguish if this was a "use error" (the device is used in a well-intentioned but incorrect manner) or "abnormal use" (the operator is deliberately acting in omission or commission intended to produce adverse results). The meeting organizers obviously had chosen the video as an example of what not to do. Once a product is created, how it is used is entirely dependent on the end user, which is why education of the end user for proper use of the medical product is so important. Health information technology system design expert Sensmeier formulated the following:

> Watch what people actually DO. Don't believe what people SAY they do. Definitely don't believe what people predict they MAY do in the future [42].

There are frameworks for specifically measuring and understanding the technological knowledge that is the knowledge of how to produce goods and services. A thorough understanding of stages of knowledge framework helps to precisely map, evaluate, and compare levels of knowledge within a team or a process. Based on this information, we can decide whether and how the team or process, the key tasks of the workforce, and other major aspects of its management can be controlled and automated. Better understanding of stages of knowledge leads to better performance without increased physical investment [43].

Stages of Knowledge [44]

- Ignorance
- Phenomenon not recognized or the variable's effects seem random
- Awareness
- Variable known to be influential but can neither be measured nor controlled
- Measure
- Variable can be measured but not controlled
- Control of the mean
- Control of the variable possible but not precise
- Control of variance around the mean not possible
- Process capability
- Variable can be controlled across the whole range
- Process characterization
- Know how small changes in the variable will affect the results.
- Know why
- Fully characterized scientific model of causes and effects, including secondary variables
- Complete knowledge
- Knowledge of all interactions such that problems can be prevented by feed forward control

3. *Facility*. This concerns not only the physical building but also the organization, management, training, and culture of a health service. To assess the proper care of the patients within the healthcare facilities, the data analyzed from the Hospital Consumer Assessment of Healthcare Providers and Systems which is a patient satisfaction survey required by CMS (the Centers for Medicare and Medicaid Services) for all hospitals in the United States asks about nine dimensions of care:

- Communication with doctors
- Communication with nurses
- Responsiveness of hospital staff
- Pain management
- Communication about medicines
- Discharge information
- Cleanliness of the hospital environment
- Quietness of the hospital environment
- Transition of care

  To maximize the best possible care for the patients, it may be important to provide specialty care. In a recent study of high-scoring hospitals, four out of five of the top-scoring hospitals were specialty facilities—surgical hospitals, orthopedics hospitals, or heart hospitals. And of the remainder, nearly all were small hospitals that were nominally general-purpose but in practice provided the same kind of focused care that the specialty hospitals did [44]. Obviously using a device in a facility not suited for it reduces the chances of better outcome for the patients. For example, a competent surgeon inserting a vaginal mesh kit in an orthopedic hospital will introduce the patient to many sources of errors that would have been eliminated if the patient was operated on by an experienced cohesive specialty women's team.

4. *Environment*. Facility and environment go hand in hand. The physical design of the healthcare environment should enhance the operations of the health services. Aspects such as lighting, heating/cooling, acoustic, adequate work and storage space, elevators, utilities, pagers, phones, etc. should be thought through carefully. Defects within a device or installation can remain undetected if only only end-user input is relied on. Conducting regular inspections and the accessibility, the availability, or the absence of policy or guidelines are important. Even when there are written policies, there can be misinterpretation or non-compliance with policies, procedures, or established practices. Once there are established policies and protocols, the availability and flow path of information (verbal, written, or electronic) among staff and with patient and family members should be evaluated regularly. Documentation of activities by the staff as well as activities and communication with the patients should be standardized. For example, chronological documentation and timing of a surgery can convey much about operating room efficiency and team dynamics [3] (Fig. 2.16) [40].
5. *Patient*. The patient's physical or mental health status when pursuing medical care will chiefly determine the outcome of treatment in contrast to the typically expected outcome. Although prognostic models can identify subgroups of patients who may have a very high risk of dying before hospital discharge (e.g., very old intensive care unit patients) [3], these models may not be validated for a new medical device. For example, using a vaginal mesh kit in a patient with severely uncontrolled diabetes will increase the risk of mesh infection, erosion, or extrusion. Or, using a vaginal mesh kit in a patient with underlying pelvic pain may exacerbate the pain. The instructions for use (IFU) by the manufacturer are meant to be a comprehensive guide for patient selection when a physician is being oriented to the new device.

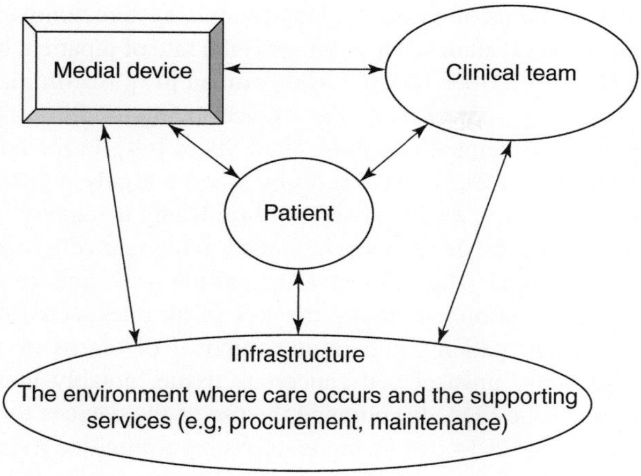

Fig. 2.16 Diagram summarizing the interactions between a medical device, the clinical team, and the patient within an infrastructure that include both the physical environment and the supporting services. Each of the elements (device, clinical team, patient, and infrastructure) interacts and depends on each other (From Amoore [40], with permission)

Examples of Medical Device Assessment Failure

A new medical device's safety concerns are detectable with meticulous comprehensive monitoring by the manufacturers but are often overlooked. The medical device manufacturers in turn are monitored for safety concerns by the FDA. Rather than duplicate efforts and collect more dilute data, focusing to better use the available data or to collect high-quality data increases the detection rate of safety events. An example in which this is readily apparent involves the monitoring of medical devices [45].

The advent, increase, and decline in the use of the laparoscopic gastric band to treat morbid obesity illustrates how examination of existing data could have changed practice much earlier. The gastric band device (commonly referred to by its brand name Lap-Band [Allergan, Irving, California, USA; now manufactured by Apollo Endosurgery, Austin, Texas, USA]) was approved by the FDA in 2001 and peaked in usage by 2008 [45]. However, use of the device gradually declined as reports emerged describing complications (e.g., band erosion, band slippage) and variable effectiveness (e.g., inadequate weight loss) that required reoperation to revise, replace, or remove the device. A recent study using Medicare claims found that of the $470 million paid for the gastric band device, $223 million (47%) was for reoperations [45]. There is broad consensus now that the use of the gastric band device should be significantly restricted [46], if not eliminated, but why did the medical device monitoring system not identify these concerns sooner?

As another example, power morcellators were laparoscopic surgical devices that used electromechanical energy to cut solid tissue specimens into smaller pieces, thereby allowing minimally invasive hysterectomy and myomectomy for large uteri and fibroids. Power morcellator devices were first described in 1993 and were widely adopted by gynecologists. Supporting their use was evidence that laparoscopic hysterectomy has advantages over abdominal hysterectomy, including less blood loss, less postoperative pain, more rapid recovery, fewer wound infections, and shorter hospitalizations. Uptake of the new technology was rapid. From 2005 to

2013, the rate of outpatient laparoscopic hysterectomy increased from 31.4 to 161.6 per 100,000 adult women, whereas the rate of inpatient hysterectomy declined from 172.1 to 72.1 per 100,000 adult women [47]. According to one report [48], at their peak usage, power morcellators were being used in an estimated 55,000 to 75,000 procedures annually in the United States [49]. In the fall of 2013, power morcellation came under intense scrutiny when a highly publicized case raised awareness that some masses diagnosed as fibroids might actually be undiagnosed cancers and the use of the devices might spread malignant cells from these tissues throughout the abdomen. The FDA investigated the issue and, in April 2014, issued a safety communication estimating the risk of an unexpected uterine sarcoma at 1 out of every 350 patients undergoing removal of uterus or fibroids. Given the risk of "spreading unsuspected cancerous tissue, notably uterine sarcomas, beyond the uterus," the FDA discouraged the use of the devices for the removal of fibroids. In November 2014, following an advisory committee meeting, the FDA immediately required a "black box" warning label on power morcellator devices [49].

Following these FDA actions, there was a rapid and steep decline in the use of the power morcellators. The largest manufacturer withdrew its device from the market, large hospital organizations across the country restricted use of power morcellators, and some insurance carriers denied reimbursement for surgeries involving the devices. An intense debate followed over whether the FDA failed to act sufficiently to protect patients or, alternatively, acted too aggressively and interfered inappropriately with patient care [49].

The similarity of gastric band, morcellators, and hundreds of other similar devices with vaginal mesh kits is illustrative of a systematic process problem. Medical devices are introduced, trialed on patients, litigated, and then withdrawn from the market. Despite the need for answers to questions like the ones posed by devices such as gastric bands, power morcellators, and vaginal mesh kits, current post-marketing surveillance studies remain infrequent and limited in scope. The FDA has envisioned a far more robust system using medical records to track device safety, to be known as the National Evaluation System for health Technology (NEST). However, NEST is years from adoption, requires additional funding, and may not survive the new administration's interest in deregulation [49].

In the case of vaginal mesh kits, in the early 2000s, FPMRS as a specialty was just in the process of board certification and rather early organizational stages. FPMRS training took three additional years after completing 12–13 years of undergraduate, medical school, and obstetric/gynecology or urology training. The surgeries were long and technical, and the number of trained specialists was few in relation to the population with disease. The industry found its "blue ocean" by creating vaginal mesh kits that were easy to place. From the industry's point of view, the business analysis was complete. From most FPMRS physicians' point of view, the outcome data was lacking. The industry's salesmen and saleswomen marketed the device to the larger in number obstetrician/gynecologists and urologists. After foiling of most vaginal mesh kit manufacturers or settlement over their products, the market corrected itself by specialists becoming dominant in the field once again and performing the procedures in ways that were safer for the patients.

The economic and financial impact of vaginal mesh kits for the patients was enormous. In a study published by the author, vaginal mesh complications had a sustained disability impact that continued despite mesh removal. The complications were associated with increased economic burden for the families of the affected individuals and a drop in family income in more than one-third of the families [50]. In this study, 29% were extremely disabled after vaginal mesh surgery, and only 8% of patients reported that they had no disability. The median for overall disability score after vaginal mesh procedure was 8, which qualifies as "marked" disability. The majority of patients missed a median of 12 months (0–80 months) of their school or work because of their mesh complications. In this study 59.6% did not return to their symptom-free condition (before their first vaginal mesh surgery) and did not have improvement in symptoms after mesh removal, and 33.9% stated that their family income dropped because of productivity loss related to mesh complications. The mean time between vaginal mesh placement and mesh removal was 4.7 years [50].

Based on the average time lost (0.8 months) from work, it can be estimated that 8700 months or 49,714 hours of wages were lost in 2010 alone due to mesh complications. Using the US minimum wage of $7.25 as a base for the value of an hour of any service, this loss of productivity in dollars equals 49,714 hours × $7.25 = $360,428. It is estimated that, in addition, 21/62 or 34% of US women's family income dropped as a result. It can be estimated that in 2010, subsequent to their surgery, 60% or 6482 US women who had complications never felt better even after their vaginal mesh was removed (Tables 2.4 and 2.5 [50, 51]).

Based on these numbers, it can be concluded that if vaginal mesh kits were an innovation to better patients' lives, not only did they not reach this objective, but they left patients much worse off financially and physically.

Federal Regulations in the United States to Monitor Adverse Events and Recalls

The FDA Center for Devices and Radiological Health (CDRH) is the regulatory entity that reviews and systematically evaluates medical device recall data. As defined at Title 21, Code of Federal Regulations (CFR), 7.3(g), "*Recall* means a firm's removal or correction of a marketed product that the Food and Drug Administration considers to be in violation of the laws it administers and against which the agency would initiate legal action, e.g., seizure." The recalls are divided into three classes as "there is a reasonable probability that use of or exposure to a violative product":

- *Will cause* serious adverse health consequences or death (*Class I*)
- *May cause* temporary or medically reversible adverse health consequences or where the probability of serious adverse health consequences is remote (*Class II*)
- *Is not likely* to cause adverse health consequences (*Class III*)

Table 2.4 Disability impact of vaginal mesh complications based on years lived with disability (YLD) questionnaires

Question	Response
How many months did your symptoms cause you to miss school or work or left you unable to carry out your normal daily responsibilities? Median (range)	12 (0–80)
How many months did you feel so impaired by your symptoms that even though you went to school or work, your productivity was reduced? Median (range)	24 (0–132)
How many months did you not go to school or work, because you needed additional medical care? Median (range)	0.8 (0–60)
How long (years) did it take for you to feel totally well (like before surgery) from the date of your original mesh surgery Median (range)	4 (0–14) 37/62 (59.6%) Never got better
Did your family's income dropped as a result of vaginal mesh complications? (yes, no) (yes % total)	21/62 (33.9%)
Years between mesh placement and removal Mean ± sd	4.7 ± 2.9
What is your family's annual income? Median (range)	45,000 (0–475,000)

From Javadian and Shobeiri [50], with permission

Table 2.5 Estimated financial impact of vaginal mesh complications in 2010 in the United States (based on FDA report [45]) (N = 10,875)

Patients' disability severity based on Sheehan questionnaire		
Not at all: 0, no. (%)	870 (8)	
Mildly: 1–3, no. (%)	1196 (11.2)	
Moderately: 4–6, no. (%)	1196 (11.2)	
Markedly: 7–9, no. (%)	4350 (40.3)	
Extremely: 10, no. (%)	3262 (29)	
How many months did your symptoms cause you to miss school or work or left you unable to carry out your normal daily responsibilities? (median, range)	12 (0–80)	130,500 months
How many months did you feel so impaired by your symptoms that, even though you went to school or work, your productivity was reduced? (median, range)	24 (0–132)	261,000 months
How many months did you not go to school or work, because you needed additional medical care? (median, range)	0.8 (0–60)	8700 months
How long (years) did it take for you to feel totally well (like before surgery) from the date of your original mesh surgery? (median, range)	4 (0–14)	
	37/62 (59.6%)	6482 patients
	Never got better	Never got better
Did your family's income dropped as a result of vaginal mesh complications? (yes, no), no. (%)	21/62 (33.9%)	3678 families

From Javadian and Shobeiri [50], with permission

Combating Unsafe or Defective Medical Device Public Health Risks

The FDA is engaged in continuous improvement of the device monitoring process. While there were 18 high-risk medical device recalls in 2008, this rate increased by 350% in 2013 when 63 high-risk devices were recalled by the FDA [52]. The annual number of medical device recalls increased by 97 percent between 2003 and 2012, which was attributed to enhanced cognizance by device firms, especially the ones previously named for reporting violations, and exact CDRH initiatives to improve medical device safety. The annual number of Class I device recalls historically associated with high numbers of device problems, such as ventilators, infusion pumps, and external defibrillators, increased partly because of joint CDRH and industry efforts to enhance safe device performance. Per CDRH reports between 2009 and 2012, medical device problems were effectively addressed, and underlying problems were resolved, as evidenced by the fact that the average classification times for high-risk Class I and Class II recalls were reduced by 9 and 26 days, respectively.

The top reasons for recalls were related to device design, software, and nonconforming material or component issues. If industry and CDRH could successfully address these problems, as many as 400 recalls could be prevented annually [52].

The medical device firms, the FDA Office of Regulatory Affairs (ORA), and the CDRH interact and collaborate to initiate, classify, and terminate the process of medical device recalls (Fig. 2.17) [52].

The recall process typically relies upon the device manufacturer acknowledging an issue that warrants a recall action. In initiating a recall, the FDA's ORA district office is notified. While it typically takes the FDA 1 day to post the classification, the annual average time from firm awareness of the problem to acknowledging the problem by recall posting between 2010 and 2012 ranged from 233.7 to 256.6 days [52].

Once the firm notifies the FDA (Phase I in Fig. 2.18), the ORA district office issues a 24-h alert to CDRH and a recall classification recommendation (Phase II). CDRH conducts a final review and classification (Phase III). Recalls are publicly posted online within a day of classification. The average number of days from firm awareness of the need to conduct a recall to FDA's posting of the recall classification is displayed in Table 2.6 [52].

The CDRH recall of radiation-emitting products and medical devices was analyzed in a 10-year study period (see Fig. 2.18) [52]. According to the FDA, between 2003 and 2012, there was an increase in the overall annual recall counts from 604 recalls to 1190 recalls, representing a 97% increase in both Class I and II recalls. Class I recalls increased from 7 (1%) in FY 2003 to 57 (5%) in FY 2012. Between 2003 and 2012, annually Class II recalls more than doubled, while the number of Class III recalls declined by approximately 35%. Recalls were associated with distinct medical specialties (Fig. 2.19) [52]. Radiology, cardiovascular, general hospital, general surgery, orthopedics, and chemistry were the six specialties that represented the majority of recalls. The radiology medical device use of identified media was the top recall item, which resulted in focusing and better monitoring for and reporting of problems by radiology industry [52].

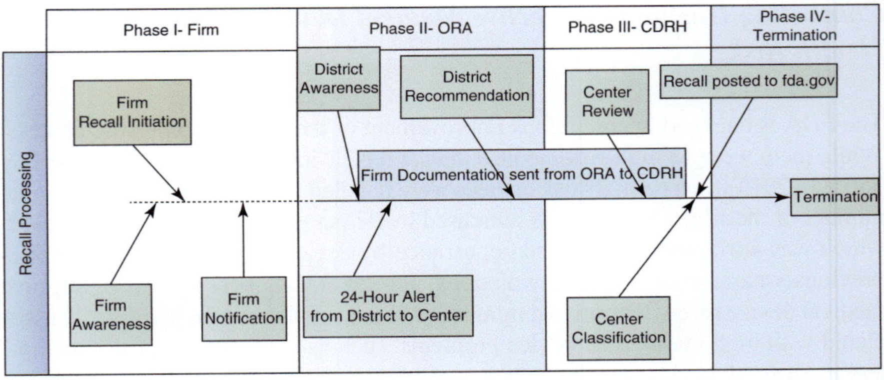

Fig. 2.17 Medical device recall processing. *ORA* Office of Regulatory Affairs, *CDRH* Centers for Devices and Radiological Health (From US Food and Drug Administration [52])

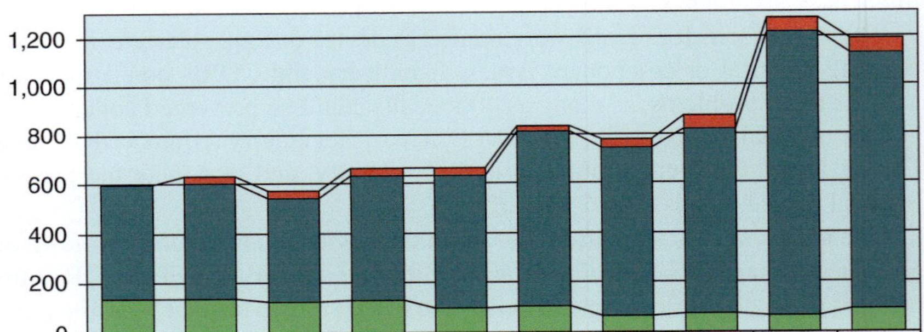

	2003	2004	2005	2006	2007	2008	2009	2010	2011	2012
Class I	7	24	26	22	26	14	32	49	50	57
Class II	460	467	422	505	540	710	677	753	1,152	1,043
Class III	137	140	124	132	96	108	67	74	69	90
Totals	*604*	*631*	*572*	*659*	*662*	*832*	*776*	*876*	*1,271*	*1,190*

Fig. 2.18 Centers for Devices and Radiological Health (CDRH) recall counts by fiscal year and class FY2003–FY2012 (From US Food and Drug Administration [52])

Device Procodes

The FDA uses a device "procode" which is composed of five components: industry, class, subclass, PIC, and product. This is a useful method of cataloging and monitoring medical devices to report industry-wide product performance problems and barriers that impact device quality, safety, and effectiveness. Between 2004 and 2012, the ten top device procodes associated with recalls (0.15% of all procodes) resulted in 20% of device recall events (Table 2.7) [52]. Given this system, the CDRH can conduct a more detailed analysis of recall data to identify trends. As an example, trend analysis of the most frequently recalled radiological device (linear

Table 2.6 Average days by phase and years

Year	Number of recalls	Phase I Firm awareness to district awareness (mean d)	Phase II District awareness until recommendation sent to CDRH (mean d)	Phase III CDRH receipt to classification and posting (mean d)	Phase I–III Total recall days to posting (mean d)
FY2010	876	85.7	99.7	48.3	233.7
FY2011	1271	98.2	111.6	37.1	246.9
FY2012	1190	99.4	135.9	21.3	256.6

From US Food and Drug Administration [52]

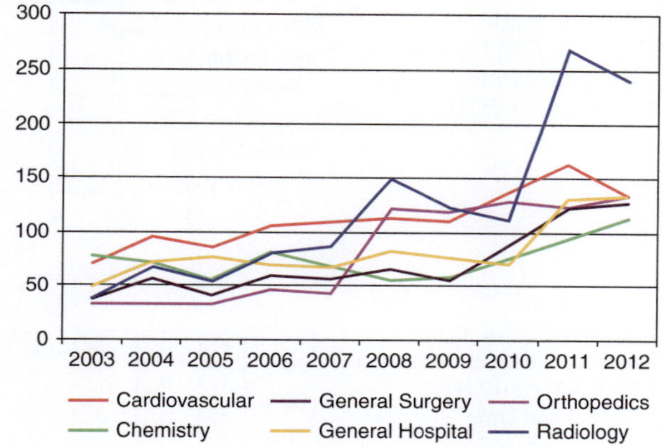

Fig. 2.19 Recalls by medical specialty (From US Food and Drug Administration [52])

Table 2.7 Most commonly recalled procodes

Recalls	Procode	Product description	Specialty
176	IYE	Accelerator, linear, medical	Radiology
153	LLZ	System, image processing, radiological	Radiology
130	FRN	Pump, infusion	Gen Hospital
115	JAK	System, X-ray, tomography, computed	Radiology
109	MKJ	Automated external defibrillators	Cardiovascular
106	GEI	Electrosurgical, cutting and coagulation and accessories	Surgery
101	JJE	Analyzer, chemistry, for clinical use	Chemistry
98	JQP	Calculator/data processing module, for clinical use	Chemistry
97	GKZ	Counter, differential cell	Hematology
96	JWH	Prosthesis, knee, patellofemorotibial, semi-constrained	Orthopedic

From US Food and Drug Administration [52]

accelerators—procode IYE, (Fig. 2.20)) demonstrated that software failures caused the majority of recalls (Fig. 2.21) [52]. Breaking down the software issues further, system compatibility (interoperability between treatment planning and treatment delivery systems), user interfaces (human factors), and dose calculation (clinical

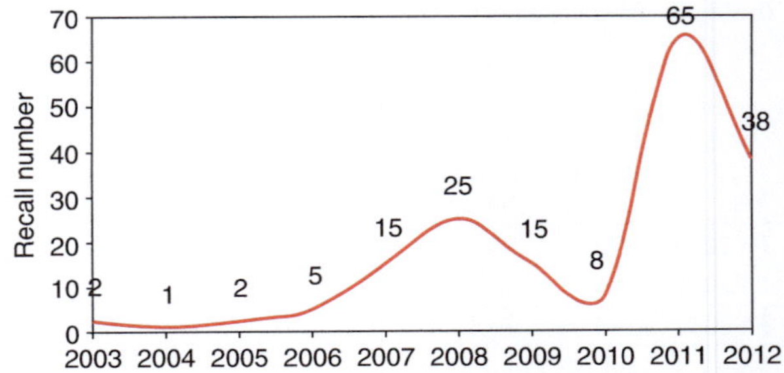

Fig. 2.20 Recalls for FDA procode IYE (accelerator, linear, medical) FY2003–FY2012 (From US Food and Drug Administration [52])

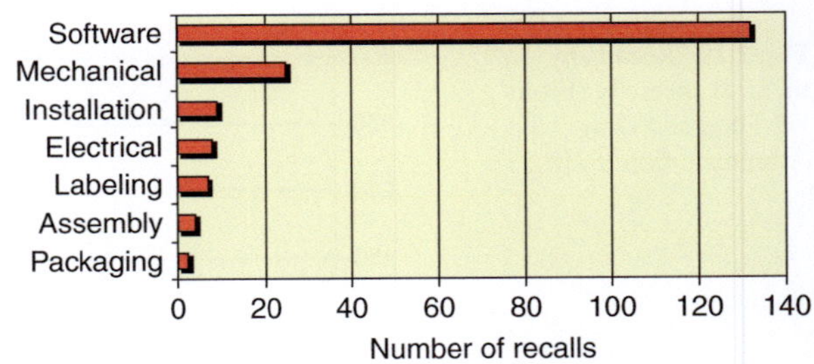

Fig. 2.21 Causes of linear accelerator recalls FY2003–FY2012 (From US Food and Drug Administration [52])

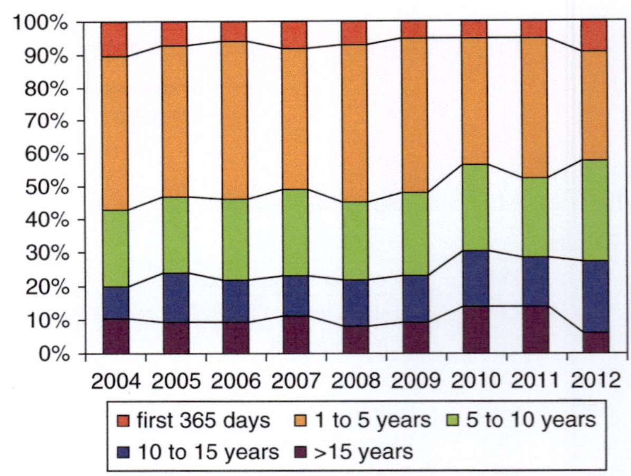

Fig. 2.22 Age of recalled devices: time on market FY2003–FY2012 (From US Food and Drug Administration [52])

decision support software) were the most frequently quoted reasons, accounting for more than 66% of these specific recalls.

Between 2004 and 2012, the percentage of recalls affecting medical devices within 1 year of FDA marketing approval held constant at around 10%. Likewise, medical devices that had been on the market for more than 15 years consistently represented around 10% of recalled devices, proving that the proportion of recalls had not increased (Fig. 2.22) [52]. No trends were recognized in respect to the time on market and medical device recalls.

Recall and Regulatory Violations

For each medical device recall, FDA decides the related Federal Food, Drug, and Cosmetic Act (FDCA) violations such that a medical device recall may be assigned one or more regulatory violation. The top ten regulatory violations for medical device recalls classified between 2010 and 2012 were all linked to Quality System Regulation (QSR) as listed by recall class in Table 2.8 [52].

Recall Reasons

Recall causes between 2010 and 2012 are listed in Table 2.9 [52] in decreasing frequency of use and also listed in Fig. 2.23 as proportions of reasons for the recalls. Each recall which uses FDA current terminology and processes has only one recall cause assigned as below [52]:

Design, which includes design of the device and related software

Change control such as component, labeling, vendor, process, packaging, software, or finished device

Process control, which includes process, packaging process, process design, or reprocessing controls

Material/component, including nonconforming material and components, component design/selection, material contamination, material mix-up, and removal or release of material prior to testing

Packaging/labeling such as mix-up of labeling, packaging, packaging design/selection, expired dating, labeling design, labeling false and misleading, or error in labeling

Table 2.8 Regulatory violations for medical device recalls classified from FY2010–FY2012 counted and ranked. The top ten, all related to Quality System Regulation (QSR), listed by recall class. A recall may have more than one regulatory violation

Number	Regulation subpart title	Class I	Class II	Class III
820.30	Design controls and related subparts	703	1759	36
820.80	Receiving, in-process, and finished device acceptance	204	1068	61
820.70	Production and process controls and subparts	119	830	58
820.90	Nonconforming product	17	415	28
820.75	Process validation	16	390	30
820.50	Purchasing controls	19	366	29
820.130	Device packaging	0	377	5
820.120	Device labeling and related subparts	2	271	29
820.25	Personnel	0	159	2
820.100	Corrective and preventive action	0	122	7

From US Food and Drug Administration [52]

Table 2.9 Recall causes assigned by FDA tabulated for recalls classified during FY2010–FY2012, by decreasing frequency of use. Note that each recall has only one recall cause determination

Recall reasons	Number
Nonconforming material/component	429
Software design (device)	429
Device design	425
Process control	266
Component design/selection	144
Employee error	134
Leveling mix-ups/errors	99
Under investigation by the firm	81
Process design	77
Packaging process control	76
Error in labeling	59
Packaging	58
Mix-up of material/components	49
Material/component contamination	47
Labeling design	42
Radiation Control for Health and Safety Act of 1968 (PL 90-602)	41
Labeling false and misleading	39
Component change control	37
Equipment maintenance	31
Process change control	31
Software change control	24
Software design (process)	22
Premarket approval: illegally marketed	21
Labeling change control	19
Packaging design/selection	18
Release of material/component prior to receiving test results	15
Expiration dating	15
Vendor change control	12
Packaging change control	8
Manufacturing material removal	8
Storage	7
Environmental control	6
Unknown/undetermined by the firm	6
Finished device change control	4
Reprocessing controls	2

From US Food and Drug Administration [52]

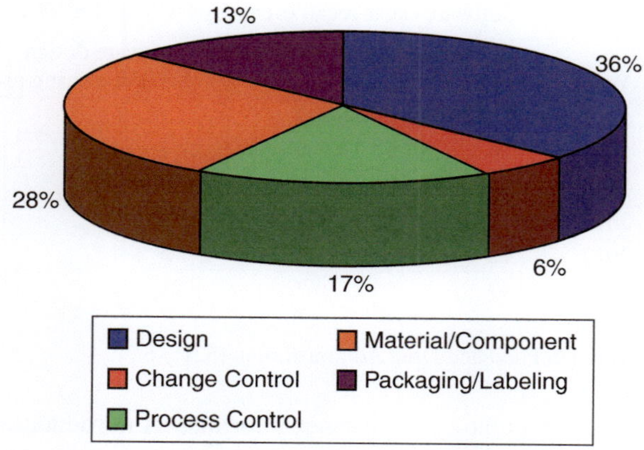

Fig. 2.23 Recall cause categories FY2003–FY2012 (From US Food and Drug Administration [52])

Software Design Failures as the Most Common Cause of Recall

Software can be part of a medical device, or alternatively, software alone may be itself a medical device, or software may be employed in the manufacture of a medical device. Medical devices more and more depend on software, and it is evident that even minor deviations to software result in significant consequences for medical device utility and clinical performance. Not implementing software design controls and testing measures, along with the increasingly complicated nature of the medical device environment, may result in software malfunction that would require correction or removal (Table 2.10) [52].

Analysis of medical device recall data can support the FDA in:

- Refinement and explanation of observed trends
- Understanding frequent reasons for device failures
- Identification of hazards posed by a specific device category
- Identification and prioritization of process improvement
- Enhancement of risk-based inspections of companies
- Reaching out to offer guidance and to provide workshops for external interested parties

Increase in the number of recalls between 2003 and 2012 was credited to better reporting by manufacturers that were named in 806 reporting violations and by producers of radiological devices. There has been better reporting by industry and additional determined exertion by the CDRH and manufacturers to collaborate to increase the quality as well as the safety of medical devices.

Table 2.10 Software cause recall events by FY2008–FY2001

Year	Software change control	Software design	Software design (manufacturing process)	Total	% of all CDRH recalls
2008	13	141	2	156	18.3
2009	9	111	1	121	15.4
2010	4	73	3	80	8.9
2011	11	182	10	208	15.8
2012	12	169	5	186	15.5
Sum/ Overall	49	676	21	746	15.1

From US Food and Drug Administration [52]

The regulatory requirements for market introduction of new medical devices differ radically around the globe. Notwithstanding a wide range of different initiatives aiming at regulatory synchronization, opposing regulatory standards for approval continue, with a rising number of countries demanding local testing before local approval. Just to give an example of differing standards and timelines, it was 10 years between European regulatory approval of the WATCHMAN™ Left Atrial Appendage Closure Device (Boston Scientific, Marlborough Massachusetts, USA) and FDA 2015 approval in the United States, and it was just in 2017 that a clinical trial was finally initiated in Japan to secure device regulatory endorsement in that country [53].

Marketing of Medical Devices

During the 1997 and 2006 period, given the evolution of market dynamics, the frequency and type of financial content observed in pharmaceutical vs medical device commercials changed. The scarcity of supportive proof in medical device ads and pharmaceutical formulary assertions are potential areas of worry that need further analysis by watchdogs, policymakers, and academia [54]. Interestingly, the types of financial assertions in pharmaceutical vs medical device commercials differed considerably. The pharmaceuticals frequently presented market share claims (12.8%), whereas the medical device commercials seldom made such claims (1.1%) ($p < 0.01$). Additionally, assertions other than market share claims were more numerous for medical devices compared to pharmaceuticals (28.3% vs 11.4%; $p < 0.01$). For example, claims concerning compensation were encountered frequently in medical device advertisements (4.9% vs 0.8%; $p < 0.01$), as were cost-effectiveness claims (6.5% vs 0.6%; $p < 0.01$). Price claims were more common for medical devices (10.3%) compared with pharmaceuticals (6.9%) (Table 2.11) [54]. Of the 561 distinctive commercials with economic content, 408 (73%) gave supportive proof of the assertions. While proof was commonly given in pharmaceuticals, it was not provided for medical device ads. Just one medical device ad that made a financial claim gave any proof (Table 2.12) [54].

Table 2.11 Economic content by advertisement type

Type of claim	Type of advertisement[a] No. (%)		P value*
	Pharmaceutical (n = 2, 205)	Medical device (n = 184)	
Any economic content	507 (23.0)	54 (29.3)	0.06
Market share claims	282 (12.8)	2 (1.1)	<0.01
Other economic content	251 (11.4)	52 (28.3)	<0.01
Price claims	152 (6.9)	19 (10.3)	0.10
Non-price claims	127 (5.8	43 (23.4)	<0.01
Co-payment	7 (0.3)	2 (1.1)	0.15
Formulary	37 (1.7)	0	0.11
Reimbursement	18 (0.8)	9 (4.9)	<0.01
Value	18 (0.8)	3 (1.6)	0.22
Cost-effectiveness	14 (0.6)	12 (6.5)	<0.01
Other	38 (1.7)	18 (9.8	<0.01

From Ackerly et al. [54], with permission
*P values from Fischer exact tests
[a]Advertisements could contain more than one kind of claim. Table does not include reminder advertisements

Table 2.12 Prevalence of verifiable claims that had supporting evidence

Type of claim	Type of advertisement			
	Pharmaceutical		Medical device	
	n[a]	No. (%) with evidence	n	No. (%) with evidence
Market share	282	276 (97.9)	2	1 (50.0)
Price	152	126 (82.9	14[b]	0
Co-payment	7	0	0[b]	0
Formulary	37	5 (13.5)	0	0
Reimbursement	3[b]	3 (100.0)	9	0
Value	18	8 (44.4)	3	0
Cost-effectiveness	14	5 (35.7)	12	0

From Ackerly et al. [48], with permission
[a]The total number of economic claims exceeds the number of advertisements because single advertisements can include multiple claims
[b]The number of claims requiring evidence represents the verifiable claims and are thus lower than the overall number of claims

Conclusions

Advances in medical device innovations often evolve from profound clinical acumen and a need-based approach to providing more efficient clinical care. It can be argued that there is a significant role for incremental improvements to existing solutions, but what if the paradigm for existing solutions is wrong? Then real shifts in clinical outcomes, population health, patient satisfaction, surgical efficiency, and a better use of economic resources dictate a transformational paradigm shift, which in the case of medical devices can only be achieved by thinking outside the box by way of disruptive innovations [55]. From the medical device industry's point of view, successful innovation and marketing require collaboration with both customers (patients and surgeons) and technology providers (academia, SMEs, and large companies). The needs of the patients and surgeons should be identified, and the innovations should translate into commercially feasible solutions, by the use of existing or evolving technologies [1].

The author believes a medical device should arise from the following general steps while complying with local regulatory standards:

1. Identify a need.
2. Ideate the responsible innovation.
3. Patent the invention.
4. Obtain financing (*first* round).
5. Build the prototypes.
6. Perform laboratory testing.
7. Obtain financing (*second* round).
8. Perform clinical trials.
9. Limited evaluation.
10. Educate the customers.
11. Obtain feedback from the customers to improve product.
12. Build second-generation devices.
13. Commercialize the device.
14. Dominate the market.
15. Educate the customers.
16. Obtain feedback from the customers to improve product.
17. Dominate the market.

Prior to introducing a medical device into the market or producing a device, all technological, societal, economic, and administrative challenges and "side effects" of the medical device from the design phase on should be thoroughly studied. A medical device is not passive in the sense that it is only used by one end user in the organization. On the contrary, a device affects the immediate team and impacts the social contexts and supporting mechanisms of organizations. From the financial perspective, a value analysis to assess milestones to be achieved at specific times is important. Adoption of the medical device by insurance providers and appropriate reimbursement is a crucial milestone before mass production. There are systematic methods for performing these tasks (Fig. 2.24) [56]. While the history of other disruptive revolutions suggests systemic transformation is occurring in healthcare, there is a crisis in medical instrument industry which requires "responsible innovation" for a medical device to succeed in the market [9].

The term "responsible" is used to denote the manufacturers' responsibility to adequately educate and provide a continuous quality control feedback loop mechanism in the field once the product is released. Many companies today provide the physicians with medical devices without proper training. Although disruptive technologies enable caregivers to move competently upward, education is needed to reach competence. For the case of vaginal mesh kits, the physicians who had little

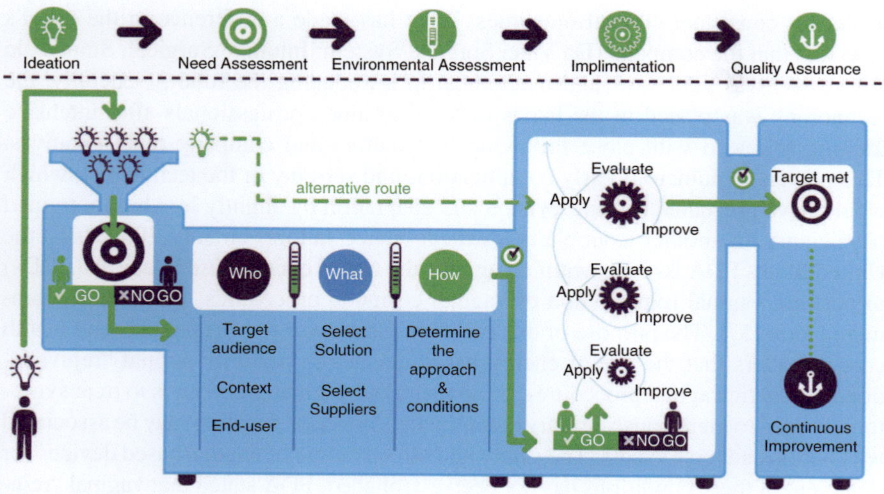

Fig. 2.24 Implementation of toolkit technology in healthcare. Adapted from (https://www.waardigheidentrots.nl/) (Courtesy of Waardigheid en Trots, Utrecht, the Netherlands)

experience with vaginal reconstructive surgery were taken to daylong cadaver courses before returning to their home institutions to perform these procedures without supervision. Or in some cases, they were given the devices to use with proctors present without a through introduction. Vaginal mesh kit innovations may have transformed the care of female patients with pelvic organ prolapse if the devices had been first used by experts. Instead, first-generation devices were released to a large number of poorly trained users in great volume, and the industry failed to create a feedback loop mechanism to keep track of complications as they arose. Although the vaginal mesh kits were more expensive than simple use of sutures to repair vaginal prolapse, the introduction of this technology made sense because the original surgeries were technically difficult to perform.

Some even more unlikely innovations have risen since the fall of vaginal mesh kits. The robot companies pushed a very expensive technology into the hands of highly skilled physicians in urology and the other subspecialties, and once these markets were saturated, they expanded by placing their devices into the hands of some highly skilled generalist surgeons. Robotic innovations have transformed healthcare by allowing surgeries to be performed more safely and efficiently but perhaps at a significant financial cost in many circumstances. Many endometrial cancer surgeries that were previously performed in morbidly obese women resulted in chronic wound infections and various complications. These surgeries are now done in outpatient setting. The economic analysis of robots is mixed, but the patients are undoubtedly doing better. The robot technology's success flies in the face of the general belief that the "blue ocean" growth markets merge when the alterations are made to products, processes, or technologies to allow less highly compensated groups of individuals to perform tasks in a more expedient settings. The robot technology has gone through many revisions through the years but still uses a highly trained expensive workforce to deliver consistent clinical outcomes. What has made a difference in the robot's case was that the company (Da Vinci Surgical System; Intuitive Surgical, Sunnyvale CA, USA) was very slow and methodical in introducing the robot. Generally, the technology was placed in the hands of highly trained professionals after intensive training followed with close follow-up by proctors and company representatives. This prevented numerous early complications and scrutiny of the technology, which would have prevented it from revision and adaptation by slightly less highly trained physicians. As another example of medical device failure, on July 30th 2018, the United States FDA issued a warning against the use of energy based devices (EBDs) to perform vaginal rejuvenation or vaginal cosmetic procedures: FDA safety communication [57]. The purpose of this communication was to alert patients and health care providers that the use of energy-based devices to perform vaginal "rejuvenation," cosmetic vaginal procedures, or non-surgical vaginal procedures to treat symptoms related to menopause, urinary incontinence, or sexual function may be associated with serious adverse events. The safety and effectiveness of energy-based devices for treatment of these conditions has not been established. FDA stated that vaginal "rejuvenation" is an ill-defined term; however, it is sometimes used to describe non-surgical procedures intended to treat vaginal symptoms and/or conditions including, but not limited to vaginal laxity: vaginal atrophy, dryness, or itching; pain during sexual intercourse; pain during urination and decreased sexual sensation. FDA further stated that "we have not cleared or approved for marketing any energy-based devices to treat these symptoms or conditions, or any symptoms related to menopause, urinary incontinence, or sexual function. The treatment of these symptoms or conditions by applying energy-based therapies to the vagina may lead to serious adverse events, including vaginal burns, scarring, pain during sexual intercourse, and recurring/chronic pain." The evolution, marketting and possible market failure of EBDs is currently unfolding.

How can the healthcare instrument industry, venture capital, entrepreneurial energy, and technology development interface with the regulators, insurers, physicians, hospitals, and medical schools so that they won't end up in litigation? The medical institutions are certainly no match for Goliaths such as Johnson & Johnson, Bard, and Boston Scientific, but they do have the responsibility of educating the next generation of surgeons to practice evidence-based medicine and to ask for long-term safety and efficacy data for a new product. The frustration of patients and physicians, however, should not be directed at the FDA alone. The agency does not bear sole responsibility for the current situation of lack of sufficient data to support and inform the use of many high-risk and implanted devices such as vaginal mesh kits. Responsibility is shared with the clinical community, which often resists requirements to report data; with manufacturers, which often oppose strong premarketing and post-marketing requirements; and with payers, which often do little with the major data assets that they control [49].

Currently, there is a significant divide in the information accessible to evaluate the value, safety, efficacy, or quality of medical devices [45]. The reporting of medical device issues is voluntary, and there is no centralized data source to obtain details on the specific brand or model of medical devices in use. It is postulated that if health insurance claims included device-identifying tracking information, researchers could [58] gauge the incidence of device malfunctions and failures to further evaluate the total costs of care connected with different medical device products. The insurance claims databases are used currently in a similar manner to monitor the safety of prescription drugs [59].

A nongovernmental organization called X12 (the Accredited Standards Committee X12) is a standards organization chartered by the American National Standards Institute in 1979, which develops and maintains the X12 Electronic data interchange (http://www.x12.org/). It manages the data submitted in typical insurance claims forms used by hospitals or health insurers. X12 has published a draft recommendation to include in claims the device identifiers that implanted device manufacturers have been placing on their packaging since early 2015. The claim forms are updated very infrequently, and the current environment provides an optimal timing for introducing this revision. A delay would mean an additional decade or more before changes can be instituted [60]. Integrating unique device identifiers (UDI) in medical devices is supported by the health insurers, hospitals, medical societies, the Medicare Payment Advisory Commission, the FDA, the CMS, and the Office of Inspector General of the Department of Health and Human Services [60].

It is unlikely that the medical device industry can completely safeguard patient safety, and it is unlikely that governments can effectively regulate the medical device manufacturers without also suffocating innovation. While some of the responsibility lies with *academic* medicine, which has been slow to teach evidence-based practice in medical schools and residency programs, the innovation, evolution, and marketing of medical devices often affect surgeons who are in *clinical* practice and not subservient to medical schools. Hospital credentialing committees ask for certificates of training, which are issued by the manufacturers. So, the decision as to which surgeon or healthcare team member may use a medical device in a competent manner depends on the education provided by the manufacturers and which surgeon or healthcare team member is a good candidate for training depends on selection by field representatives, most often with educational degrees unrelated to healthcare. To this date no standard exists on who should be trained or what constitutes adequate training for a medical device. In conclusion, the innovation of medical devices is an exciting, necessary yet costly and complex process. It should be conducted in a manner that enhances operators' ease of use, increases device safety and rewards innovators for their effort while enhancing societal benefits. This seemingly simple objective has not been achieved given the increasingly complex nature of modern medical devices and the cost associated with bringing an idea to the market. Nevertheless, patients' well being should constitute the center of all that we do to achieve Zero harm.

References

1. Bayon Y, Bohner M, Eglin D, Procter P, Richards RG, Weber J, Zeugolis DI. Innovating in the medical device industry – challenges & opportunities ESB 2015 translational research symposium. J Mater Sci Mater Med. 2016;27(9):144.
2. Abenstein JP. Technology assessment for the anesthesiologist. Anesthesiol Clin. 2006;24(4):677–96.

3. Wieringa FP, Poley MJ, Dumay AC, van der Steen AF. Avoiding pitfalls in the road from the idea to certified product (and the harsh clinical environment thereafter) when innovating medical devices. Proceedings of the IEEE Benelux EMBS Symposium/ Belgian Day on Biomedical Engineering: Brussel: TNO Industrie en Techniek 30; 2007.
4. Geertsma RE, de Bruijn AC, Hilbers-Modderman ES, Hollestelle ML, Bakker G, Roszek B. New and emerging medical technologies: a horizon scan of opportunities and risks. Report 360020002. 2 Feb 2007. Bilthoven: Centre for Biological Medicines and Medical Technology. National Institute for Public Health and the Environment (RIVM). p. 116.
5. NHS England. Design for patient safety. A system-wide design-led approach to tackling patient safety in the NHS. London: Department of Health; 8 Oct 2003. http://www.nrls.npsa.nhs.uk/resources/collections/design-for-patient-safety/?entryid45=59881. 84 p.
6. Dumay AC. Innovating eHealth in the Netherlands. Stud Health Technol Inform. 2007;127:157–65.
7. Kim WC, Mauborgne RA. Blue ocean strategy, expanded edition: how to create uncontested market space and make the competition irrelevant: Harvard Business Review Press; 2015.
8. Innovation versus science? (Editorial). [Internet]. Nature 2007;448(7156):839.
9. Christensen CM, Bohmer RM, Kenagy J. Will disruptive innovations cure health care? Harv Bus Rev. 2000;78(5):102–12. 99.
10. U.S. Food & Drug Administration. Medical devices. Premarket approval (PMA). Last updated 27 Mar 2018. https://www.fda.gov/medicaldevices/deviceregulationandguidance/howtomarketyourdevice/premarketsubmissions/premarketapprovalpma/. Accessed 24 Apr 2018.
11. World Intellectual Property Organization (WIPO), Geneva. Statistical Country Profiles. United States of America. http://www.wipo.int/ipstats/en/statistics/country_profile/profile.jsp?code=US. Last updated March 2018. Acceessed 23 Apr 2018.
12. MedTech Europe. The European medical industry in figures. [Internet]. Brussels: MedTech Europe; 2018. http://www.medtecheurope.org/medtech-industry-in-figures. Accessed 25 Apr 2018.
13. World Intellectual Property Organization (WIPO), Geneva. Record year for international patent applications in 2016; strong demand also for trademark and industrial design protection. PR/2017/804. Geneva; 15 Mar 2017. http://www.wipo.int/pressroom/en/articles/2017/article_0002.html#designs. Accessed 3 Feb 2018.
14. Murphy LM, Edwards PL. Bridging the valley of death: transitioning from public to private sector financing. NREL/MP-720-34036. Golden: National Renewable Energy Laboratory; May 2003. http://www.cleanenergystates.org/CaseStudies/NREL-Bridging_the_Valley_of_Death.pdf
15. Steinmetz KL, Spack EG. The basics of preclinical drug development for neurodegenerative disease indications. BMC Neurol. 2009;9(Suppl 1):S2.
16. Bingaman J, Simon RM, Rosenberg AL. Needed: a revitalized national S&T Policy. [Internet]. Issues Sci Technol. 2004;20(3)
17. Morrison RJ, Kashlan KN, Flanangan CL, Wright JK, Green GE, Hollister SJ, Weatherwax KJ. Regulatory considerations in the design and manufacturing of implantable 3d-printed medical devices. Clin Transl Sci. 2015;8(5):594–600.
18. Li TW, Tu PW, Liu LL, Wu SI. Assurance of medical device quality with quality management system: an analysis of good manufacturing practice implementation in Taiwan. Biomed Res Int. 2015:670420.
19. Worldwide Medtech Sales by EvaluateMedTech® Device Area: Top 15 Categories & Total Market (2016 & 2022). http://info.evaluategroup.com/MTWP2017-EMF.html.
20. Roberts EB. Technological innovation and medical devices. In: Ekelman KB, editor. New medical devices: invention, development, and use. Washington, DC: National Academy Press; 1988. p. 35–47.
21. Makower J, Meer A, Denend L. FDA impact on U.S. medical technology innovation: a survey of over 200 medical technology companies. November 2010. [Internet]. http://www.medtecheurope.org/node/246. Accessed 3 Feb 2018.
22. Sharma A, Blank A, Patel P, Stein K. Health care policy and regulatory implications on medical device innovations: a cardiac rhythm medical device industry perspective. J Interv Card Electrophysiol. 2013;36(2):107–17.

23. Long G, Mortimer R, Sanzenbacher G. Recent average price trends for implantable medical devices, 2007–2011. Sept 2013.
24. Goldman DP, McGlynn EA. U.S. health care: facts about cost, access, and quality. Santa Monica: RAND Corporation; 2005. https://www.rand.org/pubs/corporate_pubs/CP484z1.html
25. Moss AJ, Hall WJ, Cannom DS, Daubert JP, Higgins SL, Klein H, et al. Improved survival with an implantable defibrillator in patients with coronary disease at high risk for ventricular arrhythmia: the Multicenter Automated Defibrillator Implantation Trial (MADIT) Investigators. N Engl J Med. 1996;335(26):1933–40.
26. Buxton AE, Lee KL, Fisher JD, Josephson ME, Prystowsky EN, Hafley G. A randomized study of the prevention of sudden death in patients with coronary artery disease: the Multicenter Unsustained Tachycardia Trial (MUSTT) Investigators. N Engl J Med. 1999;341(25):1882–90.
27. Moss AJ, Zareba W, Hall WJ, Klein H, Wilber DJ, Cannom DS, et al.; Multicenter Automatic Defibrillator Implantation Trial II Investigators (MADITII). Prophylactic implantation of a defibrillator in patients with myocardial infarction and reduced ejection fraction. N Engl J Med. 2002;346(12):877–83.
28. Kadish A, Dyer A, Daubert JP, Quigg R, Estes NA, et al.; Defibrillators in Non-Ischemic Cardiomyopathy Treatment Evaluation (DEFINITE) Investigators. Prophylactic defibrillator implantation in patients with nonischemic dilated cardiomyopathy. N Engl J Med. 2004;350(21):2151–8.
29. Bristow MR, Saxon LA, Boehmer J, Krueger S, Kass DA, De Marco T, et al.; Comparison of Medical Therapy, Pacing, and Defibrillation in Heart Failure (COMPANION) Investigators. Cardiac-resynchronization therapy with or without an implantable defibrillator in advanced chronic heart failure. N Engl J Med. 2004;350(21):2140–50.
30. Bardy GH, Lee KL, Mark DB, Poole JE, Packer DL, Boineau R, et al.; Sudden Cardiac Death in Heart Failure Trial (SCD-HeFT) Investigators. Amiodarone or an implantable cardioverter-defibrillator for congestive heart failure. N Engl J Med. 2005;352(3):225–37. Erratum in: N Engl J Med 2005;352(20):2146.
31. Drummond M, Weatherly H. Implementing the findings of health technology assessments. If the CAT got out of the bag, can the TAIL wag the dog? Int J Technol Assess Health Care. 2000;16(1):1–12.
32. Brouwer WB, van Exel NJ, Baltussen RM, Rutten FF. A dollar is a dollar is a dollar – or is it? Value Health. 2006;9(5):341–7.
33. Reijnen MM, Zeebregts CJ, Meijerink WJ. Future of operating rooms. Surg Technol Int. 2005;14:21–7. (Review).
34. Lee K. Designing the OR of the future [Internet]. Healthcare design. Construction and engineering. 24 Sep 2015. http://www.healthcaredesignmagazine.com/trends/construction-engineering/designing-or-future/. Accessed 2 Feb 2018.
35. Kopelman Y, Lanzafame RJ, Kopelman D. Trends in evolving technologies in the operating room of the future. JSLS. 2013;17(2):171–3.
36. Gallagher AG, Smith CD. From the operating room of the present to the operating room of the future. Human- factors lessons learned from the minimally invasive surgery revolution. Semin Laparosc Surg. 2003;10(3):127–39.
37. Wieringa F.P. Pulse oxigraphy: and other new in-depth perspectives through the near infrared window [Internet]. Erasmus University Rotterdam; 2007. Available from: http://hdl.handle.net/1765/10031. Accessed 24 Apr 2018.
38. Vosburgh KG, Newbower RS. Moore's law, disruptive technologies, and the clinician. Stud Health Technol Inform. 2002;85(85):88–113.
39. Baim DS, Donovan A, Smith JJ, Briefs N, Geoffrion R, Feigal D, Kaplan AV. Medical device development: managing conflicts of interest encountered by physicians. Catheter Cardiovasc Interv. 2007;69(5):655–64.
40. Amoore JN. A structured approach for investigating the causes of medical device adverse events. J Med Eng. 2014;2014:314138.
41. AACE Health Technology Foundation, Clinical Alarm Task Force. Impact of clinical alarms on patient safety: a report from the American College of Clinical Engineering Healthcare Technology Foundation. J Clin Eng. 2007;32(1):22–33.

42. Sensmeier J. Survey says: care, communication enhanced by IT. Nurses report ups and downs of current systems. Nurs Manag. 2006;37(Suppl):2, 4, 6 passim.
43. Bohn RE. Measuring and managing technical knowledge. MIT Sloan Manag Rev. 1994;36(1):61–73.
44. Want to please patients? Maybe you should start a specialty hospital. 1 Apr 2015. [Internet]. Advisory Board (advisory.com). https://www.advisory.com/research/health-care-advisory-board/blogs/at-the-helm/2015/04/patient-experience-and-specialty-hospitals. Accessed 2 Feb 2018.
45. Ibrahim AM, Dimick JB. Monitoring medical devices: missed warning signs within existing data. JAMA. 2017;318(4):327–8.
46. Obeid NR, Pryor AD. Is the adjustable gastric band dead? Ann Surg. 2017;265(3):446–7.
47. Moore BJ, Steiner CA, Davis PH, Stocks C, Barrett ML. Trends in hysterectomies and oophorectomies in hospital inpatient and ambulatory settings, 2005–2013. HCUP Statistical Brief #214. Nov 2016. Rockville: Agency for Healthcare Research and Quality. http://www.hcup-us.ahrq.gov/reports/statbriefs/sb214-Hysterectomy-Oophorectomy-Trends.pdf.
48. Levitz J, Kamp J. How morcellators simplified the hysterectomy but posed a hidden cancer risk. The Wall Street Journal. 11 Apr 2014.
49. Redberg RF, Jacoby AF, Sharfstein JM. Power morcellators, postmarketing surveillance, and the us food and drug administration. JAMA. 2017;318(4):325–6.
50. Javadian P, Shobeiri SA. The disability impact and associated cost per disability in women who underwent surgical revision of transvaginal mesh kits for prolapse repair. Female Pelvic Med Reconstr Surg. 2017; https://doi.org/10.1097/SPV.0000000000000489. Epub ahead of print
51. U.S. Food and Drug Administration. Center for Devices and Radiological Health. Urogynecologic surgical mesh: update on the safety and effectiveness of transvaginal placement for pelvic organ prolapse. July 2011. https://www.fda.gov/MedicalDevices/ProductsandMedicalProcedures/ImplantsandProsthetics/UroGynSurgicalMesh/ucm262301.htm. Accessed 6 Feb 2018.
52. U.S. Food and Drug Administration. Center for Devices and Radiological Health. Medical device recall report FY2003 to FY2012. www.fda.gov/downloads/aboutfda/centersoffices/officeofmedicalproductsandtobacco/cdrh/cdrhtransparency/ucm388442.pdf. Accessed 2 Feb 2018.
53. Stein KM. The long and winding road after FDA approval: a medical device industry perspective. Circulation. 2017;135(20):1877–8.
54. Ackerly DC, Glickman SW, Schulman KA. Economic content in medical journal advertisements for medical devices and prescription drugs. PharmacoEconomics. 2010;28(5):429–38.
55. Ray PP, Amaral JF, Hinoul P. Innovation best practices in the medical device industry. Tech Vasc Interv Radiol. 2017;20(2):90–3.
56. Waardigheid en trots. Implementatie toolkit technolgie in de zorg. www.waardigheidentrots.nl. Utrecht. Accessed 24 Apr 2018.
57. FDA Warns Against Use of Energy-Based Devices to Perform Vaginal 'Rejuvenation' or Vaginal Cosmetic Procedures: FDA Safety Communication. 2018 August, 1 2018.
58. Reed TL, Levy D, Steen LT, Roach J, Taylor T, Call K, et al. Adverse event triggered event reporting for devices: report of a Food and Drug Administration-supported feasibility pilot of automated adverse event reporting. J Clin Eng. 2016;41(2):83–9.
59. Moscovitch B, Rising J, Daniel G, Drozda J. Time to fix the black hole in Medicare data. [Internet] 29 June 2016. Health Affairs (Blog). https://www.healthaffairs.org/do/10.1377/hblog20160629.055612/full/. Accessed 6 July 2017.
60. Moscovitch B, Rising JP. Medical device identification in claims data. JAMA. 2017;318(19):1936–7.

Chapter 3
Business Aspects of Vaginal Mesh Kits: Lessons Learned

Neeraj Kohli

Introduction

The successful and safe treatment of stress incontinence and prolapse with good long-term results continues to challenge even the most skilled female pelvic surgeon. Until the turn of this decade, the vast majority of surgical procedures for these conditions were performed using native tissue or nonspecific commercial items without any significant associated commercial interest. With a perceived need for better results and medical innovation, companies introduced the concept of vaginal mesh to augment incontinence/prolapse repairs. With clinicians' increasing experience and comfort with mesh use, commercial kits were developed and made available from a variety of companies to enable a growing group of physicians to adopt and promote these procedures in their care of patients. In addition to clinical stimuli, a variety of business principles, including medical innovation, consumer demand, market share, and shareholder value, drove this market forward. With rapid growth, increasing data and scrutiny resulted in reevaluation of these products. Increasing reports of complications prompted the US Food and Drug Administration (FDA) to reevaluate the safety and efficacy of mesh use for stress incontinence and pelvic organ prolapse (POP). This resulted in two separate public health notices with resulting change in the regulatory approval pathway, issuance of professional society recommendations, strict physician guidelines, and requirement of increasing data for continued use. In addition to the clinical factors involved in the introduction and subsequent evolution of pelvic mesh products, general business principles also guided and predicted the natural course of the pelvic mesh market. A review of business principles and lessons learned is helpful

N. Kohli
Boston Urogynecology, Newton-Wellesley Hospital/Brigham and Women's Hospital, Wellesley, MA, USA

Department of Obstetrics and Gynecology, Harvard Medical School, Boston, MA, USA
e-mail: nkohli@partners.org

S. A. Shobeiri (ed.), *The Innovation and Evolution of Medical Devices*,
https://doi.org/10.1007/978-3-319-97073-8_3

in understanding the history of pelvic mesh and potentially avoiding a similar pitfall for future innovation. It is helpful to evaluate vaginal mesh through standard business models, including the "hype cycle" and "McKinlay's seven-stage model."

The Hype Cycle

The "hype cycle" was introduced by the American research, advisory, and information technology firm, Gartner, to describe the introduction, adoption, application, and maturity of specific technologies and can be applied to a wide range of products including media, technology, and medical innovation [1]. There are five distinct phases of the hype cycle which include:

- *Phase 1 – Technology Trigger:* In response to a perceived need for limitation, a new technology breakthrough is introduced. Early proof of concept stories and media interest triggers significant publicity, and commercial viability/success is unproven.
- *Phase 2 – Peak of Inflated Expectations:* Early publicity of success stories creates enthusiasm and predictions of success without significant experience or rigorous evaluation. Companies sensing opportunity may enter the market without extensive research or historical data.
- *Phase 3 – Trough of Disillusionment:* Interest wanes and scrutiny increases as the technology may fail to deliver on expectations or may be associated with increased risk or cost. Producers and/or advocates of the technology begin to decrease an investment continues only if surviving providers improve their products to satisfaction of early adopters and future users.
- *Phase 4 – Slope of Enlightenment:* The technology with its associated risks/benefits becomes more widely understood and its application for success more specific. Second- and third-generation products appear to address previous limitations.
- *Phase 5 – Plateau of Productivity:* Increasing information regarding risks/benefits and specific application of the technology allows mainstream adoption, while criteria for assessing viability and success become more clearly defined.

Application of the hype cycle to transvaginal mesh products illustrates the opportunity, enthusiasm, scrutiny, criticism, innovation, and application that have occurred over the last 2 decades.

Phase 1: Technology Trigger

Prior to the introduction of the ProteGen preconfigured mesh by Boston Scientific (Marlborough MA, USA) in 1995 and the Gynemesh PS mesh by Ethicon (Somerville NJ, USA) in 2002, there was no significantly commercially available or successful mesh kit promoted for treatment of stress incontinence and POP, respectively. Use of mesh for vaginal use was popularized by the introduction of the Gynecare tension-free transvaginal taping, or TVT® (Ethicon) retropubic sling procedure in 1998. Prior to introduction of these commercial products, the primary surgical procedure advocated by gynecologists/urogynecologist for uncomplicated stress incontinence was an abdominal colposuspension, requiring an abdominal incision with associated postoperative hospitalization and morbidity, or laparoscopy with a steep learning curve and lengthy operative times. The traditional suburethral sling using either a synthetic or biologic (allograft vs autograft) was reserved for recurrent stress incontinence, intrinsic sphincter deficiency, or as a salvage operation. For many years, the primary surgical technique for anterior and posterior prolapse was traditional colporrhaphy with suture-based plication of the weakened fascial layer and excision of the redundant vaginal mucosa. In the 1990s, the concept of the site-specific defect repair was popularized by Richardson, who advocated the paravaginal defect repair for lateral detachment of the pubocervical fascia from the white line for treatment of displacement cystocele [2]. This pathophysiology and associated site-specific repair technique was subsequently adopted for rectocele and enterocele repair. Unfortunately, these techniques had only average long-term success rates, and most patients undergoing POP surgery had a reoperation rate of up to 30%, prompting clinicians to seek a better solution for greater durability and long-term success. Addressing the perceived needs of clinicians and market opportunity, women's health companies introduced self-contained kits for incontinence and prolapse, which included specific configuration of mesh and trocars/devices for its placement.

Phase 2: Peak of Inflated Expectations

The most established and studied kit product, the Gynecare TVT® retropubic (TVT-R) sling procedure, had overtaken Burch colposuspension as the preferred operation of choice for genuine stress urinary incontinence (GSUI) with success rates as high as 90% and complication rates as low as 5%. The introduction of TVT accounted for up to a 20% increase in the number of incontinence surgeries performed. In less than 10 years, more than 550,000 TVT procedures had been performed with an overwhelming number of papers and presentations worldwide [3].These papers were often published by experienced surgeons and sometimes sponsored by medical device companies. Based partially on these specific data, surgeon enthusiasm and expectations for transvaginal mesh increased rapidly within the surgical community, regardless of education or experience. Professional education, device-sponsored symposiums, and cadaveric training increased exposure. Based on the success of the trocar-based TVT sling kits and due to technological advances and commercial marketing, kits with precut mesh pieces for anterior or posterior prolapse repair and needle introducers were introduced by various surgical device manufacturers. As the first mesh kits were classified as class II (moderate-risk) devices, subsequent kits were given 510 K clearance, which bypasses clinical trials and requires manufacturers only to show that their product is substantially equivalent to one already on the market.

Over the 10 years following initial approval, more than 40 companies began manufacturing mesh devices for pelvic floor conditions. Combined use of synthetic mesh/biologic graft for both anterior and posterior repair commonly became referred to as the total vaginal mesh (TVM) procedure. The surgical procedure was quickly marketed to physicians and patients and adopted by pelvic surgeons in an effort to achieve higher success rates comparable to those seen by the TVT sling procedure. Initially, mesh/graft augmentation was recommended for the patients at high risk for recurrent prolapse to be performed only by qualified well-trained surgeons. According to the FDA review of market data from surgical device manufacturers, approximately 300,000 women underwent surgical procedures in the USA to repair POP in 2010 with approximately 1 out of 3 POP surgeries using mesh and 3 out of 4 mesh POP procedures performed transvaginally.

Phase 3: Trough of Disillusionment

In response to growing consumer complaints, the FDA began investigating complaints of adverse effects and issued its first Public Health Notification in 2008 [4]. This caused patients and physicians to reevaluate the procedure, safety, and outcomes. Subsequently, introduction of legal scrutiny and subsequent mass tort action was initiated bringing greater media attention and scrutiny [5]. Studies should little change in mesh use after the first notification [6]. This cycle was further enhanced by the second Public Health Notification issued in 2011 with stronger recommendations after reassessment and finding on ongoing complications.

Phase 4: Slope of Enlightenment

With increased scrutiny and data analysis, the FDA, medical device companies, physicians, and patients become more knowledgeable about the specific indications, risks, benefits, and postoperative implications regarding mesh use for incontinence and prolapse. The FDA reviews the Manufacturer and User Device Experience (MAUDE) database with belief that the overall increase in the number of serious adverse events is cause for concern. Safety, efficacy, and limitations of existing literature are reviewed in greater detail. Based on their analysis, the FDA recommends specific recommendations for patients and healthcare providers and reclassifies transvaginal POP repair from class II to class III, requiring manufacturers to submit premarket approval applications, including relevant clinical data. They also recommended further 522 clinical studies to address the risks and benefits of mesh use and to expand post market monitoring of device performance. Medical device manufacturers have revised marketing materials and instruction for use to better reflect current safety data. Based on clinical data, products with comparatively lower success rates or higher complication rates have been removed from the market.

One example includes the Uratape® or Obtape® (Mentor, Irvine CA, USA) transobturator sling procedure, which was shown to have a higher risk of vaginal erosion ranging from 1.9% to 20% with or without associated infection and/or dyspareunia mainly due to its microporous configuration. All current mesh products are Type 1 macroporous monofilament to enable tissue ingrowth and to reduce risk of infection. Lower weight meshes with improved weaves have been introduced into the market. As a result of this phase of the hype curve, products improved, patient and physician education increased, indications for mesh use became more specific, and safety/effectiveness data standards were established.

Phase 5: Plateau of Productivity

We are currently in phase 5 of the vaginal mesh hype cycle – reassessment of transvaginal mesh product use with increasing reliance on data and focus on qualified surgeons performing procedures in appropriately selected patients for specific indications. The consent and counseling process has significantly improved, protecting the physician, patient, and medical device manufacturer. Ongoing and completed studies supporting products currently in use have provided patients and physicians with better information to make appropriate clinical decisions. There are five companies currently manufacturing mesh for transvaginal POP repair. The Pelvic Floor Disorders Registry (PFDR) was established as a private and public collaboration comprising professional societies, the National Institutes of Health, the FDA, and industry. Its threefold objective includes (1) to collect, store, and analyze clinical data related to prolapse treatment, (2) to establish common data elements and quality metrics, and (3) to provide a framework for external stakeholders to conduct POP research.

McKinlay's Seven-Stage Model of Medical Innovation (TVT-Secur)

In 1981, sociologist John McKinlay described the "seven stages in the career of a medical innovation," which parallels the hype cycle and loosely maps introduction, marketing, and implementation of medical devices into complex healthcare settings [7]. The seven stages are described as follows:

- *Stage 1 – Promising Reports:* Optimistic reports about a new innovation appear either in the media, case reports, or uncontrolled observational reports in medical journals, often trying to address limitations of current treatment options.

- *Stage 2 – Professional and Organizational Adoption:* The new innovation is adopted by influential groups such as key opinion leaders or professional organizations, sometimes facilitated by professional education and company-sponsored research.
- *Stage 3 – Public Acceptance and Third-Party Endorsement:* The public accepts the innovation as "beneficial," and the healthcare system, including physicians, hospitals, and insurers, agrees to provide or fund the innovation.
- Stage 4 – *Standard Procedure and Observational Reports:* The innovation becomes part of clinical care while studies (retrospective studies, case reports, or follow-up studies of patients already subjected to the innovation) to ascertain effectiveness begin.
- Stage 5 – *Randomized Controlled Trials (RCTs):* After widespread adoption of the innovation, more rigorous studies are undertaken, often showing it to be less effective or safer than indicated by earlier observational studies.
- Stage 6 – *Professional Denunciation of RCT Findings:* RCTs are criticized because they do not support and may challenge current practice; the criticism often appears as opinion or letters to the editor.
- Stage 7 – *Erosion and Discreditation:* Professional and public opinion of the innovation declines due to increasing data, critical reports, or introduction of newer and possibly more attractive innovation.

McKinlay's seven-stage model has been used to analyze the history of previous medical innovation, including hormonal replacement therapy for menopause [8], physiotherapy [9], and previous incontinence devices [10]. Application of the seven-stage model specifically for the TVT-Secur (Gynecare, a div. of Ethicon, Inc., Somerville, NJ, USA) may provide insight into medicoeconomic aspects of transvaginal mesh. Analysis suggests that clinical practice is often not based on strong evidence but on future promise and that innovations should be objectively evaluated with adequate follow-up prior to widespread adoption and recommendations.

Stage 1: Promising Reports

Early reports of new innovation are generally small case series with poor study methodology, limited number of surgeons and patients, and short postoperative follow-up. Reports often serve as an introduction with enthusiasm regarding future potential, especially in addressing limitations with the currently available technology. Amidst an increasing competitive market with concerns about adverse effects and ease of physician adoption, TVT-Secur was introduced in 2005 with marketed benefits of being easier, faster, and safer. TVT-Secur was licensed in Europe, the USA, and Canada on the basis of a predicate licensed moderate-risk device, so no additional evidence of safety or efficacy was required prior to marketing the product. Ethicon, the manufacturer, claimed the device was substantially equivalent to the company's TVT and TVT-Obturator (TVT-O®) devices that were already on the market and released the novel single incision sling product based on safety data and outcomes of its older products and based on a limited observational report with short-term follow-up. No human studies reporting long-term safety or efficacy were done by the company prior to release. Compared to the predicate TVT or TVT-O®, there were few to no promising reports or early data available.

Stage 2: Professional and Organizational Adoption

Upon its introduction, the TVT-Secur entered a competitive urogynecologic device market with multiple manufacturers and product offerings encompassing a wide range of materials (synthetic vs biologic), designs (weave and composition), and surgical approaches (retropubic, up; retropubic, down; transobturator, inside out; and transobturator, outside in). It is difficult to say how widely the device was adopted based on its marketed benefits of single incision, quicker operative time, less postoperative pain, and less risk of complications. A large industry-funded prospective registry examining the clinical effectiveness of TVT-Secur compared to TVT-R and TVT-O® reported on 1334 women with 49% undergoing the TVT-Secur procedure.

Stage 3: Public Acceptance and Third-Party Endorsement

As the TVT-Secur was licensed as an equivalent device for readily accepted and endorsed indications of stress incontinence, there was no specific or separate assessment or cost-benefit analysis performed on behalf of third-party payers, hospitals, or professional organizations prior to widespread use. Public acceptance would be based on physician assessment/approval and patient education. Thus, stage III presents little barriers for new device use once it is cleared for marketing, and most public acceptance is based on sales representative interaction, professional education, and peer-to-peer communication, rather than on established review processes.

Stage 4: Standard Procedure and Observational Reports

The first research reports regarding TVT-Secur began to appear in 2008. The studies were limited due to their cohort design with inherent biases, small number of patients, and short follow-up. Over time, increasing studies revealed outcomes to be less favorable with more adverse effects and lower effectiveness [11–14]. The lack of large studies with longer follow-ups most likely was due to the competitive marketplace with a large variety of available surgical kits for the treatment of stress incontinence – making clinical study of a single product more difficult.

Stage 5: Randomized Controlled Trials

By 2010, better designed and more rigorous studies regarding TVT-Secur began to appear in the literature albeit still comparatively weak compared to Gynecare TVT-R, which had a significant period of market monopoly and clinical research following initial introduction. The RCTs included mainly comparison of TVT-Secur to Ethicon's TVT-R and TVT-O® and only a few comparing TVT-Secur to devices from other manufacturers. It is unclear which studies were sponsored by Ethicon. As expected, RCT results were less favorable than the previously published cohort studies.

Stage 6: Professional Denunciation of RCT Findings

Compared to the letter published in 2011 by over 600 members of the Pelvic Surgeons Network as an evidence-based response to the FDA Safety Communication, there was no documented professional denunciation of the TVT-Secur RCTs, most likely because the device did not achieve significant market penetration and adoption by most surgeons. In addition, market need for a minimally invasive surgical option for stress incontinence was adequately addressed by the variety of other devices available on the market, potentially reducing the need to support an additional surgical option.

Stage 7: Erosion and Discreditation

Since 2013, there are at least four papers providing explicit evidence of erosion and discreditation of the TVT-Secur device. Some include rigorous systematic reviews as well as a Cochrane review and comparative outcomes to other slings. All came to very similar conclusions that TVT secure was not as effective as the more traditional devices and lead to more adverse effects.

Lessons Learned from the Business of Transvaginal Mesh Similar to experiences with past medical products, including breast implants, there are valuable lessons to be learned for current practice and future decision-making. First, FDA approval does not imply safety or effectiveness of a product. The FDA regulatory pathway has many options, which can allow a product to come to market without specific and long-term safety/efficacy data. Second, provided and published data should be approached with caution. Many early studies are sponsored by medical device companies and may include very skilled surgeons and specific patient selection criteria. Widespread application of study results to the average physician and general population may not always apply. Early adopters of technology should be aware of changing guidelines, indications, and risks/benefits, and patients should be counseled and consented accordingly. The complications of most medical therapies are generally underestimated. The MAUDE database contains only those complications that are reported and most likely underrepresents the total number and type of complications associated with any medical device. In addition, the denominator that indicates total number of cases is sometimes difficult to determine in order to provide adequate prevalence and incidence of certain complications. Complications can potentially occur at any time during a patient's life, especially with implantation of a foreign body or use of chronic medications. Safety data should be assessed individually by each patient and physician when making a decision for surgical treatment.

Future Implications

Lessons learned over the last decade with our experience using vaginal mesh for incontinence and prolapse should serve us well moving forward. Future technologies currently emerging in the treatment for pelvic floor dysfunction include laser/radiofrequency energy application and stem cell therapy for vaginal laxity, overactive bladder, stress incontinence, postmenopausal symptoms, and sexual dysfunction. With patient apprehension, physician anxiety, and negative publicity regarding vaginal mesh use, these therapies are increasingly being advocated as high-benefit and low-risk alternatives. Most have yet to undergo clinical study, rigorous evaluation, or approval for pelvic floor indication by the FDA, professional societies, and third-party payers. Both are currently at the earliest stages of the hype cycle and seven-stage model of medical innovation. Hopefully, the lessons learned from transvaginal mesh will not only allow us to better offer mesh safely to patients in the appropriate circumstances but to honestly and fairly evaluate new technologies in the future for the benefit of clinical medicine and, most importantly, our patients.

References

1. Fenn J, Raskino M. Mastering the hype cycle: how to choose the right innovation at the right time. Boston: Harvard Business Press; 2008.
2. Richardson AC. Paravaginal repair. In: Benson JT, editor. Female pelvic floor disorders. New York: W.W. Norton & Co.; 1992.
3. Ward K, Hilton P. Minimally invasive synthetic suburethral slings: emerging complications. Obstetr Gynaecol. 2007;7(4):223–32.
4. U.S. Food and Drug Administration. FDA Public Health Notification. Serious complications associated with transvaginal placement of surgical mesh in repair of pelvic organ prolapse and stress urinary incontinence. 20 Oct 2008.
5. U.S. Food and Drug Administration. Center for Devices and Radiological Health. Urogynecologic Surgical Mesh: update on the safety and effectiveness of transvaginal placement for pelvic organ prolapse. Jul 2011.
6. Reynolds WS, Gold KP, Ni S, Kaufman MR, Dmochowski RR, Penson DF. Immediate effects of the initial FDA notification on the use of surgical mesh for pelvic organ prolapse surgery in Medicare beneficiaries. Neurourol Urodyn. 2013;32(4):330–5.

7. McKinlay JB. From "promising report" to "standard procedure": seven stages in the career of a medical innovation. Milbank Mem Fund Q Health Soc. 1981;59(3):374–411.
8. Wright J. Hormone replacement therapy: an example of McKinlay's theory on the seven stages of medical innovation. J Clin Nurs. 2005;14(9):1090–7.
9. Bø K, Herbert RD. When and how should new therapies become routine clinical practice? Physiotherapy. 2009;95(1):51–7.
10. Wall LL, Brown D. The perils of commercially driven surgical innovation. Am J Obstet Gynecol. 2010;202(1):30.e1–4.
11. Oliveira R, Silva A, Pinto R, Silva J, Silva C, Guimarães M, et al. Short-term assessment of a tension-free vaginal tape for treating female stress urinary incontinence. BJU Int. 2009;104(2):225–8.
12. Solà V, Ricci P, Pardo J. Third generation sub-mid urethral mesh: experience with 110 TVT-SECUR. Arch Esp Urol. 2009;62(5):376–86.
13. Debodinance P, Amblard J, Lucot JP, Cosson M, Villet R, Jacquetin B. TVT Secur: prospective study and follow up at 1 year about 154 patients. J Gynecol Obstet Biol Reprod. 2009;38(4):299–303.
14. Meschia M, Barbacini P, Ambrogi V, Pifarotti P, Ricci L, Spreafico L. TVT-secur: a minimally invasive procedure for the treatment of primary stress urinary incontinence. One year data from a multi-centre prospective trial. Int Urogynecol J Pelvic Floor Dysfunct. 2009;20(3):313–7.

Chapter 4
Medical-Legal Aspects of Transvaginal Mesh Kit Complications: A Historical Perspective and the US Food and Drug Administration Review Process

Bruce Patsner

Of each particular thing, ask: what is it in itself? What is its nature?

Marcus Aurelius

Introduction

The repair of vaginal vault prolapse has been an established part of the gynecologists' surgical armamentarium for more than half a century. As such, these surgeries enjoyed decades of significant clinical success, generated little controversy, and had a serious complication rate that was both low [1] and which resulted in negligible amounts of either medical malpractice or product liability litigation.

From the 1950s through 2000s, the earliest generation of surgical therapy revolved around use of "natural" mesh products which were originally intended for use in hernia repair. The newer synthetic mesh products, and the vaginal mesh kits using these synthetic mesh products, entered the US and overseas medical markets over 15 years ago and were both widely promoted to physicians of multiple specialties (not just ob-gyns) and were promoted for surgical indications other than just recurrent, simple pelvic organ prolapse. The impact this new surgical technology had on the female surgical population in the United States and overseas once its use became widespread was simply devastating.

B. Patsner
Department of Obstetrics and Gynecology, Virginia Commonwealth University School of Medicine, Richmond, VA, USA

Quality and Patient Safety, Inova Fairfax Women's Hospital, Falls Church, VA, USA

Department of Obstetrics and Gynecology, Inova Fairfax Women's Hospital, Falls Church, VA, USA

S. A. Shobeiri (ed.), *The Innovation and Evolution of Medical Devices*,
https://doi.org/10.1007/978-3-319-97073-8_4

At the time of this writing in 2018, there are literally thousands of medical malpractice and medical device product liability lawsuits in both state and federal courts involving use of vaginal mesh and vaginal mesh kits [2]. There are thousands of patients who have sustained significant, painful, acute, and chronic pelvic, urological, and bowel morbidity. Serious controversy surrounds how the US Food and Drug Administration (FDA) allowed these medical devices (newer types of mesh and newer methods of insertion using mesh insertion kits) to reach consumers, how they were monitored (or failed to monitor) what serious adverse events were being produced by these devices, whether they delayed timely regulatory intervention, and whether what they did do when they finally intervened was adequate [3]. There are also serious questions surrounding the marketing – direct to consumer and direct to physician advertising – by the manufacturers of these kits as well as other implantable surgical medical devices [3]. And lastly, there are lingering serious issues surrounding the training and oversight of surgeons using these kits by the medical profession, as well as the role the medical profession in general (and select medical professional societies in particular) had in "partnering" with manufacturers to promote widespread use of these kits and instruct large numbers of otherwise minimally trained surgeons to use these mesh kits on their patients [3].

The advancement of this new surgical technology based on alleged or hypothetical superior surgical results, or lower primary failure rates, in the context of a virtual absence of substantive primary or comparative data, and the virtual absence of meaningful short- and long-term safety data, still remains a problem for patients, physicians, industry, and all parties involved in the regulation of the medical profession.

The manufacturers of these kits, and in many cases the physicians who used them, can now look forward to a decade or more of costly litigation and potential monetary settlements.[1] Some of the patients in whom these devices were inserted can look forward to years of mesh-related pain and surgical procedures to remove mesh. All of which raises several critical questions:

1. How this widespread surgical debacle happen?
2. What roles did the individual players – individual physicians, medical device manufacturers, FDA, medical professional societies, and plaintiff's bar – play in creating this new population of mesh kit-related injured patients?
3. How is this surgical crisis going to resolve/resolving?
4. Lastly, what lessons can be learned moving forward so that there is not a repeat of this scenario when another new pelvic surgical technology appears?

The penultimate question just posed has already been partially answered: most of the original manufacturers have withdrawn their vaginal mesh kit products from the US market as a result of ongoing litigation and controversy [4]. As a result of this, some of the publicity over these devices has diminished. Yet there is still con-

[1] Each case being litigated can easily take 5–10 years between the filing of the initial complaint and the decision of a jury, particularly if a manufacturer elects to individually litigate the case of every single patient.

tinued availability and use of some of these mesh kit devices, and new patients continue to be harmed.

Potential solutions to the final question posed will be advanced in the final part of this chapter, with the understanding that legislative changes in the medical device regulatory environment starting in 2017 may not help prevent scenarios like this from happening again.

One important note before we delve into our regulatory/medical-legal analysis is that vaginal mesh kits have been used, and promoted, as medical devices for treatment of both pelvic organ prolapse (POP) and stress urinary incontinence (SUI). There is a great deal of controversy over the use of synthetic mesh and mesh kits treatment of the former, but there is at least a moderate consensus in the medical literature that use of the synthetic retropubic slings at present is an acceptable treatment for this latter condition both in terms of efficacy and safety [5]. There is controversy about the use of transobturator tape-type slings as they use the obturator space and are associated with pain analogous to vaginal mesh kits.

For these reasons, this chapter will focus exclusively on the controversy surrounding the use of synthetic vaginal mesh kits for treatment of pelvic organ (predominately vaginal vault but also bladder and rectocoele) prolapse.

From Manufacturer to the Operating Room: How FDA Regulates Medical Devices

Any analysis of the medical-legal issues surrounding mesh kits must begin with a close examination of the process by which a new, or "almost new", commercially manufactured medical device gets from its manufacturer to the patient; only then can we explore how the various stakeholders interact. For purposes of our discussion in this chapter on vaginal mesh kits, the term "marketing" means being able to legally sell in the United States, e.g., to hospitals, ambulatory surgery centers, or a physician medical practice, so that surgeons may insert the vaginal mesh into a patient using the kit.

The first and most critical player in this process is the US Food and Drug Administration (hereafter abbreviated FDA). A close look at how the US Food and Drug Administration regulates medical devices is essential; this includes testing, approval/marketing, advertising and promotion, post-marketing surveillance of marketed devices, and its relationship/authority to/over the medical profession and surgical practice. Some general comments first.

FDA is the federal agency primarily responsible for regulation of pharmaceuticals, medical devices, vaccines and other biologicals, food, veterinary medicines, and cigarettes through its various centers such as CDER (Center for Drug Evaluation and Research) and CDRH (Center for Devices and Radiological Health). FDA is one of a handful of federal agencies such as CMS, NIH, and CDC which are all parts of the Department of Health and Human Services. As part of the executive branch of the government, its actions (or nonactions) are to some degree an extension and reflection of presidential power, policy, and social/economic priorities, though the funding of the agency is from Congress and oversight over its regulatory actions is shared by both Congress and the federal courts.

Given the enormity of its task (FDA is directly or indirectly involved in roughly 20% of the entire US economy on a budget 1/250th that of NASA's, with fewer than 15,000 employees and largely at the mercy of Congress for its funding), there are resource limitations built into FDA's ability to thoroughly and flawlessly monitor any one of the multiple industries it has oversight over. From marketing approval to postmarketing surveillance for pharmaceutical, medical devices, and biologic drug products, FDA is also responsible for ensuring that the advertising and promotion of the prescription products it has oversight over also comply with federal law, FDA "rules," and federal court decisions. The limited control FDA has over the direct advertising and promotion of its products both to physicians and to consumers is constrained both by its limited resources and by federal court decisions which have greatly expanded First Amendment protection for commercial manufacturers of drugs and other FDA-regulated products. Consistent losses by FDA in court in cases involving the manner and content of direct to consumer advertising of medical products have created an environment in which FDA is somewhat reluctant to engage industry in this arena [6].

It is important to note that FDA does not directly regulate the medical profession; this specific restriction of FDA power or jurisdiction over physician medical and surgical practices was formally codified into federal law in the Food and Drug Administration Modernization Act (FDAMA) in 1997 [7]. FDAMA specifically codified the principle that the FDA will not regulate "the practice of medicine" with respect to medical devices. For a medical device such as vaginal mesh or a vaginal mesh kit which can only be inserted by a licensed physician (i.e., it is a "prescription" medical device), this means that FDA has no control over whether a surgeon uses an approved or cleared medical device in a manner not specifically listed in the label for the medical device, i.e., for an "off-label" or "unapproved" use [7].

The regulation of the medical profession in general, and surgical practices in particular, is predominately the purview of individual state medical boards and to a lesser degree the medical profession itself with a generous amount of "help" from the plaintiffs' bar.[2] This issue of who exactly regulates the medical profession, and how, will be returned to later in this chapter. And – with minor exceptions – FDA generally does not do independent testing of drugs or medical devices for either efficacy or safety; this is almost exclusively done by the commercial manufacturers of the medical products themselves.

---

[2] Statement of Janet Woodcock, Director of the Center for Drug Evaluation and Research, before the House Subcommittee on Oversight and Investigations, 10; "6th Congress (1990), "FDA does not generally regulate the practice of pharmacy or the practice of medicine – the States traditionally have regulated both the prescribing and dispensing of drugs." See also Peter Barton Hutt, *Regulation of the Practice of Medicine under the Pure Food and Drug Laws*, 33. J.A. Food and Drug Officials 3 (1969)

On the other hand, the *sale* of a prescription medical device may only be for the intended uses that the FDA approved or cleared and which appear in the label [8]. This apparent restriction on sale is not so narrow as it sounds, as FDA construes the term "labeling" quite broadly at least with respect to medical devices: "in practical terms, FDA may find evidence of 'intended use' in a firm's websites, sales talks, promotional brochures, journal and radio advertising, office visits, training materials, samples, demonstrations, and trade show displays. FDA considers user training to be legally equivalent to labeling and another potential determinant of intended use" [9]. Lastly, it is important to distinguish regulation of the labeling of a medical device – which FDA is responsible for – from advertising for a medical device, which the Federal Trade Commission (FTC) has jurisdiction over.

CDRH and the Regulation of Medical Devices

The regulation of medical devices is the purview of the Center for Devices and Radiological Health (CDRH),[3] a branch of FDA which is much smaller than the Centers for Drugs (CDER) and Biologics (CBER). More than FDA's other centers, the personnel resources available to CDRH have not nearly kept pace with the exponential growth of the medical device industry over the past 40 years. Many of the articles written about the workings of CDRH and its alleged shortcomings or "failures to regulate" since the mid-1970s when FDA first gained direct jurisdiction over medical devices. As a distinct entity have pointed out that the combination of significant and rapid advances in medical device technology and complexity, explosive growth of the medical devices industry, the limited personnel and resources at CDRH, and most importantly the relatively non-substantive changes to the original 1976 framework for regulating how medical devices reach patients and how they are monitored for safety have all combined to create a recurring situation in which patients are repetitively "set up" to be harmed by products poorly tested prior to marketing and whose serious safety issues emerge only after much damage has been done to thousands of patients they have been implanted in.

In short, the initially workable system developed in 1976 for ensuring the safety and effectiveness of new medical devices has not been able to keep up with the exponential growth of new surgical medical device technology nor the unforeseen serious safety events which arise. Even so, readers are urged to keep in mind that many if not most of the mesh-related problems which exist are to a very large extent not solely FDA's fault: FDA can *only* do what its 1938 enabling statute and amendments to it by Congress empower it to do. The real culprit – at the federal level anyway – is Congress. And, as will be discussed at the end of the chapter, anticipated

[3] Access to the Center for Devices and Radiological Health is open to the public at www.cdrh.fda.gov

congressional legislative actions in 2017–2018 have the potential to make the "holes" in our gynecology medical device regulatory framework and safety net which protects patients from harm even larger than they already are.

The Statutory Basis of Medical Device Regulation

The Medical Device Amendments of 1976 [10] (hereafter MDA) is the pivotal piece of congressional legislation which fundamentally changed FDA's 1938 Federal Food Drug and Cosmetic Act (hereafter FDCA) to give FDA direct statutory authority over medical devices and allowed control over if and how medical devices reached patients. Prior to 1976 FDA was only able to intervene after a device was *already on* the market, and FDA often had to argue in court that a device was somehow really a drug (as ridiculous as that sounds) in order for FDA to have jurisdiction over the matter so it could regulate it. After 1976, FDA finally had independent power to force manufacturers to prove that their devices "worked" as intended and to a lesser degree that they were safe for use in humans, before they were marketed for sale to consumers and healthcare providers.

It is fitting that it was an ob-gyn device which finally motivated the Congress to amend the FDCA. The Dalkon Shield was a first-generation intrauterine gynecologic device which was marketed in 1970 without any proof of its safety or efficacy. Incredibly, prior to 1976, it was routine – and perfectly legal – for a newly developed medical device to be inserted into thousands of patients by physicians without any meaningful data on how well the device actually worked or whether there would be life-threatening adverse events in the short or long term.

After the publicity and uproar over the Dalkon shield's significant infectious morbidity, infertility, and mortality (16 direct deaths from pelvic inflammatory disease by 1975), it became apparent that hazardous medical devices were easily being marketed and that an increase in federal regulation was needed to protect women's health. This would not be the first time that a catastrophic event had to occur before major additions to FDA's oversight over industry occurred; the history of FDA's increased control over the new drug approval process was literally built after a series of disasters throughout the twentieth century [11].

Since 1976, the FDCA has been further amended (in a major way in 1990, 1992, 1997, 2002, and 2007) with provisions related to user fees for manufacturers, timely review of medical device applications by FDA, and increased ability, and requirements, for post-marketing surveillance and databases. Even with these wide-ranging and frequent amendments, the fundamental structure and regulatory framework of the 1976 has remained unchanged [12].

The 1976 MDA defines the term "device" [13] as "an instrument, apparatus, implement, machine, contrivance, implant, in vitro reagent, or other similar or related articles, including any component, part, or accessory, which is:

1. Recognized in the official National Formulary, or the United States Pharmacopeia, or any supplement to them

2. Intended for use in the diagnosis of disease or other conditions, or in the cure, mitigation, treatment, or prevention of disease in man or other animals
3. Intended to affect the structure or any function of the body of man or other animals and which does not achieve its primary intended purposes through chemical action within or on the body of man or other animals and which is not dependent upon being metabolized for the achievement of its primary intended purposes"

As mechanical products designed and intended to cure/mitigate/treat pelvic relaxation defects in women, the synthetic meshes used for repair of vaginal vault prolapse and associated pelvic relaxation defects, and by extension the kits used to insert the mesh, are by definition medical devices.

The 1976 MDA was, at its inception, an innovative piece of legislation, which de novo created an entirely new three-tier classification system for medical devices based on the *safety risk* the device posed to humans. At the same time, the MDA created two distinctly different marketing routes by which FDA could allow medical devices to reach patients. It is critical to note that this regulatory framework created 40 years ago for medical devices is largely unchanged. Regulation of devices is a complicated area of food and drug law, and what follows is an admittedly simplified, abbreviated version of a statutory framework that has many nuances.

At the heart of the MDA regulatory system are three key concepts:

1. *Three classes of medical devices – I, II, and III* [14]: The lower the classification of the device, the easier it is for a manufacturer to get approval or "clearance" for marketing. The classes are described below. FDA has the discretion to reclassify devices as more information about them emerges once they are on the market; similarly, manufacturers may request that a device be reclassified to a lower class and may be granted such a request if they can demonstrate to FDA that reasonable assurance of the device's safety and efficacy may be provided by the less stringent requirements.

   Class II and Class III devices are subject to several mechanisms of monitoring for safety events once they enter the US market, and FDA actively collects such data. Based on the accumulation of a certain critical mass of serious adverse events (SAEs), FDA has the enforcement discretion to "up-classify" a medical device from moderate to high risk. When this happens, current and future manufacturers of that device can no longer use the 510(k) clearance mechanism described below to get their new products to the market. Instead, they must submit a premarket approval application with new, clinical trial data establishing that the device is both safe and effective for its intended use and must agree to the terms for specific post-marketing surveillance. As clinical trials may take years and cost tens of millions of dollars (to say nothing of the risk to the manufacturer that they may demonstrate that the device is neither effective nor relatively safe), up-classification of a medical device sometimes places the manufacturer in the position of having to decide whether to continue manufacturing the device for the US market or to withdraw it.

2. *Two routes to marketing* [15]: PMA (premarketing approval) vs. 510(k) clearance. There are two options manufacturers may request, or FDA may insist on, for a new medical device to get to the market. The first and by far the most widely utilized is the 501(k) clearance mechanism; it is easier for the manufacturer because of the lower financial, safety, and efficacy data requirements which must be provided to FDA in support of an application. In many instances, manufacturers have to provide little more than cursory information which merely supplements what FDA knows about similar products already on the market. This easier path for marketing cuts both ways: because of its limited resources and personnel, CDRH invariably favors the easier approval mechanism as well because it is less labor-intensive.

   The second, and more costly and complicated, route to marketing of a new device is the PMA (premarket approval) process which requires submission of substantial new clinical data on efficacy and safety. The economic factors favoring the 510(k) clearance mechanism as a route to market are offset somewhat by the loss of federal preemption protection against product liability lawsuits (and the risk of much greater awards by juries for damages) in state courts which are available to manufacturers under the MDA if their product is approved [16].
3. *The predicate medical device* and the doctrine of "substantial equivalence" – a device which is already on the market and which can be shown to be "substantially equivalent" to the newer device [17][4]. These two concepts are the main reason why most medical devices like vaginal mesh kits get to patients with little or no proof of efficacy and a virtual total absence of safety data.

   The downside of basing an easier route to marketing (501[k]) clearance on the easier demonstration of substantial equivalence to an already marketed medical device is the inevitable development of "equivalence creep": incremental changes in devices over many generations of devices can create a situation where progressively newer, more complicated, and potentially more dangerous medical devices enter the market without much efficacy or safety information.

   In the absence of a "gold standard" medical device to which all new devices must be directly compared, and the ability to allow market entry for new devices which combine two or more different previously cleared devices, it is possible and even likely that a newly cleared product may be very far afield indeed from the original predicate medical device cleared a decade or more earlier. Making matters worse, because of the personnel structure of decision-making at CDRH, in many instances, the determination of whether two devices are substantially equivalent may not even be made by a physician; it may be made by an engineer with little or no clinical medical training or experience.

   One final note of consequence is that there is no law or regulation which requires FDA to approve only prescription drugs or medical devices which are equal to, or superior to, those already being marketed. In fact, FDA has and will

[4] Note: A decision tree for facilitating the determination of substantial equivalence was developed by FDA. See Office of Device Evaluation, Guidance on the CDRH Premarket Notification Review Program (CDRH website (www.cdrh.fda.gov).

likely continue to approve prescription drugs or restricted medical devices which are either non-inferior or inferior to products already on the market. This is because the individual product approval process is a "weighing" of risks versus benefits, and if on balance a drug or device meets its efficacy endpoint(s) and poses "no" significant safety issues, it will likely get approved (whether CMS or private insurers will pay for it if its benefits are negligible is a separate issue and also a separate question as FDA has no real role in the pricing or reimbursement decision). Comparative studies between two medical devices for the same medical or surgical indication are rare.

The 510(k) clearance mechanism has the potential to routinely allow products with real, but undefined, safety risks onto the market with no meaningful efficacy or safety data for the product per se and a virtual absence of comparative efficacy and safety data to existing procedures/devices/technology.

Classes of Devices

Class I medical devices are defined in §513(a)(1)(A) as those which pose the least risk to humans for which the general controls of the MDA with respect to adulteration, misbranding, registration, defect notification, reports, good manufacturing practices, etc. are sufficient to provide a reasonable assurance of the safety and effectiveness of the device. In short, nothing special needs to be done. Examples of Class I medical devices are tongue depressors, crutches, and basic surgical instruments. After 1997 most Class I devices were exempted from the need to go through any marketing mechanism; what this means is that once designated as a Class I device by FDA, manufacturers can simply put their new device on the market.

Class II devices are more complicated, intermediate-risk devices whose safety and efficacy are not guaranteed by just the general control provisions of the MDA for which special controls may be needed. The special controls may include requirements for performance standards, patient registries, specific FDA guidance on use of the product, and/or requirements for post-marketing studies (i.e., investigations to be done once the device is on the market). To get to patients, the vast majority of Class II devices need to go through 510(k) clearance. Vaginal mesh and vaginal mesh kits are Class II medical devices.

Class III devices are those devices for which both general and special controls together are not sufficient to establish their safety and efficacy. They are defined in §513(a)(1)(C) as devices that (1) are used in supporting or sustaining human life, or (2) are used which is of substantial importance in preventing impairment of human health, or (3) present a potential unreasonable risk of illness or injury. A deep brain-implantable probe for treatment of refractory seizures, or the artificial pancreas, is a good example of Class III devices. In other words, these are the highest-risk devices; if it's lifesaving or life-threatening, it's a Class III device. Under §515 of the MDA, Class III devices are almost always subject to the premarket approval (PMA) requirement to reach the market. One could argue, in retrospect, that vaginal mesh kits should have been classified, or later reclassified, as Class III medical devices based on the surgical morbidity data which emerged once use of the these kits were widespread and complications reported in the medical literature.

How the 510(k) Clearance Works

The two different routes of marketing access for medical devices are very different paths, with enormous differences in cost, requisite amounts of supporting efficacy and safety data, administrative burdens, time FDA may take to review the application, and post-marketing regulatory requirements (Table 4.1) [13].

FDA uses the §510(k) clearance mechanism to permit marketing access for new medical devices which are claimed by the manufacturer to be similar (read: substantially equivalent) to already legally marketed Class I, II, or III medical devices for which premarket approval is not required, i.e., a predicate medical device.

The manufacturer of the medical device must submit a 510(k) notification to FDA at least 90 days prior to the intended date of introduction of the new device into the market, and once FDA finishes its evaluation of the application, FDA issues an order to the manufacturer. The FDA order simply states that the new device is substantially equivalent to a, or more than one, predicate device which is already

Table 4.1 US Food and Drug Administration (FDA): A comparison of the 510(k) premarket clearance and premarket approval (PMA)

Criterion	510(k) premarket notification	Premarket approval (PMA)
Devices subject to requirement	Some Class I Most Class II and Class III pre-amendment devices for which PMAs have not been called	All Class III post-amendment devices Class III pre-amendment devices for which PMAs have been called
Clinical data requirements	Most not supported by clinical data	Clinical studies required to support submission
Evidence of safety and efficacy required	Info and data to support the "substantial equivalence" of the device to an already legally marketed predicate device	Clinical data and/or scientific evidence supporting "safety and efficacy" claims
Marketing rights	No exclusivity	Like a product license
Average FDA review time	69 days	290 days
Regulations on device changes	Must file new 510(k) if the change "could significantly affect" the safety or efficacy of the device	Must file a new PMA or supplement or annual report, depending on the nature and effect of the change on the safety or efficacy of the device
FDA Advisory Panel Review	No review for all 510(k) devices	Review for some but not all PMAs

Adapted from Kahan and Wilson [13], with permission

legally being marketed in the United States. This determination will be reflected, and stated, in the label for the new medical device.

The 510(k) application[5] is usually no more than 30–60 pages long and may be acted upon within a short amount of time. There is no requirement for the manufacturer to submit any new efficacy or safety data since the whole point of this application is to essentially "piggyback" approval on something which FDA has already cleared and to which it has been determined the new device substantially similar to.

Even a cursory view of this process reveals the major drawback from a public safety point of view: it is possible to repetitively expose patients to progressively more complicated and potentially more dangerous generations and iterations of new devices for years, based on a brief application which contains no new evidence of efficacy or safety and with only a brief written summary of the safety and efficacy information upon which the substantial equivalence is based. This virtually never includes clinical trial data or any direct comparisons between the two medical devices. Exacerbating the problem is that the determination of substantial equivalence may be made at CDRH by someone with an engineering, not a medical, background who might not have any clinical experience which might allow them to appreciate that the submitted new device represents a clear departure in potential risk to patients.

The second major drawback is that substantial equivalence does not require that a proposed new device be compared to some "gold standard," superbly functioning, and safe medical device; rather, what is required is only that the new device be found to be substantially equivalent to one or more legally marketed devices and that it meet two requirements. Those requirements are that:

1. The new device must have the same intended use as the predicate medical device to which it is being compared.

2. (a) Either the same technological characteristics as the predicate device
   or
   (b) If it has different characteristics that the information submitted for clearance must not raise any new questions about safety or efficacy, i.e., that it is substantially equivalent. There may be some performance data submitted to "show" that the proposed new device is as same as effective as the predicate device, but this is not a requirement, and there is great flexibility in what can be submitted to show this.

Proposed new medical devices need not be cleared based on comparison to just one predicate device; a device with two or more different parts – such as a mesh kit which has both mesh and anchors for insertion – may be cleared as a new device by demonstrating substantial equivalence separately for each part even if they have not been previously combined together in an existing medical device.

---

[5]The information required in a 510(k) premarket notification appears in several section of the *Code of Federal Regulations*.

FDA is quick to point out that the 510(k) mechanism does not "approve" a premarket notification in the same way that it approves a PMA, and in an absolute sense this is correct. The PMA process is a much more complicated determination which requires clinical studies to support the submission's claims of effectiveness and safety for its intended use. On the other hand, FDA simply stating that a 510(k) notification of clearance only says whether a new device is substantially equivalent to a predicate device and *not* whether it is effective and safe for its intended use or that it is "approved" for that use is at its core an empty gesture. The fact is that it allows new medical devices to get to market/reach patients without being supported by *any* substantive clinical efficacy or safety data.

The one huge trade-off for manufacturers who go the 510(k) clearance route to get their new medical devices to market is that manufacturers lose complete federal preemption of state court tort claims for damages which devices which are approved for marketing via a PMA enjoy. In most instances, this should be of little concern since the odds are in the manufacturers favor that there will be no new serious morbidities from a new medical device substantially similar to an existing predicate medical device which may have a decade-long track record of safe and effective use in large numbers of patients.

On the other hand, if there has been substantial "predicate device drift" and the cleared new medical device actually is qualitatively different in potential safety effects from the already marketed predicate device(s), then there is great potential liability exposure for the manufacturer if they are sued in state courts by patients injured by their products, either because they were directly damaged by the product (i.e., it is inherently dangerous even if manufactured correctly, or its production was somehow defective) or because the label for the product failed to adequately warn them of the potential risks of the product.

How Did Newer Transvaginal Mesh and Mesh Kits Reach the US Market, and Why?

The best overview in the medical-legal/regulatory literature to date on the use of surgical mesh for treatment of women with pelvic organ prolapse and stress urinary incontinence is still the FDA Executive Summary [18] generated by the FDA Obstetrics and Gynecology Medical Devices Advisory Committee which met in Washington, D.C., on September 8–9, 2011. Information from this document will be used liberally in this section of this chapter. Table 4.2 presents a simplified history of the use of surgical mesh [19].

The first surgical mesh product indicated for repair/treatment of pelvic organ prolapse (POP) arrived at CDRH in 2001. FDA classified this mesh and all subsequent new meshes and mesh insertion kits as Class II medical devices. The manufacturer of this mesh claimed that their mesh was substantially equivalent to a predicate medical device already on the US market, in this case a surgical mesh

Table 4.2 Simplified history of the use of surgical mesh

Date	Development
1950	Surgeons began using surgical mesh to repair abdominal hernias
1970	Gynecologists began implanting the same surgical mesh to repair POP abdominally
1990	Surgical mesh was first used for the *transvaginal* repair of POP
1996	FDA clears the first surgical mesh designed for use in SUI surgeries
2002	The first transvaginal mesh device was cleared for use as a Class II moderate-risk device for use in POP surgeries
2016	Most transvaginal mesh kits removed from the US market

POP pelvic organ prolapse, *SUI* stress urinary incontinence

which had been used for several decades for hernia repairs. All of the initial and subsequent manufacturers of new meshes and mesh insertion kits requested that their devices be evaluated for possible marketing in the United States utilizing the previously discussed 510(k) clearance mechanism, and all of these requests were granted.

The FDA reviewed the comparison of the new POP mesh and the hernia mesh and found that the two devices were substantially equivalent based on a review of intended use, product design, intended label for use, material safety, and performance data on the material. The new mesh products, and later mesh insertion kits, were all cleared for marketing in the United States via this regulatory approval route.

Based on the previous lengthy discussion of classification of medical devices, marketing approval mechanisms, and the nuances of the 510(k) clearance mechanism, it should be clear that there was nothing unusual about the way FDA operated in this instance and nothing done by any of the manufacturers was deceptive nor substantively different from what hundreds of medical device manufacturers have done to get their products to physicians and patients.

According to the previously noted FDA Advisory Committee Report [18] "from 1992–2010, the FDA cleared 168 510(k)s for surgical mesh with urogynecologic indications. Examination … revealed a shift in Indications for Use statements from general soft tissue repair to inclusion of specific types of... repair, e.g. reconstruction of the pelvic floor…FDA found that it cleared 83 510(k)s for surgical mesh with an SUI indication, 63 with a POP indication, and 22 with both" [18].

Perhaps the only outstanding item about the entire 510(k) process for transvaginal mesh products and kits is that the original transvaginal mesh predicate device – the ProteGen sling – was cleared in 1996 but recalled in 1999 because of safety concerns. In retrospect, this clearly was a "red flag."

Because of the virtual complete lack of any meaningful primary or comparative efficacy or safety data, all of these new meshes and mesh insertion kits reached patients without clinical testing and with both short- and long-term adverse event types and incidence as complete unknowns, which raises the questions of how and why use of this new, untested surgical technology became so widespread, particularly given the high success rate enjoyed by transabdominal use of older mesh products for treatment of vaginal vault prolapse.

The answer to this question is beyond the scope of this chapter but is addressed elsewhere in this book in the chapters on product genesis and marketing, as well as in some of the medical and health law literature [20]. The fact is that new technology drives much of US medicine.

In this author's opinion, it is likely that some combination of a less rigorous approval/monitoring system for devices (compared to new prescription drugs, vaccines, and biologics), the relatively unfettered promotion of new technologies to physicians by the industry/medical profession, and the suggestion of a lower failure rate for pelvic organ prolapse with more "traditional" surgical approaches all combined to create the environment for use of new mesh and mesh insertion kits to become widespread. In addition, the absence of required post-marketing commitments for efficacy and safety data for 510(k) cleared devices – compared to new prescription drugs – ensures that the required adverse event reporting would be less vigorous and will "lag" given that the complications of these mesh and mesh kit products will be primarily the result of physician, and later patient, reporting to the manufacturer and then to FDA. The bulk of the safety information was inevitably initially going to be collected/be the result of reports in the medical literature and safety concerns reported by individual surgeons. This is addressed in the next section on post-marketing issues for medical devices.

Patient Safety and Advertising and Promotion Issues After Marketing Approval

First, some general comments on post-marketing safety data collection and monitoring.

Once a medical device has been cleared (via a 510(k)) or approved (via a PMA) for market, FDA's medical device adverse event monitoring system kicks in. In the case of a cleared product, the information will essentially be all de novo, whereas for PMA-approved devices, there will already be significant safety data on file. The post-marketing period is, at least from a medical-legal controversy point of view, where all of the action is; the collection and monitoring of adverse events are perhaps the core functions of FDA for everything from food to vaccines and lie at the intersection of manufacturers, federal and state regulators, patients, physicians, and tort law.

There are many post-marketing regulations for medical devices contained in the 1976 Medical Device Amendments [10] to the 1938 FDCA. Among them are good manufacturing practice (GMP) requirements to ensure that the medical devices are safe for their intended use. FDA has the power to inspect, and shut down, production facilities.

Even more important than manufacturing guidelines and inspection is the MDR[6] – medical device reporting requirements. This data collecting mechanism is

[6] The medical device reporting requirements are found in 21 C.F.R. § 803.

referred to as the MedWatch System. The medical device reporting regulation became effective for device manufacturers, user facilities, and importers in July 1996 and provides an early warning system to help ensure that medical devices are not misbranded or adulterated and that they are safe and effective for their intended use. FDA requires that user facilities (e.g., hospitals, ambulatory surgical centers) and manufacturers must report certain adverse events associated with the use of medical devices so that FDA can "track" the number, and characteristics, of potential device-related complications and safety issues to see if a "safety signal" may be discerned. The goal is to identify, and offer opportunity to correct, safety and/or efficacy problems in a timely manner. Because the MDR apply only to manufacturers and facilities, not individual physicians, in order to accomplish its goal to a great degree, the system necessarily relies on the good faith cooperation by medical device manufacturers and voluntary surgeon reporting.

The specific reporting requirements for manufacturers for known or suspected adverse events related to their marketed medical devices are straightforward and appear in different parts of Section 803. The MDR reportable events must be reported to FDA using FDA Form 3500A; use of the form is mandatory. Reports may now be filed electronically. Manufacturers are required to submit an MDR to FDA (specifically CDRH) within 30 days after either receiving or becoming aware of information from any source (e.g., patient, physician, healthcare facility, attorney) that reasonably suggests one of two things about the medical device marketed by the manufacturer:

1. That the device may have caused or contributed to a death or serious injury, as defined
2. That the device has malfunctioned and the device or a similar device marketed by the manufacturer would be likely to cause, or contribute to, a death or serious injury if the malfunction were to recur [21]

There are additional safety reporting requirements for the manufacturer. Manufacturers must submit a "5-day report" to FDA within 5 working days after:

1. Becoming aware (from any source, including trend analysis) that remedial action is necessary to prevent an unreasonable risk of substantial harm to public health
2. Becoming aware of an MDR reportable event for which FDA has made a written request for the submission of a 5-day report [22]

Of course, to some degree what constitutes "unreasonable risk of substantial harm to public health" for a medical device, on top of the baseline expected morbidity associated with anything implanted in the human body may be in the eye of the beholder. Since remedial action is required when this bar is reached, and the cost/consequences of remedial action for an established medical device may be prohibitive, manufacturers may be reluctant and FDA cautious in determining when this situation exists.

Lastly, manufacturers also are required to submit follow-up supplemental reports [23] as well as baseline safety reports [24].

The MDR system is not the only source of potentially important safety information FDA looks at in gathering information about safety concerns for a medical device. Although reporting for physicians (as well as injured patients) is voluntary, there is a mechanism through the CDRH website which allows patients as well as physicians and surgeons to directly report adverse events to FDA. The medical reviewers at CDRH also peruse the US and foreign medical literature (journals, textbooks), and Cochrane reviews, for case reports and clinical studies on complications of new (and older) medical devices.

The totality of all of these possible sources of voluntary (e.g., from consumers or physicians) and involuntary reporting is entered into an adverse event database called the MAUDE database – the Manufacturer and User Facility Device Experience. MAUDE is updated quarterly, and on the CDRH website, an online search is available which allows anyone to search for particular medical device reports in the MAUDE database. Should restricted information be encountered, requests for the information may be filed under the Freedom of Information Act (FOIA), though such requests typically may take 6 months or longer. If a manufacturer has been granted an exemption to normal reporting requirements or an alternative reporting mechanism was established as part of the PMA for approval, some information may not be in the MAUDE database.

In addition to adverse event reporting requirements, there are also medical device tracking provisions which require that a manufacturer of certain Class II and Class III medical devices be able to follow the device through the entire supply or distribution chain from final assembly to the user of the device. The original tracking provisions of Section 519(e) of the 1938 FDCA appeared in 1990 in the Safe Medical Devices Act of 1990 (SMDA) [25] which amended the FDCA to include the mandatory tracking provisions. These provisions applied if the manufacturer:

1. Was registered with FDA
2. Engaged in the manufacture of a device whose failure would be reasonably likely to have serious adverse health consequences
3. The device was either a permanently implantable device or a life-sustaining or life-supporting device used outside a device user facility

The 1990 medical device tracking provisions were further amended in 1997 by sections of the Food and Drug Administration Modernization Act (FDAMA) [26] which allowed FDA to have the discretion to require tracking in additional circumstances to those enacted in 1990 and which further codified when Class II and III medical devices would be subject to the mandatory device tracking requirements.

At the present time, a Class II or III medical device is subject to the current FDCA's device tracking requirements if any of the following three criteria are met:

1. The device's failure would be reasonably likely to have serious adverse health consequences.
2. The device is intended to be implanted in the human body for more than 1 year.
3. The device is a life-sustaining or life-supporting device used outside of a device user facility.

Additional factors which may be considered [27], at FDA's sole discretion, in determining whether a tracking order is necessary for a medical device even if it did not meet one of the above three criteria now include (1) the likelihood of sudden catastrophic failure, (2) the likelihood of significant adverse clinical outcome, and (3) the need for prompt medical intervention should safety issues arise with the device.

The bottom line is the medical device tracking is usually required for implanted, prescription medical devices and is a necessary complement to the adverse event reporting system in order to allow manufacturers to evaluate their products to determine possible intrinsic device-related etiologies of the adverse event.

In the absence of a series of unexpected patient deaths or an overt, obvious danger to public health from a medical device which might push FDA to mandate a product recall, it takes time for the agency to accumulate enough information about a product to act – require a label change, change the class of medical device the product is classified as, and require clinical trial data/a PMA for continued marketing. FDA's system for tracking serious adverse events from its Class II or III medical devices is far from perfect. Arguably, in the field of obstetrics and gynecology, the FDA has fallen well short of the market in timely and appropriate responses to safety signals from medical devices used in or implanted in the human abdomen or pelvis. Then again, the same could be said for issues which have arisen surrounding newer hip replacement technologies. The fact is that the 510(k) clearance system may be more efficient from an economic, industry, and regulatory point of view, but from a patient safety perspective, it virtually guarantees that newer medical devices will be marketed with a built-in "black hole" of data on the unique short- and long-term complications from implanting such devices.

A description of the timeline of FDA activity in the transvaginal mesh controversy appears in a subsequent section of this chapter and will give the reader an overview of FDA responses to the transvaginal mesh issue over the course of almost a decade of accumulating data. FDA's system for tracking serious adverse events from its Class II or Class III medical devices is far from perfect, and the absence of a mandatory reporting requirement of adverse events for physicians and surgeons, compared to the requirements for health professionals in other countries, doesn't help.

Advertising and Promotion of Medical Devices to Consumers and to Physicians

This important topic will be addressed in the chapter on marketing, and only a few brief comments will be made. Although widespread direct to consumer advertising of prescription drugs by pharmaceutical companies does not occur in any Western nation other than the United States – and receives the overwhelming amount of attention from both the media and the professional medical press – more than 75% of the dollars spent by industry on direct advertising is actually for advertising *to physicians*, not to consumers. There is some logic to this since the prescriptions must be written by healthcare professionals; even though ads to consumers are claimed to be educational, there is no question that their primary motivations are to increase patient awareness of the possibility of treatment with the prescription product and to increase demand for the same from their physician.

Direct to consumer advertising of restricted, surgically implanted medical devices does occur though it is much less common than that for prescription drugs [28]. There is little formal investigation of this topic in the food and drug literature. As far as promotion of medical devices to physicians is concerned, advertising for labeled indications is permitted by statute and accepted industry practice; what controversy exists for this (as well as for prescription drugs) surrounds off-label communications. The conflict between commercial speech rights of manufacturers under the First Amendment of the US Constitution and FDA's efforts to regulate pharmaceutical and medical device sponsors has taken up decades of time in federal courts, remains unresolved, and could easily fill all of the pages in this book. The bottom line is that off-label promotion is permitted but only if it is carried out in a scientific exchange which is first initiated by the healthcare provider [29].

As can be seen from Table 4.1, between 2002 when vaginal mesh kits were first introduced and 2017 when most of the kits were voluntarily removed from the market, the vaginal mesh kit industry was on a virtual sine wave cresting at extensive market penetration and then crashing on the litigation shoreline as patient safety events snowballed. The number of adverse events increased annually during this period of time, as did public awareness, volume of lawsuits filed, and regulatory actions by FDA. Some comments are in order to put the roles of the various stakeholders into proper perspective and to weigh the relative effects their actions, and inactions, had on the mesh controversy.

Between January 1, 2008, and December 31, 2010, 2874 urogynecologic surgical mesh complaints were filed with the FDA. The complaints included vaginal mesh erosion, dyspareunia, infection, urinary problems, vaginal bleeding, hematuria, rectal bleeding, organ perforation, pelvic/nerve pain, vaginal scarring, as well as seven deaths [30]. For purposes of comparison, more than 1000 reports of complications were filed by 9 device manufacturers between 2005 and 2007.

FDA's Response to Mesh and Mesh Kit Safety Data: Steady Progress but Slow to React to the Data

Vaginal mesh kits were first cleared for the US market by FDA in 2002, but it was not almost 4 years later in 2006 for the adverse events associated with vaginal mesh and vaginal mesh kits to first get on the agency's radar screen. When this happened, it was not because of information in the FDA medical devices safety collection system but rather because of a publication in the peer-reviewed medical literature [31].

A key question for which there is no simple answer is whether FDA waited too long to act and did too little (and perhaps continues to do too little) when it acted. FDA has been criticized for being slow to respond and failing to act decisively enough when it became aware of the problem, but FDA is only as good as its data collection systems, and in the absence of a mandatory requirement for physicians to report any and all adverse events surrounding their use of use of device (as is the case in the United Kingdom) and the absence of approval of vaginal mesh and mesh kits via the PMA process, there is a built-in delay in the medical device safety monitoring system for many potentially dangerous medical devices.

There are three primary sources of safety information for any FDA regulatory action re: medical devices. These are post-market surveillance of MDRS (medical device reports); the medical literature particularly case reports and peer review publication clinical reviews; and publications/internet postings from citizen committees, private individuals, medical professional societies, and newspapers (Table 4.3) [32–35].

As previously pointed out, the differences for a medical device manufacturer in cost, time, effort, and risk for having to submit a PMA instead of going through a 510(k) clearance to keep a product on the market are enormous, not the least of which is the real possibility that FDA will, on balance, find that the safety risks from use of transvaginal mesh kits for POP outweigh the expected benefits. With that FDA decision such kits could not be sold anymore in the United States. There is no doubt that the growing volumes of litigation in conjunction with the sea change in FDA's regulatory approach to mesh kits were pivotal factors in the decision by most manufacturers to withdraw their products from the US market (see below).

Legitimate criticisms of FDA's regulatory actions are the apparent 3-year lag between 2008 and 2011 in convening an advisory panel and the 3-year period of time it took for FDA to acknowledge that the transvaginal mesh kits posed a real potential danger to human life and should be up-classified to Class III devices so that *finally* some substantive safety and efficacy data would have to be produced. Given the fact that advisory committees are never used for Class II devices, once FDA decided in 2011 that an advisory committee was needed to review the safety situation for transvaginal mesh, manufacturers of these devices must have, or should have, known that major changes in the way such medical devices are regulated were imminent.

There was certainly ample evidence in the medical literature strongly suggesting that this action could have been taken earlier. If these PMAs are submitted and approved, the manufacturers will be immune from lawsuits in state court for damages to patients from their medical devices, something which is not the case (and never has been the case) for any mesh or mesh kit.

A final criticism of the FDA is that the few manufacturers who still market these products can keep them on the market for 2.5 years, while they submit the PMA, and it will take 6 months or more to review the application. In the author's opinion, this criticism is unfair, since it is entirely possible that the safety and efficacy data may show that these particular devices should remain on the market.

Table 4.3 Post-marketing signals and US Food and Drug Administration (FDA) response

Years	Signal	FDA action
2005–2007	>1000 MDRs	Review of MAUDE database
20 Oct 2008		FDA PHN safety communication for physicians and consumers regarding upturn in issues related to surgical mesh placed transvaginally to treat POP and SUI
Aug 2009		Researchers prematurely halt their study comparing outcomes of traditional prolapse surgery without mesh and vaginal surgery with mesh "due to predetermined stopping criteria for vaginal mesh erosion" [32, 33]
2008–2010	>2800 MDRs	Review of MAUDE database. More than half of the MDRs associated with POP repairs
2011	Literature review	PHN second safety communication. Formal evaluation of safety/efficacy of mesh. Findings: serious mesh complications not rare. Findings: no evidence that transvaginal POP repair more effective than traditional non-mesh repairs
13 Jul 2011		White paper regarding transvaginal mesh complications
3 Aug 2011		FDA recall of Pinnacle Pelvic Floor Repair Kit – Anterior/Apical Sterile and Posterior Sterile (Boston Scientific)
Sep 2011		Advisory panel sets goal to evaluate transvaginal POP
3 Jan 2012		FDA issues orders to 34 manufacturers requiring them to conduct 95 post-marketing surveillance studies to address specific safety/efficacy concerns for transvaginal POP repairs
4 Jan 2012 – May 2014		FDA considering proposed order [34] to reclassify mesh/mesh kits for transvaginal POP repair as Class III devices and to require manufacturers to submit PMA applications to continue marketing
Jan 2016		Final version of reclassification order published. Manufacturers have 30 months to submit PMA. Note: this is only for transvaginal POP, not SUI
26 Feb 2016		Publication of FDA Executive Summary: reclassification of urogynecologic surgical mesh instrumentation [35]

MDR medical device reports (MAUDE), *PHN* public health notification, *POP* pelvic organ prolapse, *SUI* stress urinary incontinence, *MAUDE* Manufacturer And User Facility Device Experience

The Medical Profession's Response to Mesh and Mesh Kit Safety Data: Somewhat Consistent but Clearly Conflicted

The medical profession's response to the mesh controversy may be charitably described as mixed. On the one hand, physicians and surgeons may be justifiably criticized for their lemming-like rush to embrace new surgical technologies, particularly when they offer the opportunity to do more expensive procedures for more "disease" indications and to enroll in short, industry-sponsored "courses" instructing them how to use complicated new medical devices they are unfamiliar with and to then return to their medical facilities and immediately begin using these devices often without adequate mentoring or supervision. The perpetuation of this system represents a collective failure by the medical credentialing and peer review process to adequately police the profession. On the other hand, the bulk of the medical-surgical literature reporting serious adverse events from transvaginal mesh and mesh kits was written by dedicated surgeons in both full-time academia and the private sector who honestly reported unexpected, common, and serious unanticipated surgical complications from untested new surgical equipment that they themselves might have used and in doing so increased their liability exposure in litigation they might be involved in.

The American College of Obstetricians and Gynecologists has lately taken a very cautious approach as the sponsor of the leading US journal in obstetrics and gynecology, publishing relevant clinical papers on mesh complications, commentary both pro and con, and recently co-authoring a joint committee opinion [36] on the management of "simple" mesh complications with the American Urogynecologic Society (AUGS).

Review of *prior* ACOG clinical practice bulletins, however, demonstrated a much more cautious approach to use of transvaginal mesh for pelvic organ prolapse. The February 2007 bulletin [37] warned patients and physicians that "given the limited data and frequent changes in marketed products (particularly with regard to type of mesh material itself, which is most closely associated with several of the postoperative risks, especially mesh erosion), the procedures should be considered *experimental* (italics added), and patients should consent to surgery with that understanding" [37].

Inexplicably, only 7 months later in another bulletin [38] issued on vaginal mesh surgery, the cautionary language of the warning had been softened, and the word "experimental" eliminated even though in the interim no significant clinical efficacy or safety data had appeared to warrant such change: "patients should consent to surgery with an understanding of the post-operative risks and lack of long-term outcomes data." The definitive reason for changing the language was never provided by ACOG; it is possible the original language was confusing to clinicians, possibly pejorative, or could be used as evidence to support a denial of reimbursement for surgical procedures using transvaginal mesh since insurance companies routinely deny coverage of experimental therapy [39].

The American Urogynecologic Society's role in the mesh controversy may have been less objective and possibly clouded by potential conflicts of interest. Every significant US and European review [40, 41] of transvaginal mesh insertion for treatment of POP undertaken since the safety concerns for these devices emerged years ago has concluded that POP repair with transvaginal mesh has not been proven to improve clinical benefit and outcomes over traditional non-mesh repairs, particularly for posterior repair, and poses both short- and long-term safety concerns that appear to far outweigh its comparative benefits. Despite this, senior urogynecologists at various institutions with conflict of interest related to transvaginal mesh manufacturers and who were prominent in the national and international societies continued to gloss over the safety issues by deflecting the argument, e.g., "the current litigious atmosphere threatens to derail any further innovation and progress in use of synthetic materials to treat the growing number of women with POP" [4]. These short articles often appear in non-peer review publications which are frequently read by practicing obstetrician-gynecologists for quick updates on clinical matters of import [4]. Withdrawal of "innovative" products from the US market due to litigation merited an entire page in the article but the fact that for some patients "a diverting colostomy may be need to excise and repair the erosion site and lead to life-long morbidity for the patient" [42]...not a word.

At the time of this writing, the national and international scientific societies have not issued a statement unequivocally rejecting the use of transvaginal mesh kit products for primary treatment of POP, particularly for anterior and posterior pelvic defects. Nor has there been a consensus statement about the precise context, and extent, of proper training for surgeons seeking to employ the few existing transvaginal mesh products remaining on the US market [43].

The issue of capture of academic medicine by the pharmaceutical and medical device industries [44], the role industry plays in education and training of physicians once they have completed postgraduate training, and how exactly industry should be allowed to promote off-label uses of prescription implantable medical devices to physicians all remain serious issues which complicate FDA and medical profession efforts to regulate new medical and surgical technologies.

Industry's Response to Safety Concerns: The Withdrawal of Vaginal Mesh Kits from the Market but Only After FDA Changed Its Approach

At the present time, there are only a couple of vaginal mesh kits still on the US market, as can be seen in Table 4.4 [4]. Why is this the case? How did this happen?

The decision to withdraw the vaginal mesh kits was a voluntary decision by the manufacturer and not a regulatory decision made by FDA even though FDA has the power to order an immediate withdrawal of either an implantable medical device or

Table 4.4 Current marketing status of transvaginal mesh kits

Manufacturer	Name	Status
American Medical Systems	Apogee	Discontinued
American Medical Systems	Elevate Anterior and Posterior Repair	Discontinued
American Medical Systems	Elevate with InteXen LP	Discontinued
American Medical Systems	Perigee	Discontinued
Bard	Avaulta Plus Anterior and Posterior	Discontinued
Bard	Avaulta Solo Anterior and Posterior	Discontinued
Boston Scientific	Pinnacle Pelvic Floor Repair Kit	Discontinued
Boston Scientific	Polyform Synthetic Mesh	Discontinued
Boston Scientific	Uphold Vaginal Support System	Available
Coloplast	Restorelle Direct Fix	Available
Johnson & Johnson	Gynecare Prolift	Discontinued
Johnson & Johnson	Gynecare Prolift + M Kit	Discontinued
Johnson & Johnson	Gynecare Prosima Pelvic Floor Repair System Kit	Discontinued

prescription drug from marketing. The bar for such a decision – that the product poses an immediate threat of great harm to patients – is a high one and clearly was not met in the case of vaginal mesh even though a decade of accumulating clinical evidence in the medical literature demonstrated a marked increase in both the incidence and severity of surgical complications related to use of the newer mesh products and mesh insertion kits.

Evidence of the importance of FDA's decision to reclassify transvaginal mesh kits as Class III devices and require PMAs for continued marketing in the United States can be seen by considering the dates in Table 4.2 and the announcement [45] on June 4, 2012, by Ethicon, a Johnson and Johnson Company, that they were notifying relevant courts that they were no longer going to be marketing four of their mesh products in the United States: Gynecare TVT Secur™ system, Gynecare Prosima™ Pelvic Floor Repair System, Gynecare Prolift pelvic floor repair system, and Gynecare Prolift + M™ Pelvic Floor Repair System. Ethicon's decision to voluntarily withdraw their products from the US market followed FDA's reclassification decision by 1 month; other device manufacturers followed suit. Although none of the manufacturers specifically stated their reason(s) for withdrawing their products from the market, consumer safety advocates hailed the announcement as a victory. "These companies know they will never be able to prove safety and efficacy of these devices in the studies mandated by the FDA in January of this year," said Lana Keeton, a Miami resident who has undergone 17 surgeries to remove mesh that was implanted in 2001. Keeton's group, Truth in Medicine, has lobbied the FDA on the risks of mesh in recent years [46].

The voluntary decision by most manufacturers to withdraw their vaginal mesh kit products from the US market was likely multifactorial: the rise in FDA manufacturer and device user experience database safety reports as a result of both improved collection of data and awareness of previous safety events, new publications in the medical literature surrounding mesh kits complications, contributions from social media, intense media attention, "catch-up" from the expected time delay in the occurrence of clinically significant safety events after use of the vaginal mesh kits, and mounting pressure from accumulating lawsuits filed on behalf of injured patients by personal injury attorneys. This latter factor – the cumulative effect of lawsuits filed in state courts against both physicians employing mesh kits and the manufacturers of these kits – deserves special attention.

The Plaintiff's Bar: Reaction Was Timely, Predictable, and Consequential

FDA is not the only entity which tracks adverse event reporting data for vaccines, pharmaceuticals, cigarettes, food, and medical devices: the personal injury lawyer community does so as well. It should come as no surprise that there has been a virtual blizzard of claims filed on behalf of patients allegedly injured by transvaginal mesh in virtually every state in the United States since thousands of adverse events have been reported to FDA and the total number of injured patients is almost certainly several times that number.

In instances where thousands of patients are filing claims against a pharmaceutical or medical device manufacturer, the cases fall under the umbrella of "mass torts," and very often large numbers of cases are consolidated into one or more larger, collective suits known as multi-district litigations or MDLs. There may be only one MDL for the entire country or several MDLs each in a different part of the United States depending in part on whether there is one or multiple manufacturers in the mix. At the time of this writing, there are six current transvaginal mesh MDLs:

1. C.R. Bard MDL 2817: In Re C.R. Bard, Inc. Pelvic Repair System Products Liability Litigation
2. Johnson & Johnson/Ethicon MDL 2327: In RE Ethicon, Inc. Pelvic Repair Systems Product Liability Litigation
3. American Medical Systems MDL 2325: In Re American Medical Systems, Inc. Pelvic Repair Systems Product Liability Litigation
4. Boston Scientific MDL 2326: In Re Boston Scientific Corp. Pelvic Repair System Products Liability Litigation
5. Mentor ObTape MDL 2004: In Re Mentor Corp. ObTape Transobturator Sling Products Liability Litigation
6. Coloplast MDL 2387: In Re Coloplast Corp. Pelvic Support Systems

Given the large number of lawsuits facing all of these manufacturers (more than 30,000 at last count), each maker of transvaginal mesh and mesh kits must ultimately decide whether to litigate each case, one at a time, or to enter into settlement talks. Johnson and Johnson, for example, has not entered into any settlement talks and is engaging each plaintiff one court trial at a time; other manufacturers such as Boston Scientific (which faces 12,000 cases and counting) have entered into settlement talks which their cases are ongoing. Those manufacturers which have already withdrawn all of their products from the market are more likely to settle these cases en masse.

In pursuing transvaginal mesh litigation, plaintiffs and their attorneys must decide whether to sue the individual surgeon, the medical device manufacturer, or both. The choice of defendant will in part be determined by multiple factors. The choice may depend on (1) who has the deeper pocket (the manufacturer with virtual certainty); (2) the willingness or usefulness of using the individual surgeon in court as a possible witness against the medical device manufacturer (in which case the physician will be dropped from the case in exchange for favorable testimony, e.g., "I wouldn't have used the device if I'd been aware or made aware of all of the safety issues compared to more traditional surgery"); and (3) the particular personal injury claims being made.

The defending surgeon may be sued for simple medical malpractice (e.g., negligently inserting an otherwise non-defective transvaginal mesh product) or failing to warn the patient about known, and possible, complications from use of the product. This latter claim may also be considered a failure to obtain informed consent. Under the learned intermediary rule, physicians are expected to be familiar with the contents, including safety information, contained in the product label. Manufacturers have frequently argued in pharmaceutical litigations that this doctrine shields them from liability for failure to inform consumers of possible adverse events from their products even if they have directly advertised those products to consumers. In most states, except New Jersey, this defense tends to work.

The manufacturer can be sued for failing to warn, both patients and physicians, about the known and potential risks of their products. And/or manufacturers can be sued for what might be considered product liability issues (separate from personal injury torts), i.e., that the transvaginal mesh device itself was not properly designed. Lastly, the manufacturer can be sued for fraudulently advertising the benefits/advantages of their transvaginal mesh products when no data supporting such claims exists.

Ironically, FDA is generally "kept out of court" in these cases. There is no point in blaming FDA, and doing so only creates a situation where it allows the defendant off the hook. It is also pointless to sue FDA in these matters; such cases – if they are allowed to proceed – must occur in federal courts where the potential monetary recovery is limited at best. State court is where the action, and the potential for large awards from juries, exists.

How Is All of This Litigation Possible? The Intersection of FDA Law and Tort Law: Statutory Protection of Medical Device Manufacturers

Patients are injured by Class II and III implantable medical devices all of the time, yet not all plaintiffs and manufacturers will end up in state court. The reason for this is that protection from lawsuits for damages in state court depends exclusively on how the device was allowed to enter the US market by FDA.

The great irony of the transvaginal mesh litigation is that the very mechanism which allowed all of these untested mesh products and mesh insertion kits to reach patients – the 510(k) clearance mechanism – is the precise reason why lawyers have been able to sue individual transvaginal mesh manufacturers in state court. A 2008 US Supreme Court decision [47] *Riegel v. Medtronic* held that medical device manufacturers whose devices are approved for marketing via the PMA approval are completely shielded from tort liability in state court. This complete preemption of possible state court claims applies to both claims of direct damages as well as "indirect" claims such as failure to warn/inadequate labeling and is a direct consequence of the complete preemption provision [10] in the 1976 Medical Device Amendments of 1976 to the 1938 Federal Food, Drug, and Cosmetic Act. Only manufacturers whose medical devices reached consumers via 510(k) clearance can be sued in state court for damages [48]. This is the reason why litigation is proceeding for transvaginal mesh and is going nowhere for injuries sustained from hysteroscopic sterilization with Essure [49].

In ruling in *Riegel*, the Supreme Court upheld, and extended, its prior ruling in *Lohr* [50] regarding tort claims: patients can sue manufacturers in state court for monetary damages for injuries sustained from Class II or Class III medical devices which FDA cleared for marketing via 510(k). Even though the overwhelming majority of Class III medical devices are approved via PMAs, "up-classifying" a device from II to III will not shield the manufacturer just by virtue of being a Class III device. The flip side of all this is that those transvaginal mesh manufacturers still marketing products and who submit to the PMA approval process will be completely shielded from state court lawsuits in the future as soon as FDA approves their PMA.

Where Do Things Stand Now? Current Status of Vaginal Mesh Kits and Current Recommendations for Use

Much of the shouting about the mesh controversy may be over because most of the transvaginal mesh kits have been voluntarily removed from the market by their manufacturers, and injured patients are getting their day in court as the individual mesh trials work their way through individual state courts. Manufacturers have won some [51] and lost some [52]. The controversy will continue on several levels. For one, as shown in Table 4.4 [4], a couple of transvaginal mesh kits remain on the US market and will likely remain so, while their manufacturers presumably conduct clinical trials over the next several years for their now reclassified Class III medical devices to support PMA applications for continued marketing. Secondly, despite proven non-superior efficacy for treatment of POP, and a safety profile which has repetitively and definitively been demonstrated to be inferior to more traditional surgical approaches, most prominent surgical subspecialty societies have been unwilling to categorically state that transvaginal mesh kits should not be used for treatment of POP.

Societies such as the AUGS have instead opted for language suggesting that only the most skilled providers should be utilizing these medical devices. The problem with this argument is that many of the studies demonstrating that transvaginal mesh kits don't work better and are more dangerous have been carried out by the very people who would ostensibly be the only ones who should be using them. Presumably, transvaginal mesh kits will – or should – continue to be employed only for select patients with vaginal vault prolapse and only by surgeons subspecialty trained in Urogynecology and Pelvic Reconstructive Surgery.

Based on the clinical experience of the past 15 years, however, some patients will suffer avoidable complications. How such patients should be appropriately counseled preoperatively is an ethical conundrum beyond the scope of this chapter. Similarly, how physicians still using transvaginal mesh for treatment of POP will defend their practice should they end up being sued for damages in civil court remains to be seen, since we are clearly in a new era at least in terms of how FDA is looking at the risks these medical devices pose to patients.

Looking Ahead: The Twenty-First Century Arrives with the 21st Century Cures Act

On December 13, 2016, President Obama signed into law the 21st Century Cures Act (hereafter abbreviated "the Act"), a massive 1000+-page omnibus spending bill which enjoyed widespread bipartisan congressional support and sponsorship by Vice President Joe Biden. A complicated piece of legislation, the Act, called for almost $5 billion of funding to the National Institutes of Health (NIH) for neuroscience, Vice President Biden's "Cancer Moonshot" program, and precision medicine studies. Also included were $1 billion for individual state grants to battle the nationwide epidemic of opiate addiction and $500 billion of extra funding for FDA for a wide variety of new and more streamlined older programs to advance biomedical innovation and bring new, potentially lifesaving drugs and medical devices to patients faster than the current FDA regulatory process allowed. The new provisions of the Act also touch on promotion of new drug development, regenerative therapies, regulation of clinical research, healthcare software, and interoperability of electronic medical records and medical devices.

Although the most controversial provision of the Act requires FDA to come up with a program to allow "real-world data" (however that is defined) to be used to approve new labeled indications for a marketed prescription drug without the inconvenience of FDA's current gold standard of the randomized, controlled clinical trial, the new provisions of the Act which directly affect medical devices are potentially no less troublesome. This is especially so in light of the already demonstrably easier pathway the 510(k) clearance mechanism provides to allow potentially dangerous implantable medical devices to be marketed and the fact that as a rule it is easier to get approval for a prescription medical device which will be permanently implanted in someone's body than it is to get a new prescription drug approved.

A full discussion of all of the new sections of the Act which impact on innovation and medical devices is well beyond the scope of this chapter, but two deserve special mention even though all of the new provisions are clearly designed to promote faster, and less burdensome, review of new medical device. The first one – "Least Burdensome Devise Review", §3058 of the Act – is clearly designed to further lower the evidentiary efficacy and safety bar below what has already been described earlier in this chapter. Section 3058 of the Act requires CDRH to consider the least burdensome means of demonstrating "substantial equivalence" or "reasonable assurance" of safety and effectiveness for 510(k)s or PMAs, respectively. Under this section, all FDA personnel involved in medical device marketing applications would be required to receive training on the meaning of, and correct use of, the new "least burdensome" review concept. It should be noted that the burden is to be minimized to the greatest degree possible for the *manufacturer* in providing data supporting a reasonable assurance of a device's safety and efficacy. Given the fact that virtually no safety or efficacy data is currently provided as part of a 510(k) clearance, it is unclear how much the burden could be lessened for this marketing route. PMAs, however, are certainly going to be easier for manufacturers to get approved.

Hand in hand with §3058 is a new "breakthrough device" provision, which is contained in §3051. This provision of the Act establishes a streamlined, specially staffed review program for medical devices (similar to that which already exists for drugs) which is designed to foster development of and prioritize review of those select medical devices which meet any one of several criteria which might loosely be described as an unmet medical device need. To qualify for this program the medical device must be:

1. Intended to treat or diagnose life-threatening or irreversibly debilitating diseases or conditions.
2. Represent breakthrough technology.
3. There exists no cleared or approved alternative on the market.
4. It offers significant advantages over existing cleared or approved alternatives.
5. The availability of which is in the best interests of patients. Importantly, the breakthrough device designation would apply to either premarket approval applications (PMAs) or 510(k) clearance applications.

Under the Act, FDA would have great discretion in deciding which new medical devices would qualify for this streamlined bench to patient process; given the broad language of "best interests of the patients" criterion, it is possible that new medical device products may reach patients well before any "real-world" data exists either on how well they will work or how safe in the short or long term they are. In the context of the problems which arose, and will continue to accumulate, from use of vaginal mesh kits, there is little good news in the 21st Century Cures Act for patient safety advocates. High-risk medical devices have always been approved with weaker evidence compared to pharmaceuticals, and this new law isn't going to make that situation any better.

A Final Note

The ultimate question was posed at the beginning of this chapter and can now be addressed. Adding all of what we've talked about above, *how* exactly did the transvaginal mesh mess happen? Is it because US medicine is new technology driven, in a partial "partnership" with the pharmaceutical and medical device industries over-sewn with a built-in federal regulatory "safety information lag" and accompanied by a hefty dose of a lack of self-regulation and discipline by the medical profession? Is the plaintiffs' bar the last resort to definitively protect patient safety? Is this our inevitable conclusion?

The 21st Century Cures Act may be a built-in annuity for litigation for the personal injury bar unless several things happen: (1) beefed-up FDA medical device safety oversight; (2) dramatically improved ability/effort on the part of the medical profession to self police, "weed out" newer technologies that don't work, vet new technologies in clinical trials even if not required by FDA, and publically reject medical devices for indications which they are on balance inferior to existing surgical procedures.

It should not be the case that we need the civil justice system, along with FDA, to really protect patients from the medical profession [3]. Physicians, and medical specialty societies, should not lose sight of their fiduciary obligations to patients and their duty to safeguard patient safety. When the evidence against select medical practices is clear, so is the obligation to take a definitive position against it (Table 4.4).

References

1. Nygaard IE, McCreery R, Brubaker L, Connolly A, Cundiff G, Weber AM, Zyczynski H, Pelvic Floor Disorders Network. Abdominal sacrocolpopexy: a comprehensive review. Obstet Gynecol. 2004;104(4):805–23.
2. Goldberg, Persky, White, P.C. Transvaginal mesh: injuries and your rights. serious complications associated with surgical mesh for transvaginal repair of POP are not rare. http://www.gpwlaw.com/practice/surgical-mesh. Accessed 2 Mar 2017.
3. Patsner B. Understanding the surgical mesh controversy. Food and Drug Law Institute Update. Jul-Aug 2012, p. 6–10.
4. Rosenblatt PL, Dessie SG. Transvaginal mesh. Past, present, and future. Contemporary OB/GYN. 2016;61(10):20–8.
5. Nager CW. Midurethral slings: evidence-based medicine vs the medicolegal system. Am J Obstet Gynecol. 2016;214(6):708.e1–5.
6. Leghorn J, Brophy E, Rother P. The First Amendment and FDA restrictions on off-label uses: the call for a new approach. Food Drug Law J. 2008;63(2):391–406.
7. The Food and Drug Administration Modernization Act of 1997 (FDAMA). 21 C.F.R. § 807.20(a)(2).
8. Federal Food, Drug, and Cosmetic Acct, Pub. L. No. 75-717, 52 Stat. 1040 (1938) (codified as amended at 21 U.S.C. §§ 331-397 [2006]).
9. Shapiro JK. Labeling and advertising of medical devices. In: Colonna TE, Shapiro JK, editors. Promotion of biomedical products: regulatory consideration. Washington, D.C.: Food and Drug Law Institute; 2006. p. 5.
10. Medical Device Amendments of 1976, Pub. L. No. 94-295, 90 Stat. 539 (1976) (codified at 15 U.S.C. §55 (1994) and 21 U.S.C. *passim* [1994]).
11. Junod S. Commemorating the 40th anniversary of the 1976 Medical Device Amendments. Food Drug Law J. 2017;72(1):26–31.
12. 21 U.S.C § 360c(1)(1)(a).
13. Kahan JS, Wilson EC Jr. Medical devices. In: Adams DG, Cooper RM, Hahn MJ, Kahan JS, editors. Food and drug law and regulation. Washington, D.C.: Food and Drug Law Institute; 2008.
14. 21 U.S.C. § 321(h). The definition was modified slightly by the Safe Medical Devices Act of 1990.
15. 21 U.S.C. § 360c(a)(1).
16. 21 U.S.C. § 360(e) and 360(h).
17. Gostin LO. The deregulatory effects of preempting tort litigation: FDA regulation of medical devices. JAMA. 2008;299(19):2313–6.
18. U.S. Food and Drug Administration. FDA Executive Summary. Obstetrics & Gynecology Devices Advisory Committee Meeting, 8–9 Sept 2011. Surgical mesh for treatment of women with pelvic organ prolapse and stress urinary incontinence. Washington, D.C.
19. Weinberg Group. FDA strengthens regulatory requirements for transvaginal mesh. https://weinberggroup.com/fda-news/regulatory-requirements-for-transvaginal-mesh/. Accessed 2 Mar 2017.

20. Elhauge E. The limited regulatory potential of medical technology assessment. Va Law Rev. 1996;82(8):1525–622.
21. 21 C.F.R. § 803.50(a).
22. 21 C.F.R. § 803.53.
23. 21 C.F.R. § 803.56.
24. 21 C.F.R.. §803.55.
25. Safe Medical Devices Act of 1990, Pub. L. No. 101-629, 104 Stat. 4511 (1990).
26. U.S. Food and Drug Administration Modernization Act, Pub. L. No 105-115, 111 Stat. 2295 (1997).
27. U.S. Food and Drug Administration. Center for Devices and Radiological Health. Medical device tracking: guidance for industry and FDA Staff 25 Jan 2010. http://www.fda.gov/MedicalDevices/DeviceRegulationsandGuidance/GuidanceDocuments/ucm071756.htm. Accessed 5 Jun 2017.
28. Patsner B. Direct-to-consumer advertising of restricted, surgically implanted medical devices: what does the advertising arena look like, and whose regulatory problem is it? William Mitchell Law Review. 2013;39(4):1207–28.
29. Henderson J, Humphrey DC. Medical devices and off-label communication: statutory amendment discussion draft defines "scientific exchange. Food and Drug Law Institute Update, Sep–Oct 2016. p. 16–20.
30. U.S. Food and Drug Administration. Center for Devices and Radiological Health. Urogynecologic surgical mesh: update on the safety and effectiveness of transvaginal placement for pelvic organ prolapse. July 2011.
31. Norton PA. New technology in gynecologic surgery. Is new necessarily better? Obstet Gynecol. 2006;108(3 Pt 2):707–8.
32. Iglesia CB, Sokol AI, Sokol ER, Kudish BI, Gutman RE, Peterson JL, Shott S. Vaginal mesh for prolapse: a randomized controlled trial. Obstet Gynecol. 2010;116(2 Pt 1):293–303.
33. Rabin RC. Trial of synthetic mesh in pelvic surgery ends early. The New York Times. 22 Oct 2010. http://www.nytimes.com/2010/10/26/health/research/26complications.html. Last accessed 25 May 2017. "The bottom line is not only there were more complications, but the mesh didn't prove any better than traditional surgery".
34. U.S. Food and Drug Administration. Department of Health and Human Services. Proposed Rule: Reclassification of surgical mesh for transvaginal pelvic organ prolapse repair and surgical instrumentation for urogynecologic surgical mesh procedures; designation of special controls for urogynecologic surgical mesh instrumentation. Document 79 FR 24634. 21 CFR 884. 1 May 2014.
35. U. S. Food and Drug Administration Executive Summary. Reclassification of urogynecologic surgical mesh instrumentation. Gastroenterology-Urology Medical Devices Advisory Committee Panel. 26 Feb 2016.
36. Committee Opinion No. 694: management of mesh and graft complications in gynecologic surgery. American College of Obstetricians and Gynecologists. Obstet Gynecol. 2017;129(4):e102–8.
37. Committee on Practice Bulletins-Gynecology, American College of Obstetricians and Gynecologists. ACOG Practice Bulletin No. 79: pelvic organ prolapse. Obstet Gynecol. 2007;109(2 Pt 1):461–73.
38. ACOG Committee on Practice Bulletins—Gynecology. ACOG Practice Bulletin No. 85: pelvic organ prolapse. Obstet Gynecol. 2007;110(3):717–29.
39. WBUR's CommonHealth (Boston University). Surgery under scrutiny: what went wrong with vaginal mesh. http://commonhealth.legacy.wbur.org/2011/11/surgery-under-scrutiny-what-went-wrong-with-vaginal-mesh. Accessed 2 Mar 2017.
40. European Commission. Scientific Committee on Emerging and Newly Identified Health Risks. Opinion on the safety of surgical meshes used in urogynecological surgery. 3 Dec 2015. https://ec.europa.eu/health/scientific_committees/emerging/docs/scenihr_o_049.pdf. Accessed 15 May 2018.

41. Medicines and Healthcare Products Regulatory Agency, MHRA. A summary of the evidence on the benefits and risks of vaginal mesh implants. 28 Oct 2014. https://www.gov.uk/government/publications/vaginal-mesh-implants-summary-of-benefits-and-risks.
42. Kudish BI, Iglesia CB. Posterior wall prolapse and repair. Clin Obstet Gynecol. 2010;53(1):59–71.
43. Worcester S. Kit-specific training is required for mesh kits: appropriate training needed for good outcome for anterior compartment prolapsed surgical treatment. Ob Gyn News (Mdedge / Frontline Medical Communications). 2 Dec 2010. https://www.mdedge.com/obgynnews/article/50906/gynecology/kit-specific-training-required-mesh-kits-appropriate-training. Accessed 15 May 2018.
44. Patsner B. Capture of academic medicine by big pharma. Health Law Perspectives (University of Houston Health Law & Policy Institute). Feb 2009. https://www.law.uh.edu/healthlaw/perspectives/2009/(BP)%20academic.pdf. Accessed 15 May 2018.
45. Rockoff JD, Wang SS. J&J to stop selling surgical mesh. The Wall Street Journal. 5 June 2012. https://www.wsj.com/articles/SB10001424052702303506404577448422586204212. Accessed 15 May 2018.
46. Perrone M. J&J to stop selling pelvic mesh tied to lawsuits. The Boston Globe. 5 Jun 2012. Boston.com. http://archive.boston.com/business/healthcare/articles/2012/06/05/jj_to_stop_selling_pelvic_mesh_tied_to_lawsuits/. Accessed 15 May 2018.
47. Riegel v Medtronic, Inc. 552 U.S. 312 (2008).
48. Patsner B. Riegel v. Medtronic, Inc.: revisiting pre-emption for medical devices. J Law Med Ethics. 2009;27(2):305–17.
49. Walter JR, Hayman E, Tsai S, Ghobadi CW, Xu S. Medical device approvals through the premarket approval pathway in obstetrics and gynecology from 2000 to 2015: process and problems. Obstet Gynecol. 2016;127(6):1110–7.
50. Medtronic v Lohr, 518 U.S. 470 (1996).
51. Strom P. Boston Scientific wins first transvaginal mesh trial. 4 Aug 2014. https://stromlaw.com/boston-scientific-wins-first-transvaginal-mesh-trial/. Accessed 15 May 2018.
52. Toutant C. NJ high court declines appeal in $11m pelvic mesh verdict. 7 Dec 2016. New Jersey Law Journal. https://www.law.com/njlawjournal/almID/1202774119961/nj-high-court-declines-appeal-in-11m-pelvic-mesh-verdict/?back=law. Accessed 15 May 2018.

Chapter 5
Medical Device Marketing and the Ethics of Vaginal Mesh Kit Marketing

Roberta N. Clarke

Introduction

The marketing of vaginal mesh kits raises many ethical questions: Did the vaginal mesh marketers place this device on the market without adequate testing? Did physicians utilize mesh kit products to treat vaginal prolapse without informing patients that these products had never been tested on people prior to being commercialized? Did physicians even know, by being cleared through a 510(k) process by the US Food and Drug Administration (FDA), that the vaginal mesh kit products had not been through the equivalent of human trials? Did the FDA have a greater responsibility to require more stringent testing of medical devices such as the mesh kits that were new to the market? Did the medical device manufacturers have a greater responsibility to provide training for obstetrician/gynecologists, urologists, and other physicians so that they could learn how to place the mesh kits product safely? Did all of these entities – physicians, the FDA, the vaginal mesh kit marketers – engage in ethically questionable activities?

There are no uncomplicated answers here. The field of ethics is messy and challenging. If it were straightforward and if there were simple yes/no answers to the above questions, the various entities would have been able to adjust their behaviors to encompass and reflect generally accepted ethical beliefs. As with most of life, however, while we might wish for the ease of a distinct dichotomy between our choices, an option of black vs. white, we find ourselves living in a world of various shades of gray.

For physicians, medical ethics is a cornerstone of medical education. It is often presented in terms of the right of patients to be given information relevant to their medical condition and the obligation of physicians to provide it to them. It is

R. N. Clarke
Health Care Management Program, Questrom School of Business, Emeritus Boston University, Boston, MA, USA
e-mail: rclarke@bu.edu

S. A. Shobeiri (ed.), *The Innovation and Evolution of Medical Devices*,
https://doi.org/10.1007/978-3-319-97073-8_5

couched in terms of transparency in physician-patient communications. However, the interweaving of ethics and marketing of medical products and procedures significantly compromises the ability of surgeons to provide the information needed by patients to give informed consent. This has become apparent in the case of vaginal mesh kit procedures.

One factor at play is the reliance on consumer behavior knowledge by vaginal mesh kit marketers to quell concerns about the products that surgeons might have had. Although they did not directly pay for the product nor were they the end recipients of the product, surgeons, as the agents for their patients, were the decision-makers to use or not use vaginal mesh; their decisions therefore determined that the product was bought and used. They, not the patients, were the de facto consumers of the product.

Had there been a better understanding of the marketing practices of the mesh kit manufacturers, a more informed perspective on the FDA's clearance protocols and subsequent ability to police medical devices once they have been commercialized, and a recognition of the range of behaviors taken by surgeons whose patient outcomes did not meet expectations, fewer articles like "Surgery Under Scrutiny: What Went Wrong With Vaginal Mesh" (on the website of WBUR, Boston University's National Public Radio news station) [1] might have been written. Instead, systemic forces within the US health-care system allowed a combination of "slippery slope" ethics and indirect and motivated blindness by marketers. This may well have been exacerbated by surgeons who interpreted poor vaginal mesh kit surgical results as being a result of their own surgical technique, a conclusion encouraged by mesh marketers, as it allowed them to deflect concerns that vaginal mesh kit products might not be safe. Patients were also sometimes implicated, as it was suggested in court proceedings by lawyers representing mesh kit manufacturers, that the patient may not have selected the "right" surgeon to carry out her procedure. It is reasonable to suggest that surgeons were not provided adequate and appropriate training by the mesh manufacturers, given the number of mesh kit court cases where the manufacturer's legal defense was poor surgical performance by the surgeon. The patient would, however, have been unable to make this judgment in her selection of a surgeon.

A clearer set of ethically egregious behaviors happened subsequent to the implantation of mesh kits in women. A *New York Times* article entitled "How Profiteers Lure Women Into Often-Unneeded Surgery" portrays physicians who profiteered from the vaginal mesh litigations by engaging in financial schemes by partnering with anti-mesh attorneys designed to remove vaginal mesh kits from usually asymptomatic women, thereby causing even further suffering to these women (https://www.nytimes.com/2018/04/14/business/vaginal-mesh-surgery-lawsuits-financing.html). This commercial scheme, according to the article, was created and managed by an assemblage of lawyers, marketers unaffiliated with mesh kit marketers, banks, private equity firms, and hedge funds, with the active involvement of the physicians performing and profiting from these surgeries. The wide scope of ethically challenged players involved in this scheme places it beyond the scope of this chapter, but the dominance of financial decision-making at the cost of protection of the patient christens this commercial machine as a poster child for bad ethical behavior.

Relevant Marketing Paradigms

Marketing Mix

The marketing mix is a set of tools relied on by marketers to analyze, to set objectives, and to design strategy. It consists of four components: product, price, place, and promotion.

- *Product*: consists of both the tangible offering by the marketer as well as the services that either support the tangible offering or are themselves the primary offering.
- *Price*: the money that customers or their intermediary agents have to pay for the product.
- *Place*: consists of the activities and actions in which a marketer must engage in order to make the product accessible to the customer. This often involves intermediaries who carry and/or sell the product.
- *Promotion*: consists of communications, sales, advertising, and social media activities that allows the marketer to sell the product to the target market.

Two of the four tools of the marketing mix – product and promotion – were at the core of the issues with vaginal mesh kits and with the lawsuits now facing vaginal mesh kit marketers. It is now recognized that, in many cases, the product itself was flawed [2–14]. The promotion of the vaginal mesh kit to physicians, most often by marketers' sales forces, has been construed as, at worst, deceptive or possibly incomplete, leaving physicians unable to judge the true performance and risks to be expected of the product. Alternatively, in the early phases of commercialization of these products, it is possible that the salespeople themselves were unaware of the risks presented by the use of mesh kits.

Communications Model

A second model that provides insight into physician behavior and their role as consumers of vaginal mesh is the *communications model* [15] (Fig. 5.1).

This model of consumer behavior differentiates consumption decisions on the basis of two factors:

1. The first is level of involvement of the individual in the purchase decision. How involved is the consumer (in the case of vaginal mesh kit, the surgeon) in the decision to use or not use vaginal mesh kits? Another way of asking this question is: how much perceived risk does the consumer have about this decision? Do they believe choosing to use vaginal mesh kits is an inherently risky decision or a low risk decision? A high level of perceived risk translates into a high level of involvement.
2. The second is level of perceived differentiation between the purchase choices. If the use of vaginal mesh was seen as roughly equivalent to a traditional prolapse

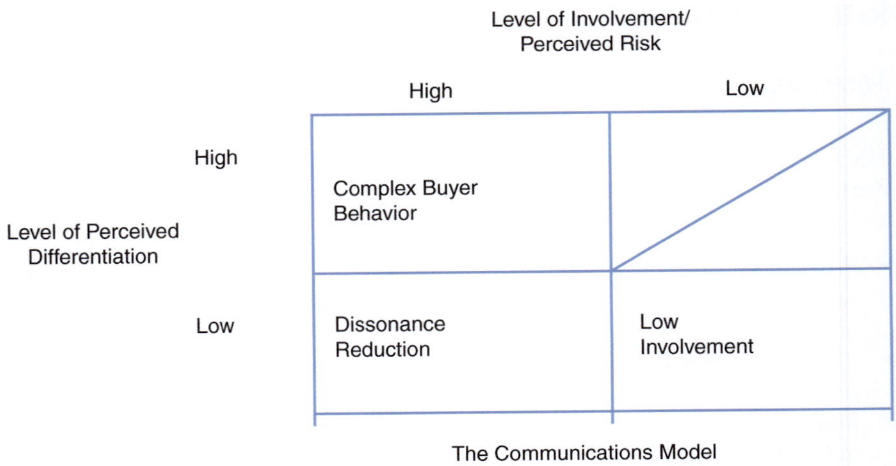

Fig. 5.1 The *communications model* of consumer behavior

repair with native tissue or with biologic graft, then there is a low level of perceived differentiation. The term "perceived" is important because there may be a true difference, but it may also be that the consumer cannot perceive this difference. Alternatively, there may be no difference, but the consumer believes that there is. The vaginal mesh kit was initially perceived as providing superior support for repairing weakened muscles and tissue, while the drawbacks of vaginal mesh kits were not yet apparent or perceived by physicians who chose to use it.

Complex Buyer Behavior Model

Each of the three consumer behavior models explains aspects of the decision to treat a patient using vaginal mesh kits. The *complex buyer behavior model* assumes that the physician views the decision as sufficiently risky that he or she is willing to spend the time to learn about the performance of the mesh kit as a medical device, to question other physicians, to question salespeople, and to search online and elsewhere for information about the benefits vs. the risks of using the product. In doing so, the surgeon becomes better able to determine the actual performance of the product. Ideally, all consumer decisions would be made this way, that is, by a fully informed consumer. However, there is a price to becoming truly informed: it takes time and effort to engage in the deep dive required to gather in-depth information, analyze it, and interpret it well enough to come to an informed decision. In the case of vaginal mesh kits, in the initial years after these products came on the market, the information was not available or at least provided no certainty to physicians who spent time searching for product performance, side effect profile, and outcome information. Given the time constraints of most physicians, it would be unreasonable to expect them to engage in complex buyer behavior for each new medical device, even if they would wish to make their decisions in this manner. This is not the consumer behavior model characterizing these types of decisions for most surgeons, particularly for those not affiliated with academic medical centers.

Low Involvement Model

The *low involvement model*, also called habitual buying behavior, is essentially the opposite of the complex buyer behavior model. The consumer views the decision as engendering so little risk that there is almost no search for information; all the alternatives are viewed as roughly similar, explaining why the decision is viewed as nearly riskless. Without solid information, it is almost impossible to make a truly informed decision. The smallest perceived differentiation allows the consumer to make a choice, even if it is based on perceived but not necessarily actual differences. Given that surgery always poses some risk, the choice to use vaginal mesh kits in the early stages of commercialization likely did not follow this model. If surgeons became very comfortable over time through continued use of the vaginal mesh kits, they might have moved more toward this behavior model. Their choice of product would then have become habitual, where they would use the same brand of kit each time, as that would be expected to keep the risk low.

Dissonance Reduction Model

The *dissonance reduction model* involves high perceived risk and high levels of involvement but no real search for information. This may happen when time is limited so severely that there is not sufficient time to carry out an information search. Alternatively, the consumer may actively search for information but find formidable barriers to accessing to information. If the consumer searches but ultimately cannot find what is viewed as a sufficient amount of credible information, the search ends, and the consumer is forced to decide without being truly informed. This model often occurs when the consumer relies on an "expert," an agent, or on someone who is expected to have the information that the consumer does not have. Thus, the agent becomes the decider of the purchase.

How does this relate to physician decision-making about the use of vaginal mesh kits? The models seem to suggest that, due to time constraints, surgeons were not fully informed when they initially made the choice to use vaginal mesh kits. A new medical device always presents a risk. However, the limited information about the device that might be found in FDA filings is not easily accessible, and physicians, although recognizing the risk inherent in a new medical device, could not take the time to locate and dig into the FDA-filed documents submitted by the medical device companies. Therefore, this is less likely to be a complex buyer behavior decision or a low involvement/low perceived risk decision, particularly in the initial years of use. The most common consumer behavior model in this situation is dissonance reduction, which denotes a recognition of the risk inherent in the decision but also a decision that must be made without full information. The most likely source of information under these circumstances is the "expert" or agent: the medical device sales representative. Other sources of information do exist: grand rounds by recognized surgeons, presentations at conferences, speaker programs for physicians (often in expensive restaurants), and so on, but the most invasive source of information is generally commercially provided.

Relevant Ethical Paradigms

Whether the patient outcome is positive or not, the normative prescription for all health-care activity is primum non nocere, first do no harm. This prescription applies to all who are charged with working in the interest of the patient, including not only physicians and other clinicians but also all who work in health-care businesses. This latter category includes medical service and product providers such as those in the pharmaceutical industry as well as in the medical device industry. Ethically, all should be held accountable for their intentional actions in the service of the patient.

The Deontology/Teleology Paradigm

Health care has traditionally used a deontological approach to ethics. Here, moral values are viewed through the lens of rightness and wrongness of actions, with norms for appropriate behavior. The power of medical science cannot provide a guarantee of a specific outcome, and factors other than the quality of medical care, including patient compliance, family support for the patient, and the patient's insurance coverage, may influence the medical outcome [16]. This suggests that outcomes may be inadequate as a measure of ethical behavior as well as of quality of care.

A reliance on the deontological approach may not exclude a teleological approach where the moral behavior is judged by the ends that are achieved or not achieved [17] (Fig. 5.2). Still, the uncertainty of medical outcomes, despite what may be viewed as excellent care, suggests that the ethics of medical decisions must be judged largely by the intentional actions of those who act, not by their results; good actions can still result in bad outcomes. However, outcomes are also determined by unintentional actions, so both deontological and teleological approaches contribute to the definition of ethical behavior in health care.

While the deontological approach arguably may or may not encompass unintentional actions, the teleological approach considers the outcome, regardless of intentionality. Given the current movement to reimburse based on clinical outcomes

Deontology: moral behavior is judged by the wrongness and rightness of one's actions, regardless of the outcome.
Teleology: moral behavior is judged by the ends that are achieved, regardless of the actions taken to achieve these outcomes.

Fig. 5.2 The *deontology/teleology* approach to ethics

either as opposed to actions or in addition to actions on the part of the clinical providers, it is reasonable to include both teleological and deontological approaches in evaluating health-care ethics. It is not a stretch to hold those who engage in health-care marketing, including those who market vaginal mesh, to this standard.

The Principles, Character, and Consequences *Paradigm*

Historically, business ethicists have examined three aspects of any ethically challenging situation through the second ethical paradigm [18]:

- The *principles* or standard of conduct that guide behavior
- The *character* of the person or company
- The *consequences* of a particular action

The Ethical Breakdown Paradigm

A third useful paradigm was introduced in a 2011 *Harvard Business Review article* on ethical breakdowns [19]:

Barriers to maintaining an ethical organization

- Overvaluing outcomes
- The slippery slope
- Indirect blindness
- Motivated blindness
- Ill-conceived goals

We will now consider the application of these marketing and ethical paradigms as they apply to the marketing of vaginal mesh kits.

Marketing as a Commercial Exchange

Marketing is based on an exchange-based model [20] where the exchange relationship exists between the company or organization and its customers. The company provides the product and/or service, and, in exchange, the customers provide payment to the company, even if indirectly through channels such as insurance companies and governmental entities. However, one has to ask if providing medical care – which involves all medical decisions, including those related to medical products – is just one more commercial exchange as opposed to being a more ethically laden interaction.

The Hastings Center, a bioethics research center, concluded in 1989 that health care is not merely a commercial exchange for three reasons [21].

First, the view of patients as being equivalent to consumers of commercial products was not reasonable due to the vulnerability of patients, their inability to judge their medical choices given the complex medical knowledge necessary, and their dependency on clinicians to make medical decisions for them. In essence the Hastings Center concluded that patients were acting by the dissonance reduction consumer behavior model, relying on the physician as the expert.

Second, the relationship with the medical provider is often intensely personal, where intimate information is shared that would not be discussed in a normal commercial exchange. Third, the physician/patient relationship represents a classic agency condition where one person (the agent) makes decisions for the other person (the principal), again arguing that this exchange is dominated by the dissonance reduction consumer behavior model. The agency dilemma arises due to the possibility that the agent might act in his own interests rather than in the interests of the principal (the patient). For example, a surgeon might select to implant a specific brand of hip in a patient due to the implant company rewarding the surgeon for choosing that brand of hip implant over another brand. The patient's best interest may or may not be served by this choice. Due to the patient's vulnerability, lack of knowledge, and sense of affinity and intimacy with the physician, however, the patient trusts the physician to act in the patient's best interests.

As we drill down into the agency issue, we see notable differences between the role of the physician in selecting a pharmaceutical product for a patient vs. selecting a medical device to be placed (as many medical devices are) inside a patient. It is rare for a medical device company to promote its device direct to consumers because patients play a particularly small role in the product or brand selection process for a device. A few, such as Medtronic and Boston Scientific, have very recently begun to engage in direct-to-consumer advertising because certain of their products compete directly with heavily advertised pharmaceutical products; the intent of the advertising is to encourage patients to consider a medical device alternative. Smith & Nephew has been engaging in direct-to-consumer advertising for even longer [22]. However, much as physicians have conflicting if not negative views of prescription pharmaceutical advertising, they hold the same reservations regarding the advertising of medical devices.

This unease was dismissed by the president of the Advanced Medical Technology Association, who stated that this concern was "misplaced" for the advertising of medical devices because patients would not and could not make a serious surgical decision based on an advertisement; he believed their influence on physicians' selection of a medical device to be more limited than it might be for pharmaceutical prescribing [23]. There is reason to believe that patients' pharmaceutical requests might be taken more seriously by their physicians than would be a medical device request. A patient might be able to provide input to the physician on the reported efficacy of a drug that they have taken in the past. They are also able on their own to make the decision to discontinue a drug that is causing them undesirable side effects. Because of their own experience with a drug and their ability to modify this experience, the patient is better able to move toward a complex buyer behavior model.

Patients are not, however, in the position to remove medical devices that have been implanted in their bodies; this can be done only by a surgeon. The role of physician as the patient's agent therefore dominates this relationship. With this role, serving as the expert in a dissonance reduction consumer behavior model, come greater ethical responsibilities.

Informed Consent by the Patient

Legal protection for the physician is provided by having the informed consent of the patient. This may be only a theoretical construct for most patients who will be receiving a medical device. True informed consent requires a number of conditions, including full disclosure by the physician, patient autonomy, and the ability of the patient to intelligently and with full understanding weigh their possible choices [24]. With the US government assessment that only 12% of the population are medically literate [25], it is highly unlikely that most patients can adequately carry out this task. Instead, as one would anticipate with an agency situation, the patient must rely on the agent, the expert – that is, the physician – to make the informed choice.

The high standards to which physicians must adhere when seeking a patient's informed consent require not merely the avoidance of deception and the avoidance of the provision of incomplete and prejudicial information but also the presentation of fair and unbiased information that is unambiguous and comprehensive relative to the decision to be made [21]. It is in this latter category that we begin to see the possibility of ethical lapses. Research has shown that the process of informed consent does not necessarily work as initially conceived. Patients often do not recall the risks with which they were presented [26]. Especially because vaginal mesh was at first experimental, a high standard of informed consent should have been required. The ability of surgeons to perform to this standard likely played a role in the subsequent history of the product.

The ability of physicians to provide patients with informed consent can be limited by the marketing efforts of the medical device companies. The ideal scenario would provide clear objective information to the physician. However, the device companies' promotional literature and sales pitches are in fact intended to sway physicians to choose their particular brand. This in and of itself is not wrong. However, they may verge toward marginally misleading statements or incomplete information intended to sway the physician to a particular product or brand [27]. Marketing tactics such as these are viewed as manipulative if they change the normal decision-making process of their intended audience. As a marketing mix tool, this type of promotion may be viewed as being ethically flawed. In this scenario, it can be expected that the outcome of the informed consent decision process would be hijacked; even an "informed" patient might make a decision that runs counter to his or her own best interests. This is a case where the deontological behavior on the part of the physician may have been ethically carried out, but the teleological result is not in the best interests of the patient.

Analysis of the Ethical Responsibilities of the Vaginal Mesh Kit Marketers

Medical device manufacturers, like most companies operating in the health-care space, fully intend to be ethical. The credo of Johnson & Johnson (J&J), a Fortune 500 company and one of the leading manufacturers and marketers of vaginal mesh kits, now being sued by more than 54,000 women [28] is "Caring for the world, one person at a time." Other vaginal mesh kit marketers have similar credos, all indicating a dedication to the patient or to the science that will serve the patient. Credos unfortunately do not protect the patient. The total number of lawsuits against vaginal mesh kit manufacturers due to product flaws exceeds 100,000 [29]. From a marketing mix perspective, this suggests that the product was defective. The vaginal mesh manufacturers' actions, if one approaches this deontologically, were intended to provide treatment and relief for women with pelvic organ prolapse (POP) and urinary stress incontinence. In retrospect, if one takes a teleological perspective where the ends are judged by the outcomes that were achieved by these actions, the companies acted immorally; that is, for a significant number of women, the outcome was poor, if not horrific. But is it really that simple?

510(k) vs. Premarket Approval [30] (Fig. 5.3)

The first vaginal mesh product was introduced by Boston Scientific (Marlborough MA, USA). Its ProtoGen mesh received FDA clearance in 1996 through the 510(k) process that oversees devices viewed as low risk and as having a predicate device already on the market; that is, the proposed device is viewed as substantially equivalent to another device that is already approved or cleared and marketed.

The predicate device for the ProtoGen was mesh used successfully to treat abdominal hernias (although by 2017, an increasing number of hernia mesh suits were being filed). The importance of distinguishing between a premarket approval (PMA) as opposed to a 510(k) clearance is that a PMA requires a much more stringent review, including the performance of human clinical trials. This makes the PMA both a more expensive route to pursue and guarantees significant delay in the introduction and marketing of the device, assuming that it is approved after lengthy clinical trials. From a business perspective, the choice of a 510(k) process is far

Premarket approval (PMA): This path requires a more stringent review of the product including the performance of human clinical trials. A product that receives a PMA is "*approved*" for commercialization.

510(k): This path requires only that there be a predicate device already on the market which is substantially equivalent to the product being introduced and that the proposed product be viewed as inherently low risk. A product that receives a 510(k) is "*cleared*" (not approved) for commercialization. No human testing is required for a 510(k) clearance.

Fig. 5.3 The two most common US Food and Drug Administration paths that companies can seek to place a medical device on the market

Table 5.1 Synthetic slings and predicate devices cleared by the US Food and Drug Administration

Sling device and FDA submission number	Clearance date	Predicate product and FDA submission number(s)
Ethicon TVT (K974098)	28 Jan 1998	ProtoGen sling (K963226)
AMS Monarc (K023516)	19 Nov 2002	SPARC (K011251, K013355, K020663, K021263)
Mentor ObTape (K031767)	17 Jul 2003	TVT (K974098)
		SPARC (K013355)

From Nosti and Iglesia [14], with permission

more attractive than a PMA process. From an ethical standpoint, if the manufacturers truly believe that the device for which they are seeking 510(k) clearance is both safe and efficacious, the choice can be supported. The ProtoGen device was withdrawn from the market in 1999 because of severe complications. However, the ProtoGen served as predicate for the next generation of sling devices for incontinence such as ObTape® (Mentor, J&J, New Brunswick, NJ, USA), which was subsequently withdrawn from the market as well (Tables 5.1 and 5.2) [14].

Most of the vaginal mesh competitors that entered the market after the introduction of the ProtoGen device used the ProtoGen technology or similar 510(k) cleared devices as their predicate devices in seeking and receiving their own 510(k) clearance. The highly successful Ethicon (Somerville, NJ, USA) Gynecare tension-free transvaginal taping, or TVT®, also used ProtoGen as its predicate. At the point of the ProtoGen withdrawal from the market, should the FDA have requested a recall or at least a reexamination of all sling mesh products that relied on the ProtoGen type and Gynecare TVT® as the predicate? This did not happen nor is it required for devices whose predicate device was recalled [31]. Up to this point, it would be difficult to assign moral lapses to the marketers of vaginal mesh kits. Subsequently, the manufacturers put the sling and mesh technology together and introduced the vaginal mesh kits as a totally untested hybrid product into the market.

The FDA finally reclassified vaginal mesh kits as high risk, and notices were sent out to this effect. However, the FDA has been unwilling to issue a full recall [32]. One can explain this failure by noting that the FDA is overwhelmed with balancing the need to review and approve (or not) the vast number of new pharmaceutical and device products being presented to it every day vs. the need to oversee all medical

Table 5.2 Synthetic transvaginal mesh for prolapse and predicate devices cleared by the US Food and Drug Administration

Mesh device and FDA submission number	Clearance date	Predicate product(s) and FDA submission number(s)
Gynemesh (K013718)	8 Jan 2002	Prolene Soft Mesh (K001122), Prolene Mesh (K962530), and Mersilene Mesh (pre-amendments device)[a]
Prolift and Prolift+M (K071512)	15 May 2008	GyneMesh PS (K013718), UltraPro (K033337), Apogee (K040537), and Perigee (K040623)
Perigee (K040623)	17 May 2004	AMS Sparc Sling System (K011251), AMS Monarc Sling System (K023516), AMS BioArc (K030123), and AMS Large Pore PP Mesh (K033636 and K040521)
Apogee (K040537)	22 Apr 2004	AMS Sparc Sling System, AMS Monarc Sling System, AMS BioArc, AMS Large Pore PP Mesh, and IVS Tunneller (K010035)
Avaulta Support System (K063712)	12 Mar 2007	Bard Collamend (K052322) and UGYTEX Dual Knit Mesh (K051503)
Uphold (K081048)	22 Aug 2008	Pinnacle (K071957) and Prolift (K071512)
Elevate (K080185)	10 Apr 2008	AMS Pelvic Floor Repair System (K051485)

From Nosti and Iglesia [14], with permission

[a]A device already on the market before the Medical Device Amendments to the Food, Drug, and Cosmetic Act was enacted on 28 May 1976

products already cleared or approved. This is not a moral issue but rather an issue of being under-resourced for the tasks that it is required to carry out. If there is an entity to be charged here with failure to act morally, it would be the US Congress whose inadequate funding of the FDA prevents it from carrying out all the tasks with which it is charged in order to protect the public.

Still, one must ask if the FDA needs to shoulder some of the blame merely for their lack of attention to the subsequent suffering their oversight failure allowed by not recalling the vaginal mesh kit products. It was not until 2008 that the FDA issued its first notification regarding the complications caused by vaginal mesh kits. It then took three more years for the FDA to issue a severe warning to the public that the use of vaginal mesh as opposed to other options to address POP not only was not superior to other options but that it in fact produced a greater risk of clinical and quality-of-life problems.

As stated earlier, after the ProtoGen withdrawal, the ObTape® was withdrawn. The direct translation from ObTape® incontinence to a device aimed at curing POP occurred when the IVS Tunneller®, an intravaginal sling placement device, was introduced and manufactured by US Surgical, a division of Tyco Healthcare, which later became Covidien (North Haven CT, USA). It was promoted both as a sling and as a prolapse product. This product was associated with significant complications. One can question, from a more judgmental perspective, if the vaginal mesh kit marketers displayed an ethical lapse in not immediately testing their own vaginal mesh products to determine if they caused patients the same problems as the ProtoGen,

ObTape®, or IVS Tunneller®. The manufacturers should have been aware of the recall of these products, as their legal or regulatory departments are charged with tracking this type of data. However, medical device manufacturers also face a daunting challenge because the predicate device may have evolved into a somewhat different product prior to its market withdrawal as the predicate device company sought to make product improvements. A company's own device might have been further developed after clearance as well. The continuous research and development invested in products, even after commercialization, may suggest that the predicate device could differ substantially from what is then on the market. Still, if these companies' primary ethical objective was primum non nocere (first do no harm), then testing their own vaginal mesh kit products to determine if they caused the same problems as the predicate device upon which they relied for clearance should have taken place. It appears that this was not the case.

Ethical Issues After the ProtoGen Withdrawal from the Market

The decisions of the vaginal mesh kit manufacturers following the recall of the ProtoGen, ObTape®, and IVS Tunneller® when viewed through the lens of "principles, character, and consequences," the second ethical paradigm detailed above [18], can be analyzed as follows.

Let us consider these in reverse order. Despite possessing the knowledge that the ProtoGen, ObTape®, and IVS Tunneller® were withdrawn from the market, the medical device companies may not have known what the *consequences* would be of allowing their similar products to remain on the market. They likely were affected by optimism bias, the belief that their product was less likely to pose a risk to the patients. This is a common bias, subject to being enhanced by the corporate objectives of sales and profits [33]. However, as time progressed and more reports of complications from the use of vaginal mesh kits became public, these companies could have been charged with acting immorally (not illegally), not merely by allowing their products to stay on the market without further testing but by continuing to market their products to physicians without sufficient warning regarding the complications that could be anticipated with the use of the products. This was a lapse involving the marketing mix tool, *promotion*.

The *character* of the person or company is more difficult to analyze. Little information escapes from most companies about their culture or their individual employees unless the companies wish to share this. When they do, the purpose is to promulgate a positive image of the company. Their credos and their public relations celebrate admirable virtues that they would very much like to characterize their companies' activities. It is unlikely that any large company, having achieved a significant size as was characteristic of most of the vaginal mesh kit manufacturers, sought to do anything other than serve the patient well. The disconnect exists due to the incentives that these companies tout to their employees; the incentives may not reflect the publicly stated culture or company mission. If employees are rewarded according to the company's top priority, revenues, market share, profitability, or some other business objective, then by definition service to the patient is not the top priority – there can be only one top priority – and will not come first in the eyes of the employee, even if that employee is a "good person" or an individual of good character. Company incentives may motivate employees to make decisions about their products and the marketing of these products that serve the interests of the company above the interests of the patient. From a corporate perspective, the employee is a good employee when sales and profit targets are achieved, not necessarily when no harm comes to the patient.

Because clinicians and patients cannot know what the future consequences of a particular action by a medical device company will be and because they cannot know the true culture that provides incentives to employees, they have to rely on the first guideline, the *principles* or standards that steer a company's behavior. Almost all companies, particularly those in the medical market space, claim standards that adhere to patient service, safety, and solutions. J&J's highly publicized response to the Tylenol crisis when seven people died due to poisoned Tylenol capsules has served as the epitome of good crisis management [34]. By withdrawing all Tylenol from distribution channels and retail stores, J&J gained the trust of the American public by demonstrating that they were unwilling to risk the public's safety. This became the standard that the public then associated with J&J. The public as a result assumed that J&J was ethically principled and would always, in the future, protect the public interest as any ethical company would do.

The second set of ethical guidelines by which we should judge the vaginal mesh kit manufacturers' ethical choices following the recall of the ProtoGen, ObTape®, and IVS Tunneller® examines the barriers to building and maintaining an ethical organization [19]. These guidelines, already listed previously, can be further explained.

- Overvaluing outcomes: This is the teleological approach where a successful outcome excuses unethical behavior.
- The slippery slope: The slow slide into unethical behavior begins with the slightest of ethical breaches that becomes viewed as acceptable. The next breach is only slightly more egregious, and the slide continues to allow the person to redefine what is and is not ethical with each subsequent breach.
- Indirect blindness: When the unethical action is outsourced to a third party, the ethical breach is not viewed as one's own, even though one knows of it and may have encouraged it.
- Motivated blindness: As Upton Sinclair notably observed: "It is difficult to get a man to understand something when his salary depends upon his not understanding it" [35]. As noted above, even the "good person" may make unethical decisions when the employer's incentives for the employee overwhelm the employee's ethical instincts.
- Ill-conceived goals: Although the goals are admirable, the achievement of those goals may encourage unethical behavior.

The behavior of the vaginal mesh kit companies would not be faulted in terms of *overvaluing outcomes*. If the outcomes had been largely positive, no discussion of this sort would be necessary. It may be that the *slippery slope* effect began with the first reports of the ProtoGen, ObTape®, and IVS Tunneller® recalls; the remaining mesh manufacturers may have thought that this was an isolated problem and would not recur in their own mesh devices. Once reports of problems with their own product appeared, they may have allowed it to be interpreted as "just a few patients" or as being the result of the rare incompetent surgeon, and thus the slow slide began. The fact that surgeons made the choice to use the vaginal mesh when non-mesh alternatives existed allowed the mesh manufacturers to engage in *indirect blindness*, outsourcing the blame to the surgeons for either their decision to use mesh when an alternative might have been superior for that particular patient or, more likely, for poor surgical technique. Still, as the number of reported complications grew, this perspective became more appalling, as the mesh manufacturers did little to alert surgeons to the building data on vaginal mesh kit complications. *Motivated blindness* is certainly one explanation for the unethical behavior of the vaginal mesh companies. Employees working on vaginal mesh products were rewarded for actions that contributed to sales of the products, so they would likely be blinded to the patient harm to which they were contributing.

The most significant barrier to ethical behavior that underlies most of the others is the primary *goal* of the company: to be a successful business, with financial and market performance metrics being the prime determinant of success. Are these *ill-conceived goals*? Certainly not, if one is a shareholder of these companies. The question becomes one of balance between the medical ethics of primum non nocere and the business imperative of operating profitably and successfully from a financial standpoint. The latter goals, in and of themselves, are not inherently bad. They become questionable only when the goals fail to encompass ethical and moral considerations. In contrast, physicians took an oath to do no harm, and, as such, being successful in business is a secondary consideration.

An example that is commonly used to symbolize this paradigm is the Ford Pinto [19], where minor rear-end collisions resulted in the car exploding into flames and fatally burning the passengers in the car. Ford had conducted rear-end collision tests only a few months after the car was in production and had identified three possible solutions to the explosion issue. These remedies would have required closing down production and retooling. Ford determined that these options were too expensive. A damning document surfaced from a researcher analyzing Ford's choice not to retool: this cost analysis focused on corporate liability in the event that Ford had to compensate crash victims, and apparently (and appallingly) was the defining criterion in the company choosing to continue selling a defective product [36]. They chose to pay off the incinerated crash victims' families as the preferred alternative over costly retooling to prevent there being incinerated crash victims at all. This was clearly a business decision in which ethical considerations were absent.

One sees similarities regarding the vaginal mesh kit companies, particularly once the products had been on the market for a number of years, resulting in a growing stream of harmed patients and related lawsuits. J&J, one of the major vaginal mesh kit marketers, appears to be the vaginal mesh competitor manifesting the most aggressive anti-litigation streak. Although it faced the largest number of vaginal mesh federal lawsuits (60,000 by the end of 2016) and had already lost a number of them, unlike many of its competitors, it continued to refuse to agree to a legal class settlement [37]. J&J has also simultaneously faced large numbers of lawsuits due to its talcum powder and Pinnacle hip implants. J&J's strategy was to refuse to settle, at least with regard to mesh lawsuits. Professor Elizabeth Burch of University of Georgia School of Law stated that J&J's strategy was "to generate the most closure possible for the least amount of money…so (their) best strategy is to play hardball and convince plaintiff's attorneys to stop bringing cases…even though you have these huge verdicts for juries, plaintiffs' lawyers have to spend lots of money on jury cases (and on appeal) J&J can negotiate down the value of the settlement" [38]. From a business perspective, this is the rational choice. From the ethical perspective of primum non nocere, this is abhorrent. Additionally, to this day no one knows exactly how many vaginal mesh kits were sold by J&J. Taking legal settlements into account as the cost of doing business, the vaginal mesh kit manufacturers still take home significant profit despite harm and injury to the patients.

Analysis of the Interaction Between the Vaginal Mesh Kit Marketers and Physicians

One clear ethical issue that arises when the interaction between the medical device marketers and physicians is examined is the flow of industry-provided gifts, trips, and temporary consulting opportunities to physicians. Some of these legitimately fall into the categories of promotion or research. However, these gifts engender a sense of reciprocity among physicians, a sense that they must reciprocate for these gifts by choosing and using the manufacturer's particular brand of device. The pharmaceutical industry is now facing legal and regulatory actions that call into question the legality, and with this, the ethics, of these marketer-initiated activities. The standards to which the pharmaceutical industry is currently being held will likely be reflective of the standards to which the medical device industry will eventually be held. Physicians should consider their own role in accepting gifts, in whatever form, offered by device companies, as the gifts likely influence their behavior in ways that do not necessarily serve the interests of their patients.

Less identifiable but no less valid as an ethical issue is the role of training and education tied to new and modified medical devices. Tangible products, as noted in the explanation of the marketing mix, are often accompanied by services that support these products. These can include warranties and after-sale "post-marketing" support if and as product issues arise. For medical devices, the most important service to accompany the sale of the product itself is the training and education in how to implant and/or utilize the medical device. If the device marketer fails to provide sufficient and timely training and support, or if the sales representative encourages use of the device with only limited training, then the surgeon might undertake the use of a device without enough knowledge to carry out the surgery properly. This is exacerbated by the ever-present pressure to use the newest and best devices, even if, as happened in this case, the full benefit-to-risk profile was not known. The surgeon has an ethical duty not to utilize a device with such support, and the device company has not only an ethical duty but a business-based responsibility to provide adequate training to all surgeons who adopt the device.

A defense frequently used by vaginal mesh marketers in the legal cases brought against them was that the product itself caused no harm. Rather, they stated, it was the incompetent or poorly trained physicians who were responsible for the poor outcomes. While there may have been validity to this in some cases, in other instances, key opinion leaders with greater knowledge of the product also carried out surgeries that resulted in poor outcomes. The convenient finger-pointing by the device companies appeared to have deflected legal blame from them initially. This strategy may also have delayed the reporting of problems with the mesh kits as surgeons may have questioned their own abilities rather than questioning the safety of the product itself. In these instances, leaving aside legal considerations, there were ethical issues on both sides. Surgeons might have chosen to delay using mesh products if they did not feel themselves to be fully trained. If they were uncertain that a poor outcome might have been caused by their own lack of ability, did they then fail to report the possibility that instead this might be a product failure? This would then have also postponed a more critical and needed examination of the safety of the product.

Alternatively, should the mesh marketers not have devoted greater resources to training for vaginal mesh kits? Or did they assume, since the mid-urethral slings had become so popular, that they did not need to invest greater resources to support surgeons in the adoption of vaginal mesh kits? A final question arises as to whether they truly believed that the harm caused by mesh kit use was due to surgeon incompetence. It is quite possible that they hoped that the tactic of blaming the physician instead would decrease the number of lawsuits against them, as patients would be less likely to sue their physician than they would be to sue a large device company.

Again, one can ask: were these easy questions for either surgeons or marketers to answer? Again, it is wise to remember that ethical dilemmas arise when circumstances are unclear and decision criteria are messy. The mesh manufacturers may have judged their own mesh products to be safer than those of the competitors, even if they relied on a competitor's mesh product for their predicate device. They may have believed that research and development had continued to modify the mesh products on the market, making them difficult to compare, such that the failure of one mesh product did not signify the failure of other mesh products. They may also have judged the product itself not to be at fault, but rather the surgical technique of the surgeon. They could further have thought that the expectations of the patients were beyond the level of symptom alleviation that vaginal mesh kit surgery could provide. Uncertainty often underlies ethical conundrums.

Analysis of the Ethical Responsibilities of the Surgeon

Trial testimony has revealed a second source of unthinking and potentially unethical behavior: the level of informed consent obtained by the surgeons placing vaginal mesh in their patients. In one of the trials against J&J, one of the company's experts, a urogynecologist, admitted that the company did not provide any information to surgeons about patient complications, about additional surgeries that were often necessary to remove the mesh, and about the impossibility of removing all the mesh in some of the cases [39]. It is reasonable to assume that the other vaginal mesh kit companies acted similarly in this regard.

The result of this behavior by companies manufacturing and marketing mesh is that the surgeons who chose to use vaginal mesh in their patients were themselves, through no fault of their own, acting without proper information and were therefore not providing correct and complete information when they carried out their informed consent duty with the patient. The heavy reliance of surgeons on medical device salespeople for information on the medical devices, not to mention the salesperson's presence in the operating room [40, 41] is well covered in the press [42] and is an example of surgeons operating by the dissonance reduction consumer behavior model. For the surgeon, the salesperson becomes the medical device expert.

Given motivated blindness, indirect blindness, the slippery slope, and corporate goals that may encourage unethical behavior, this activity on the part of the medical device representatives – not providing information about patient complications, additional surgeries needed to remove the mesh, and the difficulty of removing all the mesh when called for – can be expected to continue. If surgeons do not seek out additional information on their own, they are choosing to allow patients to make life-changing medical/surgical choices based on incomplete and possibly incorrect information.

However, to expect surgeons to demonstrate complex buyer behavior – the seeking out of truthful, honest, and complete information that is not available in public databases – is unreasonable. This raises the ethical question: how are surgeons to provide this fair, impartial, and complete information to the patient for informed consent when the primary source of data for the surgeon are the medical device representatives who finds themselves challenged to act ethically?

A second question is: what additional information should the surgeon present to the patient prior to seeking informed consent? Either a PMA or a 510(k) must always precede the commercialization of a medical device. Given the difference between PMA approval that requires clinical trials vs. 510(k) clearance requiring no human trials, does the surgeon have an ethical imperative to be fully aware of the distinction between the two? Currently, the difference between an approval vs. a clearance is not taught in most medical school curriculums. In 2015 the FDA approved only 47 devices with a PMA approval compared to 3006 clearances with the 510(k) designation [43]. It seems likely that most surgeons did not know into which category the medical device they used or were implanting fell. Hayes, Inc., a health technology and consulting company, felt the need to explain the distinction in a December 2016 blog [43] to physicians and providers, presumably because the company accepted that this distinction was not widely recognized.

Ideally, as a follow-on to learning this distinction, the surgeon would want to make the determination for each medical device he or she would use which of the two forms of approval allowed the device to appear on the market. A clearance based on a 510(k) application should cause the surgeon to further question if the predicate device has performed well over a reasonable time period and with a limited history of complications. Even PMA-approved medical devices are sometimes asked to conduct post-approval studies to assure that the product is safe and effective. Often, however, these studies are not conducted because the FDA is under-resourced and cannot follow up on every approval. In this milieu of incomplete and unavailable information, the term "informed consent" becomes an arguable term.

The FDA publishes a list of recalled devices [31]. However, for a physician to determine what the predicate device is for, a 510(k) medical device is at present not simple. From the perspective of the consumer behavior models, the ideal situation requires that the surgeon act according to the complex buyer behavior model, the one that is highly time consuming, requiring that the consumer (the surgeon) conduct a high level of analysis on data that requires heavy information search. This seems both unreasonable, given the other demands on the time of surgeons, as well as unrealistic. Yet, without this information, the surgeon is knowingly presenting what could be misleading information to the patient in the informed consent process.

It is easy to point fingers at medical device companies for both the flawed product and promotion of vaginal mesh kits that have led to so much suffering on the part of patients. It is somewhat less easy but still tenable to point fingers at the FDA for failing to communicate with medical device companies the news that the predicate device, by which their own product received 510(k) clearance, was subsequently recalled, placing their own device in jeopardy. Surgeons are the least at fault, as it is nearly impossible for them to access all the information they would need to make a fully informed (a complex buyer behavior) decision. Still, they should hold themselves accountable to the extent possible to present the best and most complete evidence to their patients in order to uphold the ultimate ethical objective in medicine: First do no harm.

References

1. Zimmerman R. Surgery under scrutiny: what went wrong with vaginal mesh [Internet]. WBUR's Common Health Reform and Reality. 2011 Nov 4. http://commonhealth.legacy.wbur.org/2011/11/surgery-under-scrutiny-what-went-wrong-with-vaginal-mesh. Accessed 1 Mar 2018.
2. Gonzalez R, Fugate K, McClusky D 3rd, Ritter EM, Lederman A, Dillehay D, et al. Relationship between tissue ingrowth and mesh contraction. World J Surg. 2005;29(8):1038–43.
3. Margulies RU, Lewicky-Gaupp C, Fenner DE, McGuire EJ, Clemens JQ, Delancey JO. Complications requiring reoperation following vaginal mesh kit procedures for prolapse. Am J Obstet Gynecol. 2008;199(6):678 e1–4.
4. Iglesia CB, Sokol AI, Sokol ER, Kudish BI, Gutman RE, Peterson JL, Shott S. Vaginal mesh for prolapse; a randomized controlled trial. Obstet Gynecol. 2010;116(2):293–303.
5. Feiner F, Maher C. Vaginal mesh contraction, definition, clinical presentation, and management. Obstet Gynecol. 2010;115(2):325–30.
6. Zimmerman CW, von Theobald P, Braun NM. Exposure and erosion of vaginal meshes: etiology and treatment. In: von Theobald P, Zimmerman CW, Davila GW, editors. New techniques in genital prolapse. London: Springer; 2011. p. 217–30.
7. Gomelsky A, Dmochowski RR. Vaginal mesh update. Curr Opin Urol. 2012;22:271–5.
8. Chermansky CJ, Winters JC. Complications of vaginal mesh surgery. Curr Opin Urol. 2012;22(4):287–91.

9. Richter LA, Carter C, Gutman RE. Current role of mesh in vaginal prolapse surgery. Curr Opin Obstet Gynecol. 2014;26(5):409–14.
10. Unger CA, Abbott S, Evans JM, Jallad K, Mishra K, Karram MM, et al. Outcomes following treatment for pelvic floor mesh complications. Int Urogynecol J. 2014;25(6):745–9.
11. Javadian P, O'Leary D. Vaginally placed meshes: a review of their complications, risk factors, and management. Curr Obstet Gynecol Rep. 2015;4(2):96–101.
12. Manonai J, Rostaminia G, Denson L, Shobeiri SA. Clinical and ultrasonographic study of patients presenting with transvaginal mesh complications. Neurourol Urodyn. 2016;35(3):407–11.
13. Javadian P, Quiroz LH, Shobeiri SA. In vivo ultrasound characteristics of vaginal mesh kit complications. Female Pelvic Med Reconstr Surg. 2017;23(2):162–7.
14. Nosti PA, Iglesia CB. Medicolegal issues surrounding devices and mesh for surgical treatment of prolapse and incontinence. Clin Obstet Gynecol. 2013;56(2):221–8.
15. Ray M, Sawyer A, Rothschild M, Heeler R, Strong E, Reed J. Marketing communications and the hierarchy-of-effects. In: Clarke P, editor. New models for mass communication research. Beverly Hills: Sage; 1973. p. 147–76.
16. Donabedian A. Evaluating the quality of medical care. Milbank Q. 2005;83(4):691–729.
17. Macdonald JE, Beck-Dudley CL. Are deontology and teleology mutually exclusive? J Bus Ethics. 1994;13(8):615–23.
18. Harris JD, Parmar BL, Wicks AC. Ethical business decisions: the lens. 2015 Jul 24 [Internet]. Darden ideas to action. University of Virginia Darden School of Business. https://ideas.darden.virginia.edu/2015/07/ethical-business-decisions-the-lens/. Accessed 2 Mar 2018.
19. Bazerman MH, Tenbrunsel AE. Ethical breakdowns. 2011 Apr. Harv Bus Rev [Internet]. https://hbr.org/2011/04/ethical-breakdowns. Accessed 2 Mar 2018.
20. Kotler P, Clarke RN. Marketing for health care organizations. Englewood Cliffs: Prentice-Hall, Inc; 1987.
21. Nelson LJ, Clark HW, Goldman RL, Schore JE. Taking the train to a world of strangers: health care marketing and ethics. Hastings Cent Rep. 1989;19(5):36–43.
22. Dickinson J. Medical devices head for pharma-type public ads [Internet]. Medical Device + Diagnostic Industry (MD+DI). 2016 Feb 26. http://www.mddionline.com/blog/devicetalk/medical-devices-head-pharma-type-public-ads-02-16-16. Accessed 1 Mar 2018.
23. Mitka M. Direct-to-consumer advertising of medical devices under scrutiny. JAMA. 2008;300(17):1985–6.
24. Beauchamp T, Childress J. Principles of biomedical ethics. 5th ed. Oxford: Oxford University Press; 2001. p. 79–80.
25. U. S. Department of Health and Human Services. Office of Disease Prevention and Health Promotion. Quick guide to health literacy; 2006 [Internet]. https://health.gov/communication/literacy/quickguide/. Accessed 1 Mar 2018.
26. Knifed E, Lipsman N, Mason W, Bernstein M. Patients' perception of the informed consent process for neurooncology trials. Neuro-Oncology. 2008;10(3):348–54.
27. Sher S. A framework for assessing immorally manipulative marketing tactics. J Bus Ethics. 2011;102(97):97–118.
28. Lopez McHugh LLP. Product news and recalls. Litigation continues over defective Johnson & Johnson transvaginal mesh. 2017 May 24 [Internet]. http://lopezmchugh.com/2017/05/24/litigation-continues-defective-johnson-johnson-transvaginal-mesh/index.html. Accessed 2 Mar 2018.
29. ClassAction.com. Transvaginal mesh lawsuit settlement. Updated 2018 Mar 12 [Internet]. https://www.classaction.com/transvaginal-mesh/settlement/. Accessed 31 Mar 2018.
30. Smith J, Barrett S. What are 510(k) clearance and premarket approval? Device Watch 12 Apr 2008. https://www.devicewatch.org/reg/reg.shtml. Accessed 31 Mar 2018.
31. U.S. Food & Drug Administration. Medical devices. Recalls, corrections and removals [Internet]. https://www.fda.gov/MedicalDevices/DeviceRegulationandGuidance/PostmarketRequirements/RecallsCorrectionsAndRemovals/default.htm. Accessed 3 Apr 2018.

32. Elkins C. Transvaginal mesh recalls & discontinued products. 2013 Apr 30 [Updated 2017 Nov 1]. [Internet]. DrugWatch. T. https://www.drugwatch.com/transvaginal-mesh/recall/. Accessed 2 Mar 2018.
33. Lovallo D, Kahneman D. Delusions of success: how optimism undermines executives' decisions. 2003 Jul. Harvard Business Rev [Internet]. https://hbrorg/2003/07/delusions-of-success-how-optimism-undermines-executives-decisions. Accessed 3 Mar 2018.
34. Rehak J. International Herald Tribune. Tylenol made a hero of Johnson & Johnson: the recall that started them all. 2002 Mar 23. *The New York Times* [Internet]. http://www.nytimes.com/2002/03/23/your-money/tylenol-made-a-hero-of-johnson-johnson-the-recall-that-started.html. Accessed 2 Mar 2018.
35. Krugman P. The conscience of a liberal. The greatness of Keynes... 2008 Nov 20 [Internet]. *The New York Times*. https://krugman.blogs.nytimes.com/2008/11/30/the-greatness-of-keynes/. Accessed 3 Mar 2018.
36. Auto Editors of Consumer Guide "1971–1980 Ford Pinto". 9 Aug 2007. HowStuffWorks.com. InfoSpace Holdings LLC. https://auto.howstuffworks.com/1971-1980-ford-pinto.htm. Accessed 2 Mar 2018.
37. Elkins C. Transvaginal mesh verdicts and settlements [Internet]. Drugwatch. 2013 Sept 25 [Last updated 2017 Dec 22]. https://www.drugwatch.com/transvaginal-mesh/verdict-settlement/. Accessed 2 Mar 2018.
38. Bronstad A. J&J looking to rebound from series of megaverdicts. 2016 Dec 7. Nat Law J [Internet]. http://www.nationallawjournal.com/id=1202774155233/JampJ-Looking-to-Rebound-From-Series-of-Megaverdicts. Accessed 19 Jul 2017.
39. Mesh Medical Device News Desk. Kavaler expert witness for J&J on stand in Beltz mesh trial. 2017 May 17 [Internet]. Sundown Legal Marketing. Available from: http://www.meshmedicaldevicenewsdesk.com/kavaler-expert-witness-jj-stand-beltz-mesh-trial/. Accessed 2 Mar 2018.
40. O'Connor B, Pollner F, Fugh-Berman A. Salespeople in the surgical suite: relationships between surgeons and medical device representatives. PLoS One. 2016;11(8):e0158510.
41. Rabin RC. Salesmen in the surgical suite. 2013 Mar 25. *The New York Times* [Internet]. http://www.nytimes.com/2013/03/26/health/salesmen-in-the-surgical-suite.html. Accessed 2 Mar 2018.
42. Boodman SG. Why is that salesman in the operating room for your knee replacement? 2016 Nov 24. *The Washington Post* [Internet]. https://www.washingtonpost.com/national/health-science/why-is-that-salesperson-in-the-operating-room-for-your-knee-replacement/2016/11/14/ab8172fa-78e6-11e6-beac-57a4a412e93a_story.html?utm_term=.36124727f876. Accessed 2 Mar 2018.
43. Bontemps B. 510(k) vs PMA: do you know the difference? 2016 Dec 21 [Internet]. Hayes Evidence Blog. http://blog.hayesinc.com/blog-what-is-the-510k-exemption-process-for-devices. Accessed 2 Mar 2018.

Chapter 6
Medical Device Innovation and Errors: The Patient Perspective

Sherrie J. Palm

Pelvic organ prolapse (POP) evades the female wellness spotlight, despite estimates indicating that a significant number of women experience this condition at some point in their lives. A report written on behalf of the "Surgical Management of Pelvic Organ Prolapse" Committee from the 5th International Consultation on Incontinence held in Paris, February 2012, and published in 2013, reports that POP "when defined by symptoms has a prevalence of 3–6% and up to 50% when based upon vaginal examination." The report concludes with the caution that "significant variation exists in the prevalence and incidence of pelvic organ prolapse surgery and how the outcomes are reported. Much of the variation may be improved by standardisation of definitions and outcomes of reporting on pelvic organ prolapse surgery." [1]. The evolution of healthcare typically follows a long and winding road, often under construction, with insufficient or ineffective signs to enable the driver to navigate appropriately. It is imperative that clinicians and patients alike openly engage in discussion regarding POP, a common, cryptic women's health issue that continues to remain shrouded in silence.

Patient voice plays an integral role in the advancement of healthcare practice. Today's healthcare-literate women seek forward-thinking healthcare professionals for both surgical and nonsurgical treatments of POP, and they should be encouraged to disclose symptoms and concerns that may be embarrassing or awkward to discuss. We must get past the discomfort zone and recognize that at its most basic level, POP is a treatable health concern that we have barely cracked the surface of exposing, regarding awareness, prevalence, research, best practice, and policy.

POP has been on medical record for nearly 4000 years dating back to the *Kahun Gynaecological Papyrus*, 1835 B.C. (Fig. 6.1) [2]. Discovery upon diagnosis is the status quo for the majority of women experiencing POP. In 2018, most women, even those whose mothers underwent surgery for POP, have never

S. J. Palm
Association for Pelvic Organ Prolapse Support, Mukwonago, WI, USA
e-mail: sjpalm@wi.rr.com

S. A. Shobeiri (ed.), *The Innovation and Evolution of Medical Devices*,
https://doi.org/10.1007/978-3-319-97073-8_6

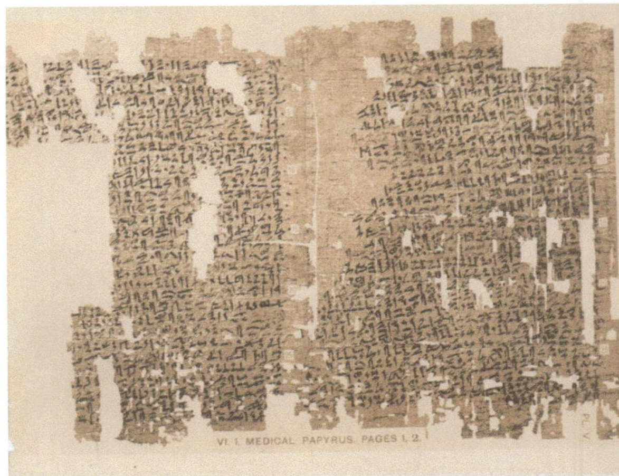

Fig. 6.1 The *Kahun Gynaecological Papyrus* (shown here, page 1 and part of page 2) is estimated to be the oldest known medical text in Egypt. Dated to the Twelfth Dynasty (1800 BCE), the tome addresses women's health, gynecological diseases, fertility, pregnancy, and contraception. (From Griffith [2])

heard of this condition until they are diagnosed with it themselves. Documentation exists of multiple POP treatments from the time of Hippocrates, such as inserting a pomegranate into the vagina as a pessary to hold the prolapsed uterus in position, rubbing the uterus with a mixture of petroleum and manure, or a treatment utilized by Euryphon, a contemporary of Hippocrates – "succussion," the practice of tying a woman upside down by her feet to a fixed frame, bouncing her repetitively until her prolapse reduced, and then leaving her bedbound for 3 days with her legs tied together [3].

A noteworthy diagnostic clinician practice gap permeates women's health despite widespread prevalence of POP and thousands of years of medical documentation. Clearly, we've come a long way since the time of Hippocrates. Considering the significant physical, emotional, social, sexual, fitness, and employment quality of life (QOL) impact of POP, and the vast mid-teenage through end of life POP patient demographic, there remains much to do to stimulate forward momentum in education of generalist healthcare providers who feel vaginal conditions should be discussed only with a gynecologist. Data was captured on January 6, 2018, from 7602 members of an online, closed, POP Facebook-based support forum, to clarify the diverse impact to women of all ages (Fig. 6.2) [4]. (Open access to "POP" patient support forum is available to POP patients and physicians upon entry request and screening. Note that the reliability of demographic data is difficult to determine due to inability to confirm birth dates posted by Facebook membership.)

POP prevalence data is widely varied in the literature [1]. Despite childbirth and menopause being the leading causal factors, women may not be screened for POP during routine pelvic exams by gynecologists or non-gynecologists alike. Even among obstetricians and gynecologists who identify POP, the misdiagnosis of the exact pelvic floor compartment is common. Simmering under the surface of women's wellness is a groundswell of patients, whose voices are growing loud and strong, wanting to know why they were not informed of or screened for POP sooner.

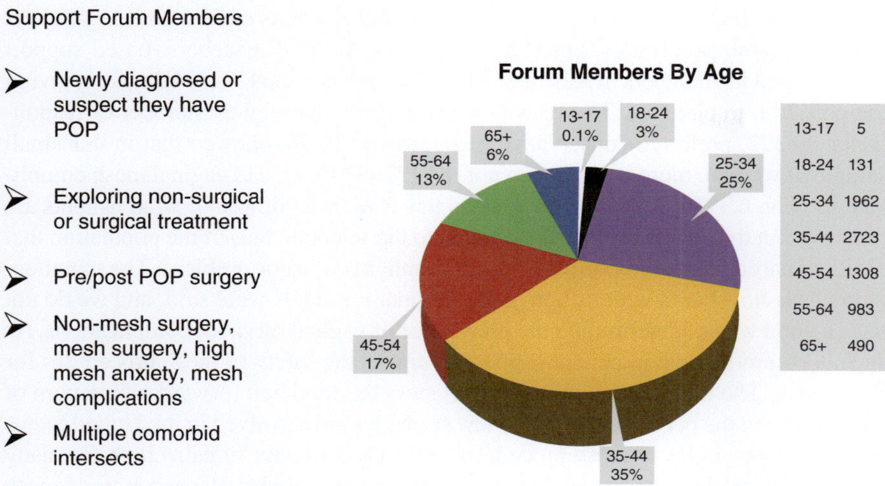

Fig. 6.2 Demographic range and aspects of pelvic organ prolapse impact vary significantly within online patient support forum structure. Note that the reliability of demographic data is difficult to determine due to the inability to confirm birthdates posted by Facebook membership

The reality is that POP can be nonsurgically treated in the majority of cases in early stage, but is often undiagnosed. It often becomes symptomatic when the prolapse has advanced to a degree that nonsurgical treatments may be less successful.

Why Mesh Turned into a Mess

Understandably, given the lack of common knowledge in the general population and among healthcare professionals, the patients may not know whom to trust with their care. I have yet to meet an individual who was not nervous heading into surgery. Patients hope their health concerns will be addressed and resolved with surgical repair. Patients hope procedures will be complication-free. Every surgical procedure comes with risks; thus the significance of appropriate surgical training, patient screening, and evaluation of the most suitable treatment to optimize patient results and satisfaction.

Patients and families report that when surgical complications occur, they are often met with a wall of silence, denial, and/or hostility. In these circumstances, patients can quickly lose confidence and trust in their clinicians. In addition to any physical impact, patients may also suffer emotionally from knowing that they have been harmed. Patients should be provided with information, support, and advice after a medical error occurs. Australia, New Zealand, and the United Kingdom are currently undergoing considerable mesh controversy and litigation, similar to what occurred in the United States (US) between 2011 and 2013 [5]. Given the engagement of support forum members from these countries, it is valuable to assess current patient mind-set regarding mesh procedures. On March 20, 2018, the POP Facebook-based support forum polled its members in Australia, New Zealand, and the United Kingdom, giving the poll 24 h to circulate. The response revealed that the highest number of respondents, 49/172, preferred conservative management. It also showed that in this small sample of women, more women than not, 17/172 vs. 3/172, had vaginal mesh complications (Fig. 6.3) [4]. Online polls such as this give us a glimpse of what patients are thinking, but the results may be skewed due to the selection bias of the population that elects to participate in an online forum. It highlights a major problem. The manufacturers have not shared with us how many vaginal mesh kits were sold, and we do not have a good way of determining the prevalence of vaginal mesh kit complications. As such, a common topic in patient support forums is the safety of mesh procedures for POP repair. The transvaginal mesh (TVM) mess has hindered forward momentum of innovations in the pelvic floor arena. New strategies have evolved in the United States to improve outcomes of mesh procedures, yet the fear factor remains high for many women who read online reports of patient anger or who review the accounts of mesh complications posted on the websites of personal injury lawyers. The benefits should be evaluated by both patient and practitioner. Seldom do women who have had successful vaginal mesh kit procedures talk about them; they simply get on with their lives, so the written word seldom imparts balanced input of the value and concerns of mesh, and a fear factor remains high in many areas.

Much has shifted forward in the United States regarding the TVM debate since the US Food and Drug Administration (FDA) Obstetrics and Gynecology Devices Panel of the Medical Devices Advisory Committee Meeting in September 2011 [6, 7]. The world at large did not replicate the FDA's action simultaneously. It was

POP Online Support Forum 24-Hour Poll

How do you feel about mesh surgery? If you don't see a category that fits, add one sentence responses. (172 responses)

I have not had surgery yet and would like to avoid it for as long as I comfortably can. I will consider all options when the time comes. 49
I have not had surgery yet, and want native tissue repair because I am afraid of mesh complications. 41
If mesh surgery would give me the best option for normalcy I might consider it. I would seek only a urogyn highly trained in mesh repairs. 18
If its mesh or nothing I would choose mesh for the chance of normality. 18
I consider my mesh surgery successful. 17
I had native tissue repair, but will choose mesh if I need another surgery. 10
I had mesh surgery and am happy knowing my success rate is so much higher. 8
If mesh gave better results for people with EDS/HSD, I wouldn't rule it out if Urogyn was highly experienced in all the issues involved. 4
I have or had mesh complications and do not consider my surgery successful. 3
I have or had mesh complications, but they were addressed and I feel my surgery was a success. 2
I did not have mesh complications, but the repair did not resolve my bowel problem - the problem probably contributed to the rectocele. 1
Mesh was my only option to improve success rate after previous surgeries in which sutures/staples failed. 1
I did not have mesh complications, but the rectocele returned within months and is worse than it was before surgery. 1
I did not have mesh complications, but had other surgical complications. 1

Fig. 6.3 Results of a closed pelvic organ prolapse (POP) patient online support forum 24-h quick poll, 172 responses indicate that POP patients' sentiments regarding mesh are extremely variable

not until January 2018 that the International Urogynecological Association (IUGA) released an update on bans and/or restrictions of TVM in Australia, New Zealand, and the United Kingdom [5]. The good news is that the currently modified standard of practice in countries experiencing a significant level of TVM complications outside of the United States now includes informed consent, recognition of the need for improved surgical self-regulation, and addressing complications at multidisciplinary centers with the appropriate expertise. The bad news is that many women in these countries suffered as a result of the use of TVM in the hands of surgeons without appropriate training or skill set, replicating what occurred here in the United States, despite significant US-based TVM media exposure from 2011 to 2013. How could companies that were actively settling close to a billion dollars in litigation in the US market concurrently sell the same products in other countries? It is important to study this and investigate what are the driving factors behind corporate behavior.

It truly takes a specializing surgeon to repair POP within the intricate female pelvic cavity, a diverse mass of multiple organ systems, soft tissue, muscle, ligaments, tendons, boney structures, and nerves, fitted tightly within a compact space. To complicate the complexity of prolapse surgery, women with POP typically have more than one type of POP in need of simultaneous repair. POP procedures should be left to the fellowship-trained experts in urogynecology. According to the Bloomberg Law Database, over 73,000 claims regarding TVM complications were filed between 2000 and 2014. Of these claims, 63.3% involved sling mesh for stress urinary incontinence, 13.3% involved POP mesh, and 23.2% involved mesh for both procedures. The number of cases increased from 730 in 2011 at the onset of claim filing to 11,798 in 2012 and then almost tripled in 2013 to 34,017. It is of considerable interest to note that only 12% of implanting surgeons were or became board-certified in Female Pelvic Medicine and Reconstructive Surgery (FPMRS)/urogynecology. It bears repeating, TVM procedures are best left to the experts with appropriate education and training [8].

It is imperative that POP surgeons utilizing mesh seek appropriate training, as well as extensive mesh experience. Preoperative evaluation, small but sufficient incisions, proper mesh insertion location, proper preparation of mesh insertion site, use of estrogen cream pre- and postsurgery, degree of mesh tension, and a two-layer closure are significant considerations for a quality mesh repair, whether the surgeon utilizes transvaginal, robotic, or abdominal technique.

Patients often express that they feel their clinicians do not believe them when they express POP symptoms, as well as do not believe them when expressing surgical complications. They often feel dismissed. To evaluate patient sentiment regarding surgical complications, a 24-h poll was posted online on the POP Facebook-based support forum on March 17, 2018, which captured 124 responses (Fig. 6.4) [4]. The questions asked were:

Which quality do you feel is most valuable in a surgeon? Obviously, patients want it all, but if you had to choose one, which would it be?

1. The ability to admit he/she made a mistake.
2. The ability to fix the mistake.
3. The ability to listen to and guide you compassionately?

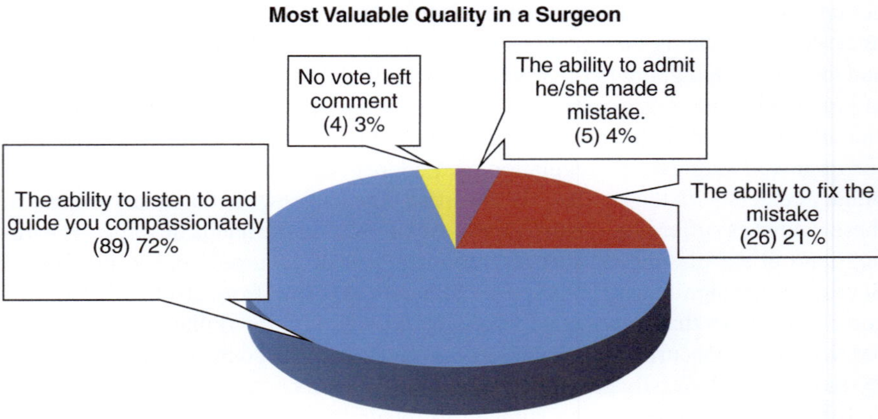

Fig. 6.4 Results of a closed pelvic organ prolapse (POP) patient online support forum 24-h quick poll, 124 responses indicate POP patients prefer compassionate clinicians over capacity to address complication efficiently

Unique patient responses were:

- "If a doctor doesn't care about you as a human being, he isn't going to care about the quality of treatment and care you get."
- "The ability to admit to a mistake is lovely, but means nothing if you can't fix it."
- "Each patient is an individual, and a 'standard fix' approach doesn't work without listening to what patient needs or wants."
- "The ability to tell you the truth of the situation. No waffle or not answering the question asked."

Tunnel Vision

Patients frequently feel dismissed when voicing concerns about POP symptoms or when discussing postoperative complications with their physicians. Their message is pretty simple; patients need clinicians to believe them when they tell them about pain, pressure, discomfort, and impact to intimacy, whether prior to or post mesh or native tissue surgery. POP invades the normalcy of women's lives in a major way. It is imperative that women disclose symptoms in entirety and insist on healthcare professionals spending the time they deserve to discuss concerns. All too often women with POP are dismissed as hysterics.

While it is imperative to address patient needs, it is also imperative that patients recognize that healthcare professionals are human beings, have good days and bad days just like everyone else, and are incredibly busy treating a multitude of patients

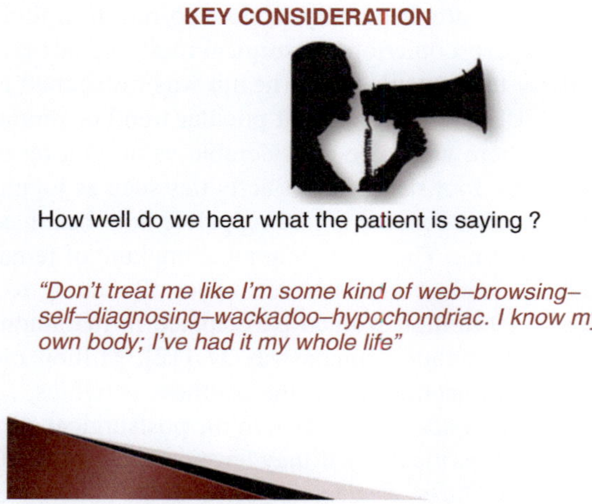

Fig. 6.5 Patients express frustration at healthcare disregarding their voices as insignificant

simultaneously. Like any other field of practice, clinicians can get stuck in tunnel vision, treating all patients with POP the same, when needs are unique from woman to woman. A clinician who listens to and encourages patient feedback is a priceless commodity (Fig. 6.5) [9].

The medical student curriculum covers a dizzying array of conditions. Significant emphasis is placed on listening to patients' feedback. As is true with so many health conditions, educators seldom experience conditions they treat, and unless given significant deep training in the condition, they may not recognize the impact of a multitude of lifestyle, behavioral, and comorbid conditions compounding severity, multiplying the impact to daily QOL. That is why seeing a specialist who understands is so very important. Women with POP simply want their clinicians to listen to them, to believe them, and to treat them with respect. Sometimes what the patient wants is not the best thing for them, but it is their body, and it is for them to make informed decision about their condition. It is imperative that both healthcare providers and patients look beyond their immediate tunnel vision and have an open evidence-based conversation about the condition and what the patient believes would be best for her. The management options for the same POP condition in a 25-year-old marathon runner vs. a mother shuttling kids to schools vs. a newly retired professional wanting to travel vs. an 85-year-old who has not been sexually active for 30 years are vastly different.

Lifestyle and behavioral activities frequently compound risk for or degree of POP severity, but what is seldom recognized is their additional potential to impact postsurgical healing. Women are often advised to return to their normal activities once they are beyond the surgical healing curve advised by their clinicians. Women seldom feel normal at the 6-week point; few women feel close to normal at the 8-week point; and while most are relatively leveled off at the 12-week point, they continue to express that it takes up to a year for their bodies to completely adjust to their new normal.

Women are frequently advised to return to their running fitness activities post POP laparoscopic/robotic surgical mesh repair (sacrocolpopexy). Impact of fitness activity to women's pelvic health was researched extensively by Kari Bø in years past [10]. Given the current popular trend of running activities, particularly marathons, there would be considerable value in a research reboot in this sector. Hard pavement foot strike fitness activities such as jogging and marathon running are of considerable concern regarding pelvic floor health and can certainly impact postsurgical healing. The most common complaint of female runners is not joint pain; it is leakage, a clear indicator of impact of running to the pelvic floor [10]. In 2016, nearly 10 million women participated in marathon runs [11]. The average age of female marathon runners was 37 [12]. Million more women jog. The hard foot strike that occurs during these fitness activities, so beloved by enthusiasts, is of particular concern in women in the postsurgical curve for any POP surgery, including TVM, particularly if they have compounding POP risk factors that may predispose them to a weakened pelvic floor, such as childbirth, age-related estrogen depletion, or tissue integrity conditions.

Heavy lifting is a documented POP causal factor, and women may experience POP as a result of either heavy lifting fitness or employment activities. What is seldom acknowledged, however, is the heavy lifting women engage in daily related to their children. Picking up a sleeping toddler is heavy lifting. Women are not educated to contract their pelvic core or floor prior to heavy lifting. Women are often distressed about how they will care for their children postsurgery, when a 10-pound load limit may be imperative to healing. Advising a mother to resist picking up her distressed toddler postsurgery will seldom result in 100% success. Will lifting toddlers postsurgery impact mesh success? There are multiple factors related to mesh procedures that we simply don't know at this point.

Comorbid conditions complicate care, whether or not mesh is utilized for surgical POP repair. Comorbid conditions that POP may cause or complicate, such as overactive bladder, underactive bladder, dyspareunia, stress urinary incontinence, urge urinary incontinence, coital incontinence, urinary tract infections, and embedded bladder wall infections, do not always magically disappear post mesh surgery and may at times compound if mesh is not used appropriately. Comorbid conditions that may cause POP or that may shift in both cause and effect directions, such as spinal cord injury or spina bifida depletion of pelvic floor function, interstitial cystitis-related pain, and the complex management of anterior support and pelvic angle in women with bladder extropy, are all concerns that could benefit from deeper analysis. Women suffering with Ehlers-Danlos syndrome, a seldom recognized or screened for genetic condition that may cause joint flexibility and hyperelastic tissue integrity, have a particularly difficult path to navigate (Fig. 6.6). Nonsurgical treatments are seldom effective in this sector of women; mesh-free surgery may fail quickly, and they seem to be at greater risk of mesh complications. It is imperative both patients and clinicians ask the right questions [9].

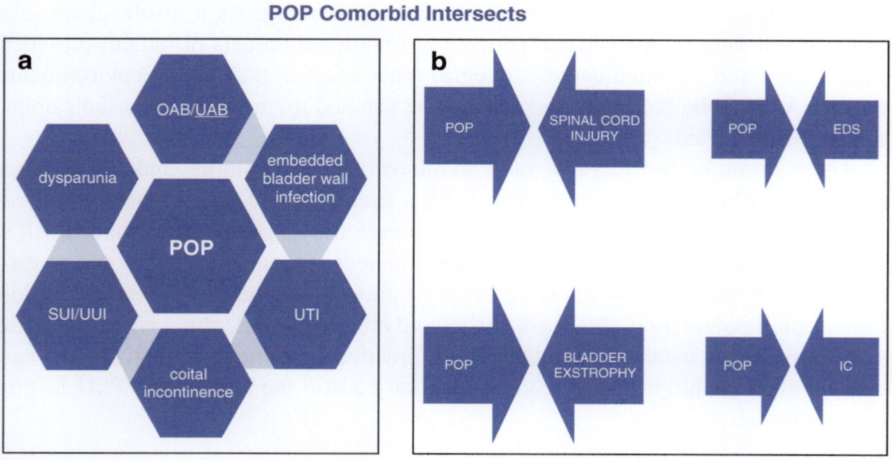

Fig. 6.6 (**a**) Possible comorbid intersects instigated by pelvic organ prolapse (POP). OAB, overactive bladder; UAB, underactive bladder; UTI, urinary tract infection; SUI, stress urinary incontinence; UUI, urge urinary incontinence. (**b**) Possible comorbid conditions that may cause POP, complicate care, or may flow back and forth between cause and effect. EDS, Ehlers-Danlos syndrome; IC, interstitial cystitis

The POP Workforce

As POP awareness surges, the demand for services worldwide will simultaneously increase significantly. Who will address the POP needs of the women of the world? Based on a study addressing discrepancies in the urogynecologic workforce of 2013, there were 6.7 practicing specializing urogynecologists for every 1 million post-reproductive women in the United States at that time, with 88% of counties in the United States lacking female pelvic surgeons [13]. Currently, the number of FPMRS specialists falls far short of demand, and undoubtedly this trend will take some time to regulate to the market demands [1]. It is likely to get worse before it gets better, because specialists currently cluster in urban areas. Patients in rural areas seldom have access to FPMRS specialists who provide quality laparoscopic mesh procedures. The potential for a women's pelvic healthcare train wreck looms large. The author hopes that, as pelvic health literacy grows with expanding discussions of this condition on TV and radio and in magazines, there will be a growing recognition of symptoms that women have quietly and privately endured for years and that this enhanced awareness will advance screening and treatment.

In the Geynisman-Tan et al. study exploring referral pattern shift in women's pelvic floor disorders, 5799 new patient visits were analyzed, disclosing that 44% of participants were referred to urogynecology by obstetrician/gynecologists, 32% were referred by primary care providers, 14% were patient self-referrals, and 9% were referred by other specialists [14]. Today's proactive patient is Internet informed and participates more directly in health decision making. As a result, given this trend in self-help Internet health education, traditional models of patient-provider relationship and communication strategies must adapt to a changing environment. Patients want to be believed, they want to be listened to, and they want their opinions to be respected.

There would be considerable value in the recruitment, training, and certification of urogynecologic advanced practice nurses, such as nurse practitioners, certified nurse midwives, and physician assistants, to ease the responsibilities that FPMRS specialists currently deliver, such as general patient assessment, history and physical examination, point-of-care tests, ordering diagnostic laboratory tests and radiological studies, and providing medications and other therapies, along with written or verbal orders per established collaborative practice agreement. Potential urogynecologic allied health evolution could potentially buffer the upcoming FPMRS specialist shortage.

Regulatory Evolution

Patients seldom have a working knowledge of FDA oversight, clinical guidelines, research flow, medical device development, or procedural technique. Research is often closed source, disabling patient access. Clearly patients trust their clinicians to guide them appropriately, and many lessons were learned at noteworthy cost to patient welfare regarding the TVM mess. Patient suffering is never an appropriate price for healthcare lessons. Unfortunately, in medicine, we don't know what we don't know, and the nature of healthcare, as in any other system, is to evolve step by step. It is imperative throughout the process that patient voice continues to be enabled and respected, to effectively and efficiently recognize issues that must be addressed.

Technology

The United States leads the world production and consumption of medical devices, housing a medical device market capturing 45% of the global market with an approximate value of $140+ billion [15]. Nearly 5000 types of medical devices are used by millions of healthcare providers in countries around the world. US exports of medical devices in key product categories identified by the Department of Commerce exceeded $44 billion in 2015 [16].

Considering the magnitude and diversity of medical device use, it's relatively obvious that device-related issues are inevitable, particularly when devices first come to market. Government regulatory agencies are not perfect, just as healthcare is not perfect. Technology can be both part of the problem and part of the solution regarding the evolution of improved healthcare. The inadvertent consequences of technology are not always possible to recognize beforehand and have been the norm in medical device development industry. In an ideal world, medical device design flaws don't harm patients. However, in the real world, technology failure typically leads to evolution of technology development. Problems may emerge related to the volume or complexity of medical devices as well as appropriate training for proper use, as well as related to fast-tracking based on patient need.

The US and European medical approval processes are unique, with fundamental differences within the regulatory agencies. According to Dr. Gail Van Norman, "The FDA historically developed as a consumer protection agency, whereas the regulations from the European Commission arose out of a need to harmonize inter-state commercial interests while preserving national autonomy" [17]. The difference in US (Fig. 6.7) [17] and European (Fig. 6.8) [18] agencies may clarify why as the United States has moved forward with navigation of medical mesh device concerns, it was not addressed proactively outside US borders. International mesh scrutiny continues in Australia, New Zealand, and the United Kingdom.

While injuries and unintended consequences of technology are not always possible to know beforehand, steps can and should be made to more efficiently address the occurrence during device development at industry, research, healthcare, and regulatory levels. Complications can and should be fast-tracked to resolution, and patient voice is a significant facet of the process.

If a new medical device is being used, a climate of trust and support between the patient and clinician should be achieved by having a frank discussion regarding the physician's experience and expertise in managing medical device complications. Addressing patient injuries and adverse events, treatment satisfaction, clinician competency, errors, goal attainment, and organizational outcomes such as care quality are imperative priorities regarding mesh or any other POP surgical difficulty.

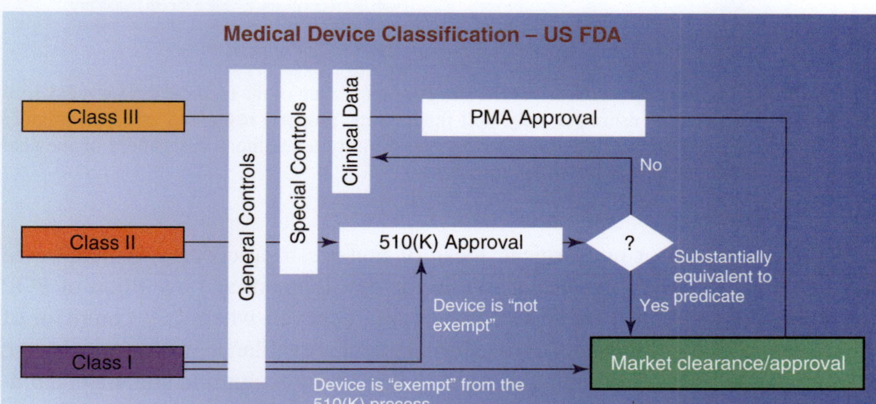

Fig. 6.7 The US Food and Drug Administration medical device approval process. The FDA was historically developed as a consumer protection agency, responsible for protecting the public health by ensuring the safety, efficacy, and security of human and veterinary drugs, biological products, and medical devices. (From De Langen [18], with permission)

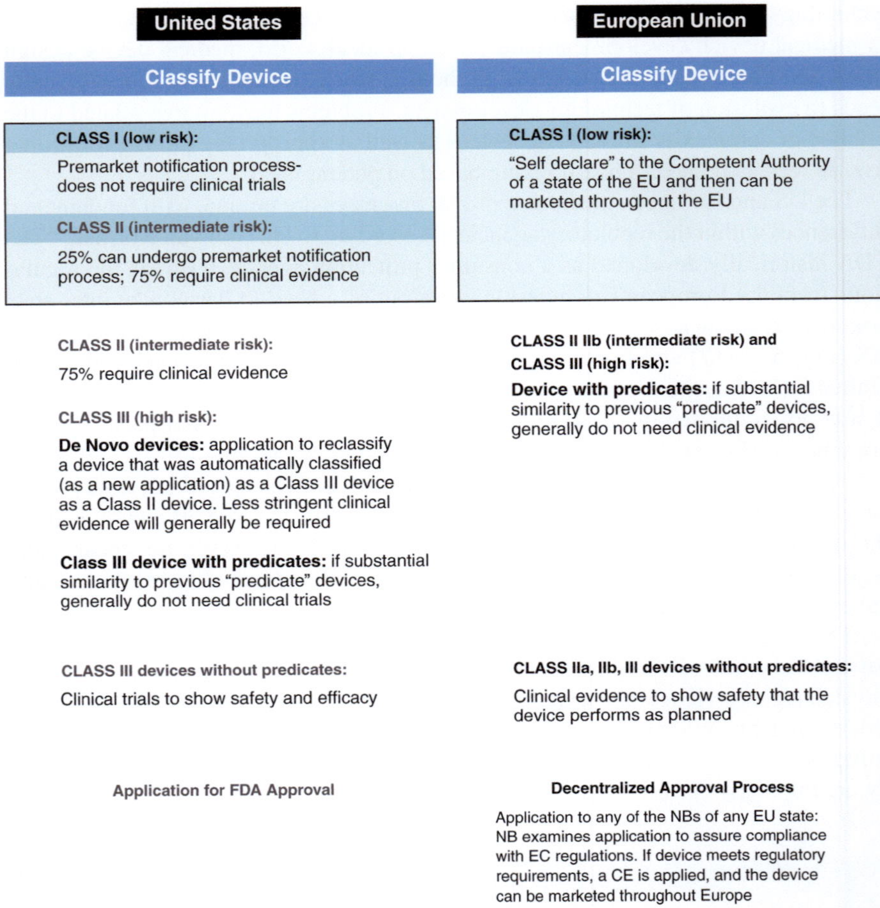

Fig. 6.8 European Commission oversees the smooth functioning of the medical device regulatory framework, by helping to ensure that only well-functioning, properly resourced and appropriately staffed notified bodies are authorized to conduct conformity assessment in the field of medical devices. (From Van Norman [17], with permission)

Whether surgical or nonsurgical, mesh or non-mesh procedures, patient voice must continue to play a significant role in the development and evolution of POP treatments. Patients must be acknowledged and believed when they complain of pain or return of symptoms post procedure. Patient surveillance postsurgery by the industry would have been a valuable asset to fast-track recognition and understanding of TVM complications. TVM patients must continue to be queried about surgical mesh outcomes. If patient voice is not appropriately utilized and included in the device evaluation process, patient outcomes and satisfaction are not optimized.

Clinician experts provide input during design, procurement, implementation, and maintenance phases. Technology end-user input is vital to appropriately measure device success and/or failure. Clinical decisions related to treatment for health conditions lean heavily on research data. POP is a relatively young specialty field, and necessary facts and figures lag behind other fields. Which surgical procedures are most effective? Which have long-term results? Which are least invasive? Which eliminate all symptoms? Since there are five types of POP, four grades of severity, and a multitude of lifestyle, behavioral, and comorbid conditions that compound and complicate impact, every woman's case has aspects of similarity, and every woman's case has aspects of uniqueness. Tracking surgeon volume, long-term surgical outcomes, and QOL treatment results are all pivotal. Identifying risk factors associated with complications, both those that can be modified and those that are more difficult to address, is pivotal. There are no simple answers.

Patient Safety

Greater awareness of patient safety is needed at international, national, and institutional levels. To many patients, the risk of unsafe healthcare is far from their thoughts when they consult a physician. Patients hope and expect that healthcare workers will provide them with safe and appropriate care. It can be very tempting to assume surgical complications are the result of action by a specific entity or person. But this mind-set presupposes that it is always possible or appropriate to implicate a single contributing factor.

> Making health care safer has to focus on the patient. I am continually moved by the accounts of medical error that affect the lives of real people. The consequences are far-reaching: they can destroy lives, affect human relationships and threaten trust in the health-care system as a whole. Patients are too often the victims of unsafe care and their points of view need to be heard within health care.
>
> Sir Liam Donaldson
> Chair, World Alliance for Patient Safety,
> World Health Organization
> Former Chief Medical Officer for England [19]

Identifying issues that contribute to TVM complications would have been critical to the development of viable solutions aimed at making POP procedures safe. At times surgical procedures, particularly early in development, have potential flaws and/or design blemishes, which may occur repetitively or as one-off events. Sadly, organizational responses to address these contributing factors have, upon occasion, been slow to occur in healthcare.

Medical device errors should not occur. Would any of us willingly and knowingly board a plane not thoroughly tested? Would any of us board a thoroughly tested plane whose pilot has not undergone 1000 h of simulation training? Errors should not occur, and internal systems that are ready to deal with errors are essential with medical device evolution. New procedures and devices at times may indicate a need for development of new sets of standards. If appropriate nonbiased monitoring does not occur at inception of utilization of new treatments, complications may go unrecognized or unacknowledged. A case in point are the TVM complications that occurred in the United Kingdom, Australia, and New Zealand. Why didn't the corporations or the regulatory bodies at large address TVM issues simultaneously with the United States in 2011? This could have hypothetically saved many women from experiencing TVM complications.

A lack of motivation to change practice behaviors is an indicator of the need for systems review. Product failure, caregiver error, comorbid complications, inappropriate postsurgical instruction, and inefficient patient educational resources (Fig. 6.9) are areas in need of continual TVM complication evaluation [4]. Some pivotal areas of focus to reduce errors are:

- Routine evaluation of standard operating procedures and guidelines with new device development
- Valid and up-to-date training, with emphasis on specialist training requirements
- Effective patient/clinician communication pre- and postsurgery

Questionnaires are often closed format (patient response is yes/no or limiting multiple choice), disallowing open patient communication and information sharing. Patients may find written health information difficult to understand. Clearly patients could benefit from better use of videos or informational wall posters and rack cards.

Patients should be empowered by clinicians to speak out. Immediate management of incidents is critical to patient trust; communication is a pivotal aspect of adverse event management and plays a key role in all aspects of surgical complication. Lack of clinician empathy is a noteworthy reason patients initiate legal action.

Sharing patients' experiences with healthcare workers in training encourages a culture in which patients are valued and their active participation in the decisions about their treatment is the normal practice. Patients' own stories of unsafe care are an important source of information and insight and can be used effectively to better understand potential causes of error and the devastation that can follow.

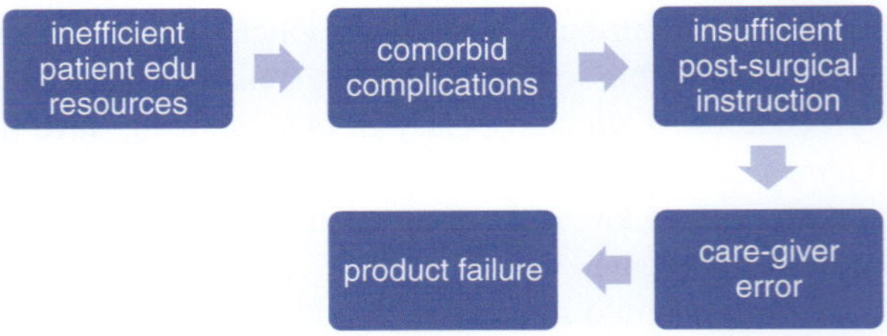

Fig. 6.9 Areas in need of transvaginal mesh (TVM) complication evaluation. Quality TVM repairs require evolution of best practices in sufficient patient education pre- and postsurgery, suitable comorbid screening protocol, surgical best practices, and appropriate product development and testing

Quality of Life

POP impacts women's QOL in multiple substantial layers, dissecting physical, emotional, social, sexual, fitness, and employment aspects of day-to-day navigation. Clearly, when mesh complications occur, the QOL impact is compounded. Asymptomatic is a term that should be eradicated from POP discussion. Considering that women are seldom aware of the existence of POP prior to diagnosis, they have no understanding that the symptoms they experience may be POP-related. However symptoms due to POP and man-made symptoms due to preventable medical device errors are vastly different.

POP symptoms such as vaginal tissue bulge, urinary or fecal incontinence, urine retention, chronic constipation, pain with intimacy, lack of sexual sensation, pain, pressure, and tampons pushing out are clearly enough to make an ogress out of a normally tranquil woman. The physical, emotional, social, sexual, and fitness impact of POP to QOL are relatively well documented. However, there is a need to explore on a deeper level the impact to employment.

Impact of TVM complications on employment is an area that to date has received little attention and is of significant concern to women embedded in the POP dynamic. Women with TVM complications initially made the difficult decision to proceed with surgery to address POP, hoping to ease POP symptoms and improve QOL. Mesh complications then turned their lives upside down, resulting in debilitating pain, impact to intimacy, and often impact to employment, including financial ramifications. A 2017 study by Javadian and Shobeiri analyzed the dynamic, utilizing a phone survey, the Sheehan Disability Scale (SDS), the years of life lived with disability (YLDs) questionnaire, and inclusion of a separate question "What do you score your disability with after vaginal procedure?" Results indicated that the majority of women missed a median of 12 months (0–80 months) of school or work because of mesh complications. A notable 59.6% of women did not return to the symptom-free condition that existed prior to first vaginal mesh surgery and did not have improvement in symptoms after mesh removal. Additionally, 33.9% stated that family income dropped because of loss of productivity related to mesh complications. Clearly ramifications of mesh complications go far beyond pain [20].

As a woman who in 2018 crossed over the 10-year anniversary of uncomplicated TVM repair, I continue to encourage women to do their homework. I was one of the lucky patients who was referred to a qualified urogynecologist. It didn't occur to me back in 2008 to ask my surgeon how experienced she was at POP repair. It didn't occur to me to ask questions about TVM. It didn't occur to me to ask about the success rate of mesh-free procedures. And it didn't occur to me to ask about nonsurgical treatments. I was lucky that my primary care clinician sent me to someone she knew to be skilled at POP repair. It is imperative that women with POP proactively understand what questions to ask and continue to dig until they receive appropriate answers, whether their questions are related to nonsurgical or surgical treatments.

Next Steps

There is a swelling trend of greater access to research funding for projects that include ongoing, long-term patient participation, a pivotal piece of the study dynamic. Health research must consider how the patient's environment impacts health. It is important to look at patients through a wide lens and to identify where both health assets and health detriments may occur.

Community-Based Participatory Research

Community-based participatory research (CBPR) is a collaborative effort that includes patients, healthcare, and industry working side by side, with long-term objectives to evolve continual research arms. Patient community partnerships may initially be difficult to capture but are tremendously valuable for long-term vision in healthcare. At onset, while relationships are in development, patients may feel research is irrelevant to their needs and may be an invasion of privacy, or engagement with researchers may feel awkward or authoritarian. Researchers may feel patient communities lack the capacity to effectively engage, particularly in long-term vision. However, the method and approach of CBPR research benefits both healthcare and patient communities tremendously by creating a climate of mutual trust and support for the benefit of all engaged in the process.

CBPR principles:

- Recognizes patient community as a unit of identity
- Builds on strengths and resources within the community
- Facilitates collaborative equitable involvement of all partners in all phases of the research
- Integrates knowledge and intervention for mutual benefit of all partners
- Promotes a co-learning and empowering process that attends to social inequities
- Involves a cyclical and iterative process
- Addresses health from both positive and ecological perspectives
- Disseminates findings and knowledge gained by all partners
- Involves long-term commitment by all partners

POP in the Twenty-First Century

POP in general is a common, cryptic health concern considered "not that big of a deal" by some members of the medical community. If asked, every single woman navigating POP will assure clinicians that it is a big deal. Within patient support spaces, communications occur between women in multiple types and various stages of this multi-faceted health condition. It is imperative these women are assured that there are treatment options that can return their lives to balance. It is imperative to let them know they are not alone and that millions of other women are experiencing the same frustration the symptoms of POP generate. As a pelvic floor health advocate, I'd like to encourage healthcare professionals who view POP as "not that big of a deal" to truly listen to their patients. And as a woman who has been surgically treated for POP and continues an informed personal regimen to maintain pelvic floor ballast postsurgery, I am hopeful that at some point, patients and healthcare professionals will be able to meet in the middle for the optimal balance of pelvic floor healthcare treatment. We have a long journey ahead of us.

The evolution of POP treatment will continue to expand considerably over the coming years. POP awareness, healthcare practice, research, device development, and both diagnostic and specialist practice policy will progress side by side. There is little doubt that POP will stimulate the next significant shift in women's health directives. As POP awareness increases, the demand for services worldwide will undoubtedly increase simultaneously.

Continual evaluation of best practices in medicine is a core aspect of healthcare evolution. Research is priceless. The value of patient voice to clarify reality and need is equally priceless. It is essential that patients, advocacy, healthcare, academia, research, industry, and policy makers come together for the greater good. As each sector explores and evolves needs, systems, and tooling, it is crucial that we cooperatively share insights captured individually in order to collectively optimize patient outcomes.

We have so much more to do; we have so much more to learn. Women with POP are hungry for hope. POP is without a doubt the biggest secret in women's health. As POP becomes widely recognized and acknowledged by the general public, the stigma of symptoms will soften. Women who have been navigating those symptoms for years, with little understanding of the cause, will find the answers they seek. Awareness, acknowledgment, and understanding of POP is one of the greatest challenges women will address in our efforts to attain health balance for our gender.

The history of healthcare, like every other industry, social enterprise, or individual initiative, is littered with the corpses of innovative visions and treatments, which at inception seem groundbreaking, yet with time and testing proved to be less than stellar. It is important that we recognize that the nature of health evolution has involved both success and failure and that rather than getting wedged in the drama, we continue to move forward, engendering progression of best practices. Patients and practitioners will collectively amplify recognition of the reality of POP. Time and experience are incredible educators.

> If we knew what we were doing, it would not be called research, would it? (Albert Einstein)

Every voice matters.

References

1. Barber MD, Maher C. Epidemiology and outcome assessment of pelvic organ prolapse. Int Urogynecol J. 2013;24(11):1783–90.
2. Griffith FL. Papyrus Kahun VI. 1, pages 1 and 2; medical papyrus 12th Dynasty. F PD-US. Wikipedia. Kahun Gynaecological Papyrus [Updated 2017 Sept 2]. https://en.wikipedia.org/wiki/Kahun_Gynaecological_Papyrus. Accessed 31 Mar 2018.
3. Downing K. Uterine prolapse: from antiquity to today. Obstet Gynecol Int. 2012;2012:649459.

4. Association for Pelvic Organ Prolapse Support. POPS online Facebook patient support forum. https://www.facebook.com/groups/184143085606/. Accessed 6 Jan 2018.
5. International Urogynecological Association. Three countries ban the use of vaginal mesh in prolapse surgery. IUGA. 2017;12(4). Released 2018 Jan 19. www.pelvicorganprolapsesupport.org/s/IUGA-mesh-ban-statement.pdf. Accessed 20 Mar 2018.
6. United States Food and Drug Administration. Urogynecologic surgical mesh: update on the safety and effectiveness of vaginal placement for pelvic organ prolapse; 2011. http://www.fda.gov/downloads/medicaldevices/safety/alertsandnotices/UCM262760.pdf. Accessed 31 Mar 2018.
7. United States Food and Drug Administration. FDA safety communication: UPDATE on serious complications associated with transvaginal placement of surgical mesh for pelvic organ prolapse; 2011. http://www.fda.gov/MedicalDevices/Safety/AlertsandNotices/ucm262435.htm.
8. Souders CP, Eilber KS, McClelland L, Wood LN, Souders AR, Steiner V, Anger JT. The truth behind transvaginal mesh litigation: devices, timelines, and provider characteristics. Female Pelvic Med Reconstr Surg. 2018;24(1):21–5.
9. Palm S. Association for Pelvic Organ Prolapse Support. Pelvic organ prolapse: help and hope. http://www.pelvicorganprolapsesupport.org/pelvic-organ-prolapse-help-and-hope/. Accessed 2 Apr 2018.
10. Bø K. Urinary incontinence, pelvic floor dysfunction, exercise and sport. Sports Med. 2004;34(7):451–64.
11. Running USA. U.S. Road race trends. Road race finisher total experiences slight year-over-year decline in 2016. http://www.runningusa.org/2017-us-road-race-trends, Accessed 31 Mar 2018.
12. Competitor Running. New U.S. marathons and halfs report reveals participation is declining 2017 Jun 19 [Updated 2017 Jun 20]. http://running.competitor.com/2017/06/news/new-report-2016-marathon-half-participation_165419. Accessed 31 Mar 2018.
13. Muffly TM, Weterings R, Barber MD, Steinberg AC. Discrepancies in the female pelvic medicine and reconstructive surgeon workforce. Female Pelvic Med Reconstr Surg. 2015;21(2):99–105.
14. Geynisman-Tan J, Brown O, Mueller M, Leader-Cramer A, Dave B, Bochenska K, et al. Changing referral patterns to urogynecology. Female Pelvic Med Reconstr Surg. 2018;24(1):48–50.
15. Zambare S. Serum Institute of India Pvt. Ltd., Slide 11. Medical developments. Size and shape of the US medical device industry. http://www.todaysmedicaldevelopments.com/article/size-and-shape-of-the-us-medical-device-industry/. Accessed 23 Mar 2018.
16. SelectUSA. Medical technology spotlight. https://www.selectusa.gov/medical-technology-industry-united-states. Accessed 22 Mar 2018.
17. Van Norman GA. Drugs and devices: comparison of European and U.S. approval processes. JACC. 2016;1(5):399–412.
18. De Langen J. Medical device reporting. Pharmacovigilance Elsevier Life Sciences. 2016 Sept 27. https://www.slideshare.net/rocheam/medical-device-reporting-27-sep2016. Accessed 1 Apr 2017.
19. Donaldson, L. Foreword. In: World Health Organization. Patient safety workshop: learning from error. WHO/IER/PSP/2008.09. Geneva: WHO Press. p. 3. www.who.int/patientsafety/activities/technical/vincristine_learning-from-error.pdf. Accessed 21 Mar 2018.
20. Javadian P, Shobeiri SA. The disability impact and associated cost per disability in women who underwent surgical revision of transvaginal mesh kits for prolapse repair. Female Pelvic Med Reconstr Surg. 2017;13 https://doi.org/10.1097/SPV.0000000000000489. [Epub ahead of print].

Chapter 7
Pelvic Floor Anatomy as It Relates to the Design and Development of Vaginal Mesh Kits

Jonia Alshiek and S. Abbas Shobeiri

Introduction

Pelvic floor disorders, including urinary incontinence (UI), fecal incontinence, and pelvic organ prolapse (POP), represent a major public health issue in the United States [1]. Pelvic floor disorders, including POP and urinary incontinence, are debilitating conditions; 24% of adult women have at least one pelvic floor disorder [2], which results in surgery in one of nine women [3]. In the United States, the National Center for Health Statistics estimates 400,000 operations per year are performed for pelvic floor dysfunction, with 300,000 occurring in the inpatient setting [4]. A study of Australian women found that the lifetime risk of surgery for POP in the general female population was 19% [5]. In an Austrian study, an estimation of the frequency for post-hysterectomy vault prolapse requiring surgical repair was between 6% and 8% [6]. A single vaginal birth has been shown to significantly increase the odds of prolapse (OR 9.73, 95% CI 2.68–35.35). Additional vaginal births were not associated with a significant increase in the odds of prolapse [7].

It is forecast that the number of American women with at least one pelvic floor disorder will increase from 28.1 million in 2010 to 43.8 million in 2050. During this time period, the number of women with UI will increase 55% from 18.3 million to

J. Alshiek
Department of Obstetrics and Gynecology, Gynecologic Subspecialties, Inova Women's Hospital, Virginia Commonwealth University, Falls Church, VA, USA

Tel Aviv Sourasky Medical Center, Sackler Faculty of Medicine, Tel Aviv University, Tel Aviv, Israel

S. A. Shobeiri (✉)
INOVA Health System, Falls Church, VA, USA
e-mail: Abbas.shobeiri@inova.org

S. A. Shobeiri (ed.), *The Innovation and Evolution of Medical Devices*,
https://doi.org/10.1007/978-3-319-97073-8_7

28.4 million. For fecal incontinence, the number of affected women will increase 59% from 10.6 to 16.8 million, and the number of women with POP will increase 46% from 3.3 to 4.9 million. The highest projections for 2050 estimate that 58.2 million women in the United States will have at least one pelvic floor disorder, 41.3 million with UI, 25.3 million with fecal incontinence, and 9.2 million with POP. This forecast has important public health implications. Understanding the causes of pelvic floor disorders is in its infancy. But what is known is that prolapse arises because of injuries and deterioration of the muscles, nerves, and connective tissue that support and control normal pelvic function. Conventionally, the surgical repair of pelvic floor disorders including stress urinary incontinence and pelvic organ prolapse was done using the patient's native tissue to restore the injured pelvic structure. However, the failure rate of this conventional treatment was high due to the reduced native connective tissue and musculature integrity, requiring repeated surgery in approximately 40% [3, 8, 9]. Therefore, a better method was required for a higher operative success rate. Both biological and synthetic grafts were introduced in order to provide such a purpose and decrease the failure rate [10].

The idea of using synthetic meshes as a treatment of pelvic floor organ prolapse originates from the general surgery field where they have used meshes for abdominal hernia repair. According to abdominal hernia studies, mesh repair-related outcomes were found to be superior to native tissue repair [11, 12]. Therefore, in the 1970s, gynecologists had assumed that similar outcomes would be achieved using meshes of abdominal hernia repair for abdominal pelvic floor organ prolapse or incontinence repair and had begun cutting hernia meshes and adjusting them for usage in abdominal pelvic organ prolapse repair. In 1990s, hernia meshes were first used for vaginal pelvic floor organ prolapse repair and for stress urinary incontinence repair. There were no specifically designed vaginal meshes, instead, gynecologists were using abdominal hernia meshes after cutting and fitting them to the specific pelvic repair that was required. In 1996 the first mesh for the treatment of SUI was introduced (ProteGen Sling, Boston Scientific Corporation, Marlborough MA, USA). Afterward, tension-free vaginal tape (TVT) followed by synthetic vaginal mesh kits which were introduced for vaginal repair of pelvic floor disorders. Understanding the anatomy will help us in understanding the rationale behind vaginal mesh kits usage and in which disorders it might be indicated. This chapter focuses on the *functional* anatomy of the pelvic floor, and how the anterior, posterior, apical, and lateral compartments are supported, as it relates to the design of vaginal mesh kits in women.

Support of the Pelvic Organs: Conceptual Overview

The pelvic organs rely on (1) their connective tissue attachments to the pelvic walls and (2) support from the levator ani muscles that are under neuronal control from the peripheral and central nervous systems. In this chapter, the term "pelvic floor" is used broadly to include all the structures supporting the pelvic cavity rather than the restricted use of this term to refer to the levator ani group of muscles. The anterior and posterior vaginal mesh kits were designed to enhance or replace the underlying pubocervical or rectovaginal tissue, respectively. These kits could be used only after identifying precisely the underlying pathology that leads to the prolapsed organ; this will be discussed later in this chapter.

To convey the pelvic floor supportive structures' 3D architecture to the reader, we can use the "room analogy." Using this analogy, the reader can conceptualize the pelvic floor hiatus as the door out of a room (Fig. 7.1). Using this very simplified analogy, if you view the pelvic floor hiatus from where the sacrum is, the door frame for this room is the perineal membrane, the walls and the floor the levator ani muscle, and the ceiling the pubic bone. However, the pelvic floor is artificially separated into three compartments (Fig. 7.2). We arbitrarily call these anterior, middle, posterior, and lateral compartments (Fig. 7.3). The tissue separating the anterior and middle compartments is pubocervical fibromuscularis or pubocervical fascia. The

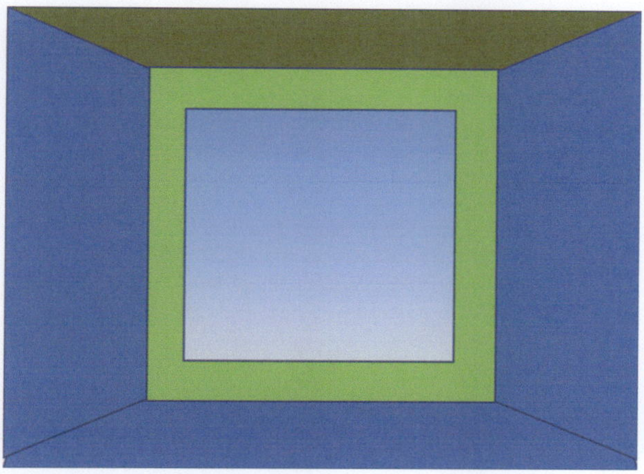

Fig. 7.1 Pelvic floor room analogy. (© Shobeiri 2013)

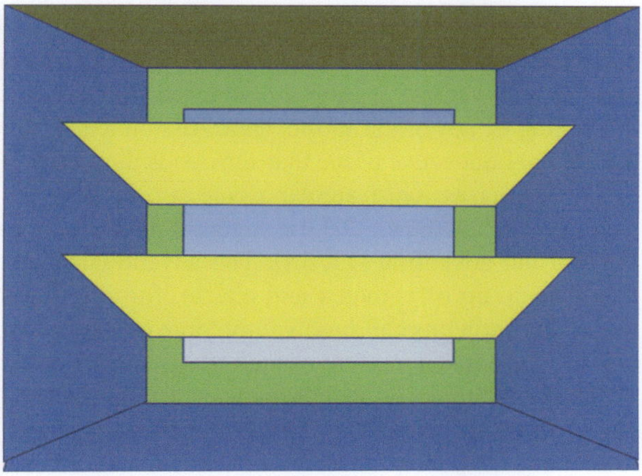

Fig. 7.2 Pelvic floor room analogy with three compartments separated. (© Shobeiri 2013)

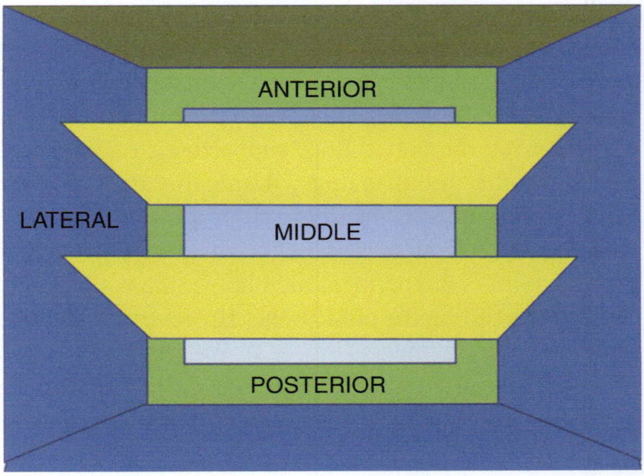

Fig. 7.3 Pelvic floor room analogy with anterior, middle, and posterior compartments and the lateral walls marked. (© Shobeiri 2013)

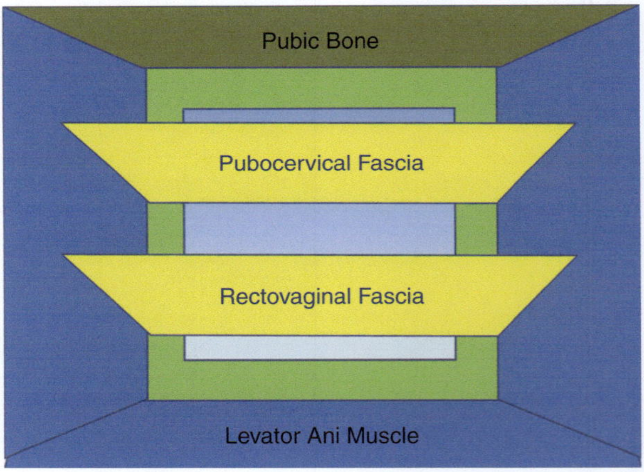

Fig. 7.4 Pelvic floor room analogy: pubocervical fibromuscularis and rectovaginal fascia separating the three compartments. (© Shobeiri 2013)

tissue separating the middle and posterior compartments is rectovaginal fibromuscularis or rectovaginal fascia or septum (Fig. 7.4). The pubocervical fibromuscularis and the rectovaginal septum are attached laterally to the levator ani muscle with thickening of adventitia in this area. Anatomically, the endopelvic fascia refers to the areolar connective tissue that surrounds the vagina. It continues down the length of the vagina as loose areolar tissue surrounding the pelvic viscera. Histologic examination has shown that the vagina is made up of three layers: epithelium, muscularis, and adventitia [13, 14]. The adventitial layer is loose areolar connective tissue made up of collagen and elastin, forming the vaginal tube. Therefore, the tissue that surgeons call fascia at the time of surgery is best described as fibromuscularis, since it is a mixture of muscularis and adventitia.

Anteriorly, pubocervical fibromuscularis is attached to the levator ani using arcus tendineus fascia pelvis (Fig. 7.5). Posterior attachment of rectovaginal septum to the levator ani is poorly understood, but we will refer to it as the posterior arcus

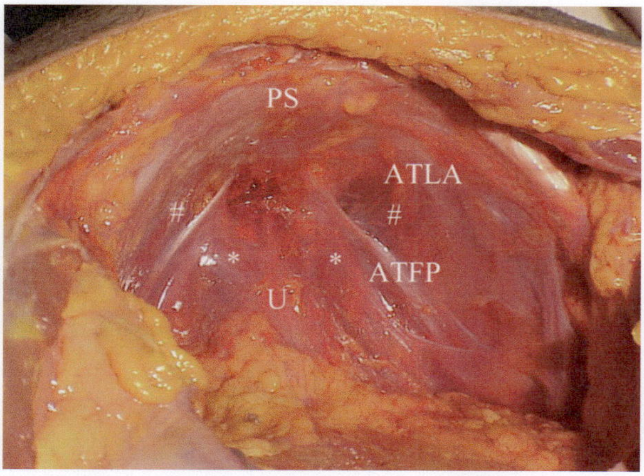

Fig. 7.5 Retropubic anatomy showing points of attachments of the arcus tendineus levator ani and the arcus tendineus fascia pelvis. The urethra sits on the hammock-like pubocervical fibromuscularis. # denotes the levator ani attachment to the obturator internus muscle. (© Shobeiri 2013)

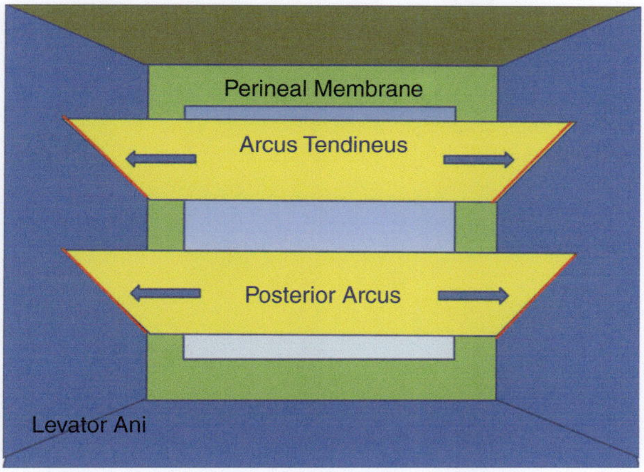

Fig. 7.6 Pelvic floor room analogy: the line of attachment of the pubocervical fascia to the levator ani is arcus tendineus fascia pelvis. The line of attachment of the rectovaginal fascia to the levator ani is the posterior arcus. Both are shown as *red lines*. (© Shobeiri 2013)

(Fig. 7.6) [15]. The anterior compartment is home to the urethra and the lower part of the bladder. The middle compartment is the vagina, and the posterior compartment is home to anorectum (Fig. 7.7). This analogy is not far from reality. When one looks at the pelvic floor structures, the three compartments are clearly separated as described (Fig. 7.8). Compartmentalization of the pelvic floor has led to different medical specialties looking at that specific compartment and paying less attention to the whole pelvic floor (Fig. 7.9).

If one looks at the middle compartment from the side, he or she can appreciate different levels of support as described by DeLancey (Fig. 7.10) [16]. Looking at these supportive structures from the sagittal view exposes the connective tissue elements that keep the room standing. Generally, a "suspension bridge" analogy is useful for describing these structures (Fig. 7.11). Although in the room analogy, the anterior, middle, and posterior compartments house the pelvic organs, in reality, the pelvic organs are part of the pelvic floor and play an important supportive role

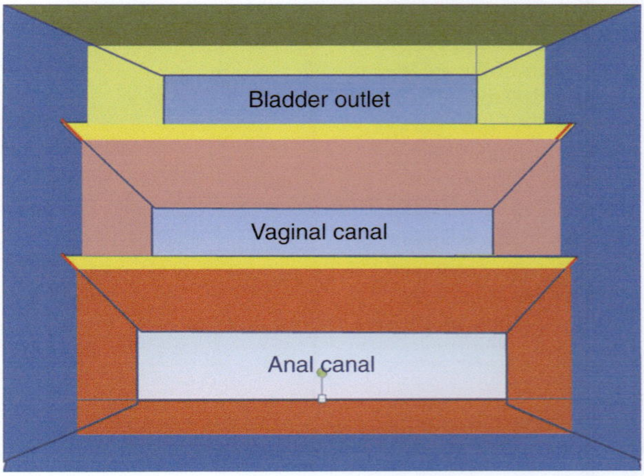

Fig. 7.7 Pelvic floor room analogy: three compartments separated. (© Shobeiri 2013)

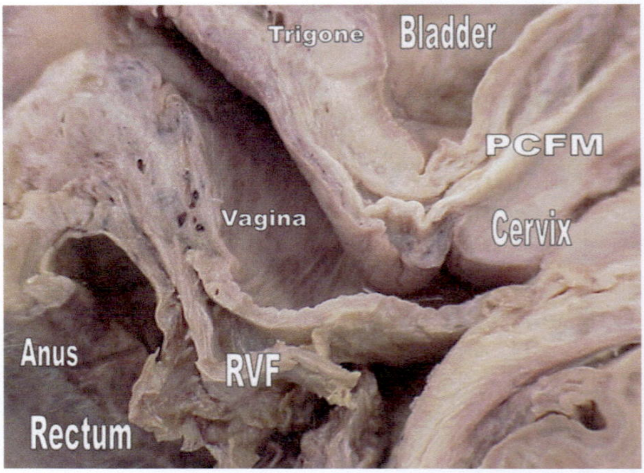

Fig. 7.8 Midsagittal anatomy of an intact cadaveric specimen demonstrating the three different compartments. (© Shobeiri 2013)

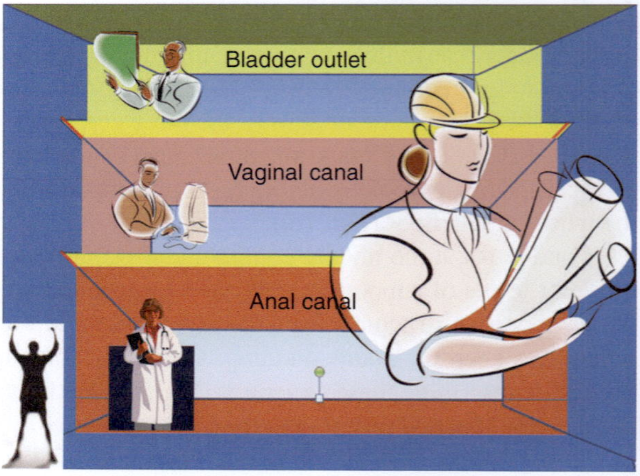

Fig. 7.9 Pelvic floor room analogy: each area or compartment may be managed by a different specialist. There is a great need for one specialty that understands the interaction between different compartments and manages them concurrently as much as possible. (© Shobeiri 2013)

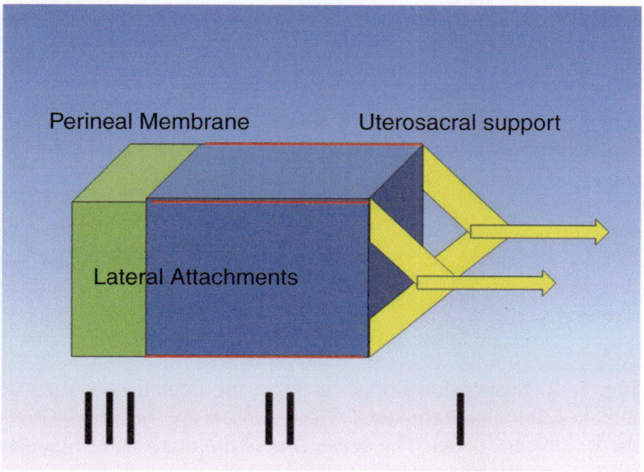

Fig. 7.10 Pelvic floor room analogy: Level 1 supports are provided by the uterosacral-cardinal ligament complex (*yellow arrows*), which keep the "room" upright. Level II supports are provided by the lateral tendineus attachments (*red lines*). The support is provided by perineal membrane (*green area*). (© Shobeiri 2013)

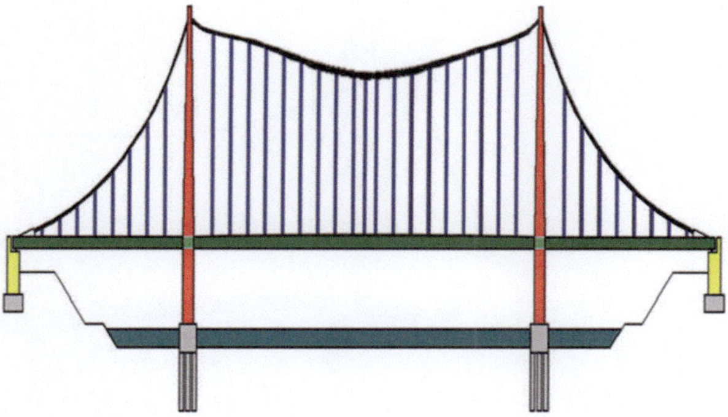

Fig. 7.11 Suspension bridge analogy; the depiction of a normal bridge. (© Shobeiri 2013)

through their connections with structures, such as the cardinal and uterosacral ligaments. Adapting this suspension bridge to the human body and the perineal body and the sacrum become the two anchoring points of the bridge. The perineal membrane (Level III) and the uterosacral and cardinal ligaments (Level I) form the two masts of the suspension bridge (Fig. 7.12). The lateral wires are the levator ani muscles of the lateral wall (Fig. 7.13), and the attachments of the vagina to the levator ani muscles laterally in the mid-part of the vagina form Level II support. The anterior and posterior vaginal mesh kits were designed to enhance or replace this Level II support mainly and Level I slightly. The levator ani muscles and the interconnecting fibromuscular structures support the bladder and urethra anteriorly, the vaginal canal in the middle, and the anorectal structures posteriorly (Fig. 7.14).

Like a room or a suspension bridge, the pelvic floor is subjected to loads that should be appropriate for its design. Should these loads exceed what the pelvic floor is capable of handling, there would be failure in one or multiple supportive elements. The pelvic floor is not a static structure. The levator ani works in concert with the ligamentous structures to withstand intraabdominal pressure that could predispose to POP and urinary or fecal incontinence during daily activities (Fig. 7.15).

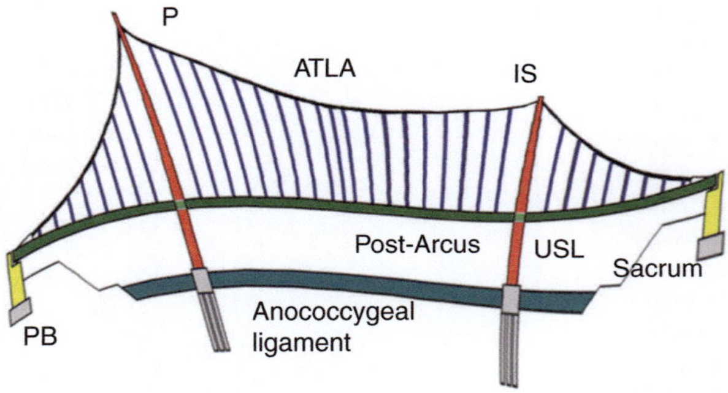

Fig. 7.12 Suspension bridge analogy; the depiction of a suspension bridge adapted to human female pelvic floor structures. The *red masts* are the ischial spine and the pubis. The *blue lines* are the levator ani fibers. The *green line* is the uterosacral ligaments continuous with the posterior arcus line. The anococcygeal ligament provides anchoring point for the posterior structures. (© Shobeiri 2013)

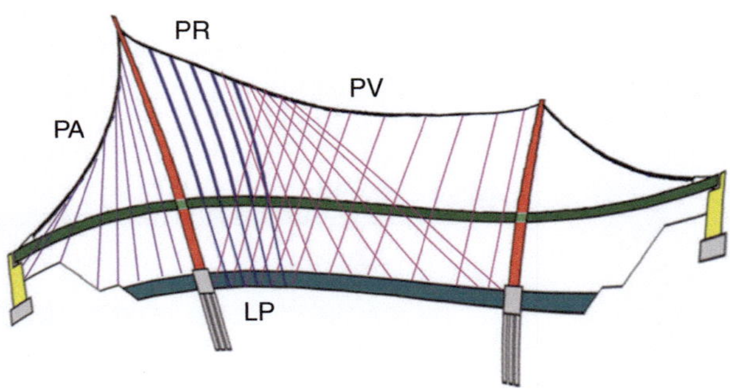

Fig. 7.13 Suspension bridge analogy; the depiction of a suspension bridge adapted to human female pelvic floor structures. The levator ani fibers have intricate and overlapping paths. The puboanalis (PA) and puboperinealis form some of the supportive structures of the perineum. The puborectalis (PR) fibers form the sling behind the rectum. Pubovisceralis (PV) is a collective term we have applied here to the iliococcygeus and pubococcygeus fibers. The levator plate (LP) is formed by overlapping of the iliococcygeus/pubococcygeus (PV) and the puborectalis (PR) fibers. (© Shobeiri 2013)

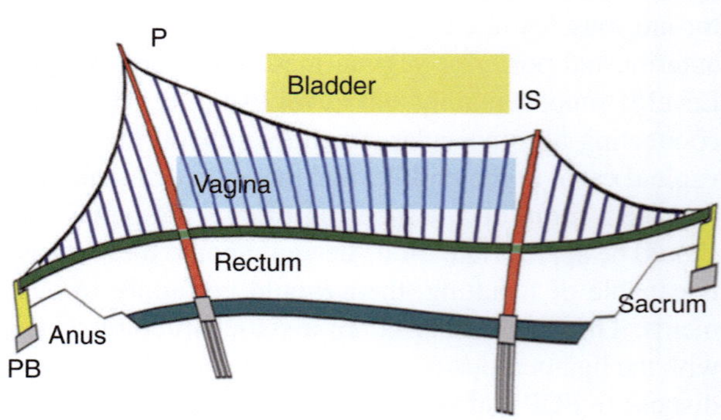

Fig. 7.14 Suspension bridge analogy; the depiction of different compartments of pelvic floor. (© Shobeiri 2013)

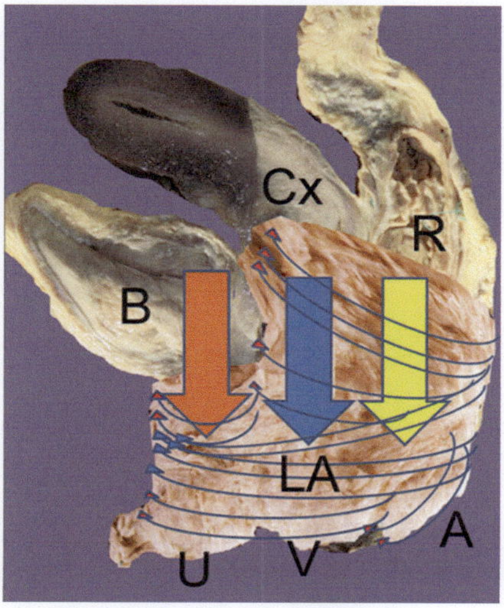

Fig. 7.15 Right lateral standing anatomic depiction of the three compartments exposed to intraabdominal pressure, which results in activation of the muscles to prevent prolapse or urinary and fecal incontinence. Bladder (B), cervix (Cx), rectum (R), levator ani (LA), urethra (U), vagina (V), anus (A). (© Shobeiri 2013)

The lower end of the pelvic floor is held closed by the pelvic floor muscles, preventing prolapse by constricting the base. The spatial relationship of the organs and the pelvic floor are important. Pelvic support is a combination of constriction, suspension, and structural geometry.

The levator ani muscle has puboperinealis, puboanalis, pubovaginalis, puborectalis, pubococcygeus, and iliococcygeus subdivisions (Fig. 7.16) [17]. The pubococcygeus is a functional unit of the iliococcygeus. These two collectively are known as the pubovisceralis muscle in our prior publications. In the older studies that utilized MRI for visualization of the levator ani muscles, pubovisceralis denotes puboperinealis, puboanalis, and pubovaginalis together. Due to the fact that ultrasound can see these subdivisions clearly, and the fact that the newer MRIs can see some of these subdivision better, the term pubovisceralis is falling out of favor. We will be using the exact terms when referring to these subdivisions. The relationship of these muscles to each other is interesting, as they crisscross in different angles to each other (Figs. 7.17 and 7.18).

Practical Anatomy and Prolapse

Overview

Level I support is composed of the uterosacral and cardinal ligaments that form the support of the cervix and upper one third of the vagina by attaching them to the pelvic wall. Stretching and failure of Level I can result in pure apical prolapse of the uterus or an enterocele formation. The cephalad arms of the vaginal mesh kits are meant to recreate the Level I support by attachment to the sacrospinous posteriorly

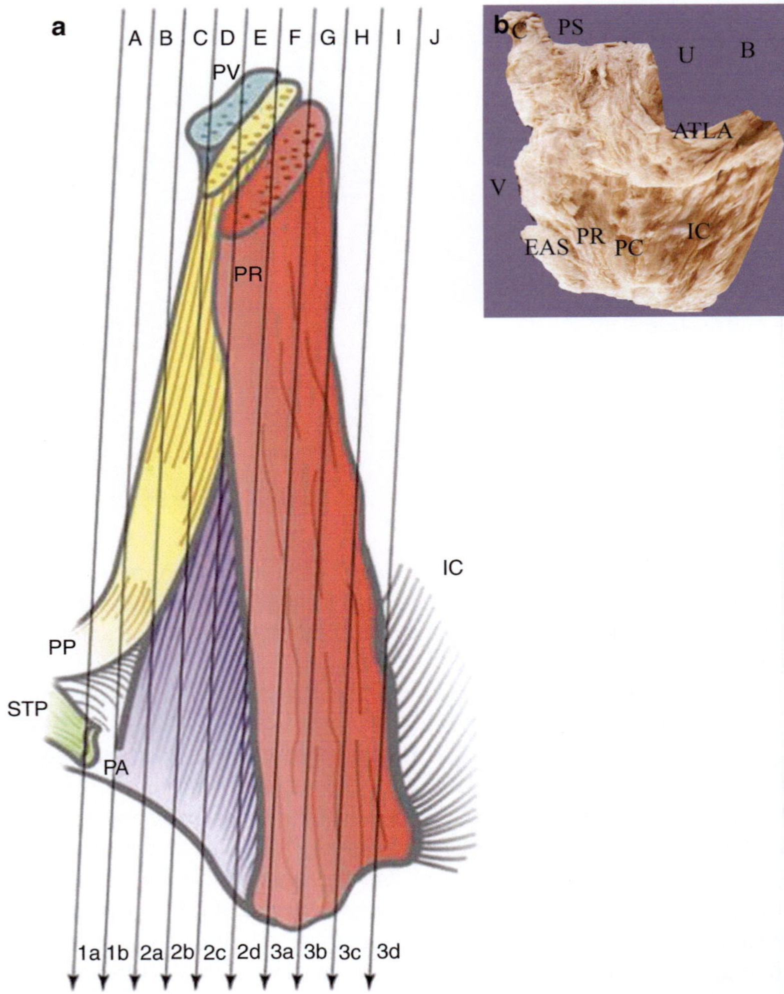

Fig. 7.16 (**a**) The relative position of levator ani subdivisions during ultrasound imaging. Iliococcygeus (IC), puboperinealis (PP), superficial transverse perinei (STP), puboanalis (PA). Illustration: John Yanson. (From Shobeiri et al. [17], with permission). (**b**)The left lateral view of the left hemipelvis. Arcus tendineus levator ani (ATLA), bladder (B), external anal sphincter (EAS), iliococcygeus (IC), pubococcygeus (PC), puborectalis (PR), pubic symphysis (PS), urethra (U). (© Shobeiri 2013)

or attachment to the cephalad aspect of arcus tendineus anteriorly. At Level II, there are direct lateral attachments of the pubocervical fibromuscularis and rectovaginal fibromuscularis to the lateral facial compartments formed by the levator ani muscles. The variations of defect in this level will be described in the following sections. Anterior mesh was designed mainly to restore and enhance Level II. In Level III the

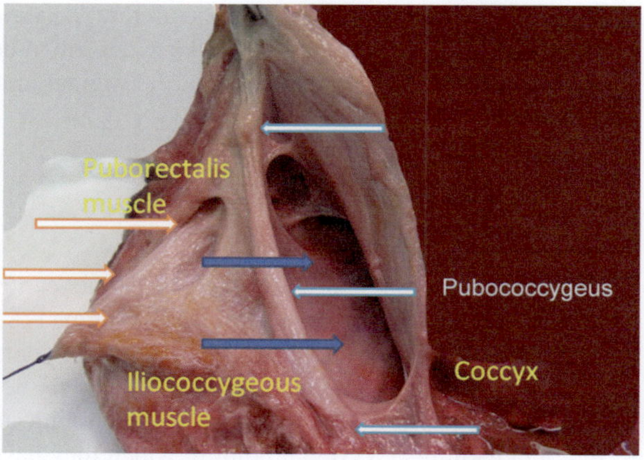

Fig. 7.17 Right hemipelvis of a fresh frozen pelvis showing the overlapping of the levator ani subdivisions fibers. *Orange arrows*, puborectalis; *blue arrows*, iliococcygeus; *white arrows*, pubococcygeus. Note the relationship between the iliococcygeus and pubococcygeus fibers. (© Shobeiri 2013)

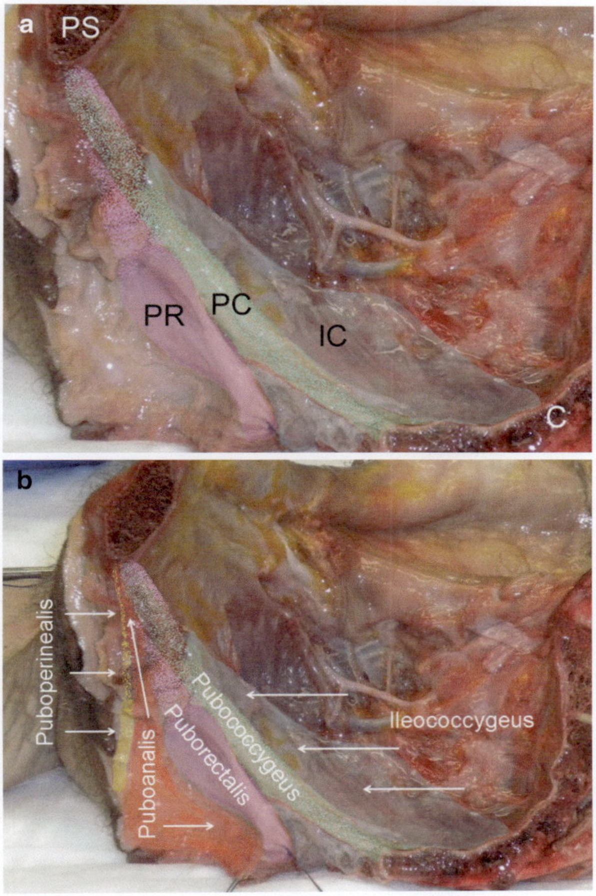

Fig. 7.18 (**a**) Right hemipelvis of a fresh frozen pelvis with the organs removed. The puborectalis (PR), iliococcygeus (IC), and pubococcygeus (PC) form the lateral sidewall. Note the relationship between the iliococcygeus and pubococcygeus fibers. (**b**) The same right hemipelvis of a fresh frozen pelvis with the organs removed. The puboanalis and the puboperinealis are outlined. These fibers are involved in the stabilization of the anus and the perineum, respectively. (© Shobeiri 2013)

vaginal wall is anteriorly fused with the urethra, posteriorly with the perineal body. Levator ani muscles in this area are poorly described but mostly consist of fibrous sheets that envelop the lateral aspects of the vaginal introitus.

Apical Segment

While Level I cardinal and uterosacral ligaments can be surgically identified supporting the cervix and the upper third of the vagina [18, 19], as they fan out toward the sacrum and laterally, they become a mixture of connective tissue, blood vessels, nerves, lymphatics, smooth muscle, and adipose tissue. The uterosacral ligaments act like rubber bands in that they may lengthen with initial Valsalva but resist any further lengthening at a critical point in which they have to return to their comfortable length or break (Fig. 7.19). Level I and levator ani muscles are interdependent. Intact levator ani muscles moderate the tension placed on the Level I support structures, and intact Level I support lessens the pressure imposed from above on the pelvic floor.

Anterior Compartment

Anterior compartment support depends on the integrity of vaginal muscularis and adventitia and their connections to the arcus tendineus fascia pelvis. The arcus tendineus fascia pelvis is at one end connected to the lower sixth of the pubic bone, 1–2 cm lateral to the midline, and at the other end to the ischial spine. A simple case of a distension cystocele could result from a defect in pubocervical fibromuscularis (Fig. 7.20). This disorder is repaired by suturing the defect and plication of the torn fascia. Such a repair could be performed by general ob/gyn surgeon, without the need of anterior mesh.

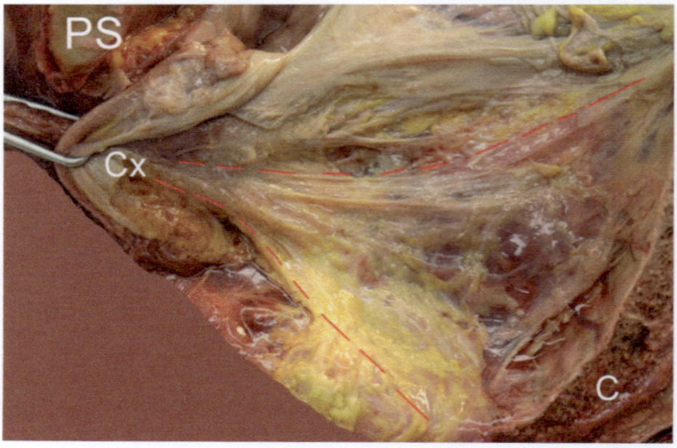

Fig. 7.19 Right hemipelvis of a fresh frozen pelvis showing the uterosacral fibers. The borders of the ligament are shown in *dotted line*. Cervix (Cx), coccyx (C), pubic symphysis (PS). (© Shobeiri 2013)

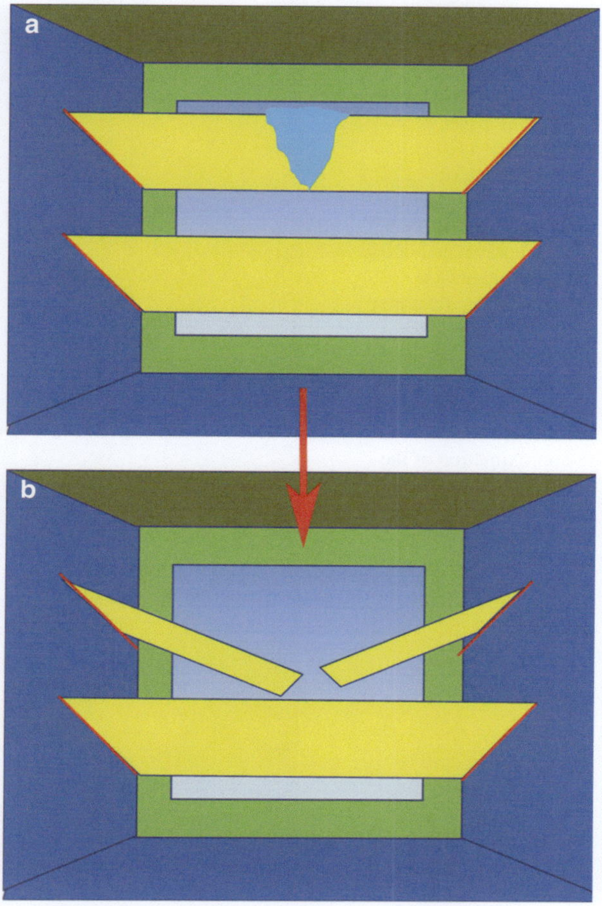

Fig. 7.20 Pelvic floor room analogy: (**a**) an occult pubocervical fibromuscularis defect can result in an overt cystocele (**b**). (© Shobeiri 2013)

The anterior wall fascial attachments to the arcus tendineus fascia pelvis have been called the paravaginal fascial attachments by Richardson et al. [20]. Detachment of arcus tendineus from the levator ani is associated with stress incontinence and anterior prolapse. The detachment can be unilateral (Fig. 7.21) or bilateral (Fig. 7.22), causing a displacement cystocele. In addition, the defect can be complete or incomplete. The surgeon who performs a traditional anterior repair in reality worsens the underlying disease process. In this case, a subspecialist surgeon should perform the surgical repair of the paravaginal detachment defect laparoscopically or vaginally. In this type of disorder, the primary repair shouldn't be anterior mesh repair. Moreover, using anterior mesh and suturing it to the detached arcus tendineus will worsen the patient's condition and might result in complications, including shrinkage of mesh, as the lateral side in not intact (see Figs. 7.21b and 7.22b).

The cephalad portions of the anterior vaginal wall can prolapse due to lack of Level I support and failure of uterosacral-cardinal complex. Over time this failure may lead to increased load in the paravaginal area and failure of Level II paravaginal

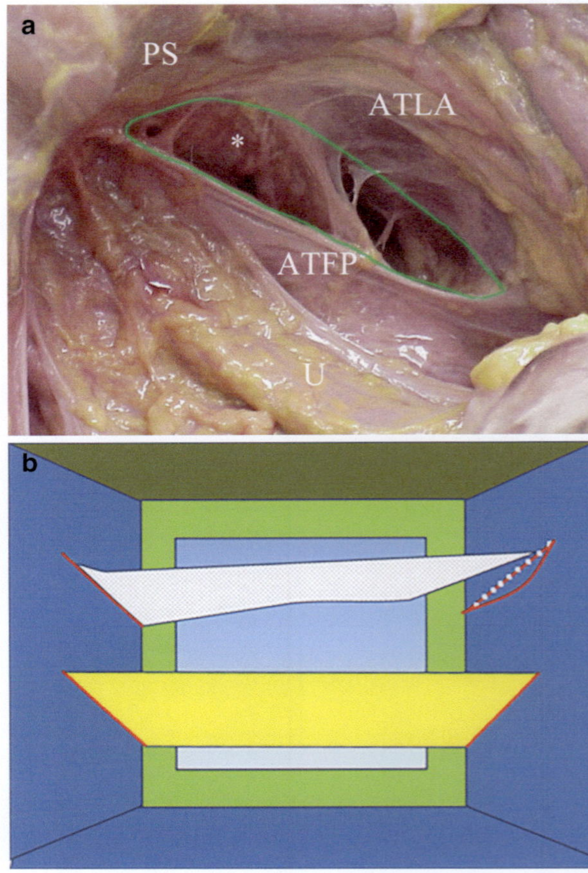

Fig. 7.21 (**a**) Right hemipelvis of a fresh frozen pelvis showing a paravaginal defect repair *outlined in green*. © Shobeiri 2013 (**b**) Pelvic floor room analogy: Left side is an intact lateral tendinous compartment, while a paravaginal defect (pubocervical fascia detachment) is illustrated in the right side of the patient (*red convex line*). The first step in this case should be repairing of this detachment by re-approximation of the detached tissues. Mesh usage without appropriate lateral repair will lead to complications in this case. (© Shobeiri 2013)

support. A study of 71 women with anterior compartment prolapse has shown that paravaginal defect usually results from a detachment of the arcus tendineus fascia pelvis from the ischial spine and rarely from the pubic bone [21]. Resuspension of the vaginal apex at the time of surgery, in addition to paravaginal or anterior colporrhaphy, may help to return the anterior wall to a more normal position or at least to prevent future failures. Another scenario that the surgeon faces is the lack of any tangible fibromuscular tissue in the anterior compartment (Fig. 7.23a). Plication of the available tissue may cause vaginal narrowing and dyspareunia. The knowledge of this condition is essential, as it will require bridging of the anterior compartment with biologic graft mostly by autologous fascia lata graft [22] or synthetic anterior mesh. The commercially available biologic tissue has had high failure rates for the anterior compartment and no improvement in the posterior compartment. The anterior mesh and vaginal mesh kits may have been an ideal product for this scenario as long as the levator ani muscles are intact and the pubocervical fibromuscularis is lacking (Fig. 7.23b). Yet, if the patient doesn't have muscles, the anterior mesh won't have lateral walls for appropriate attachment, and the mesh arms of the

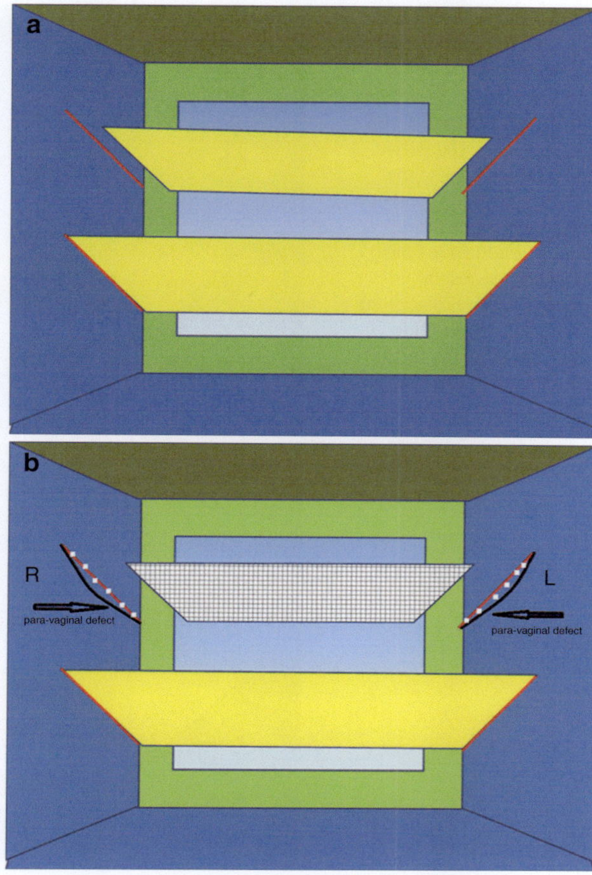

Fig. 7.22 (**a**) Pelvic floor room analogy: bilateral detachment of the pubocervical fibromuscularis can result in a cystocele. (**b**) Pelvic floor room analogy: Bilateral defect of tendinous compartments, a paravaginal defect (pubocervical fascia detachment), is illustrated in both left and right sides of the patient (black convex line). The first step in this case should be repairing of this detachment by re-approximation of the detached tissues in both sides. Mesh usage without appropriate bilateral repair will lead to complications in this case including shrinkage of mesh. (© Shobeiri 2013)

anterior mesh kits won't have an anchoring point, and if the muscles are intact, the mesh arms may cause pain traversing through muscles that move constantly.

Various grading systems such as Pelvic Organ Prolapse Quantification (POP-Q) system [23] used to describe prolapse do not take into account the underlying cause of the prolapse. Different clinical- and imaging-based modalities have been used to pinpoint the location of defect, and pelvic floor ultrasound has become valuable in the skilled hands to diagnose levator ani defects.

Perineal Membrane (Urogenital Diaphragm)

A critical but perhaps underappreciated part of pelvic floor support is the perineal membrane as it forms the Level III support (Fig. 7.24) [16] and one of the anchoring points in the suspension bridge analogy. On the anterior part caudad to the levator ani muscles, there is a dense triangular membrane called the urogenital diaphragm.

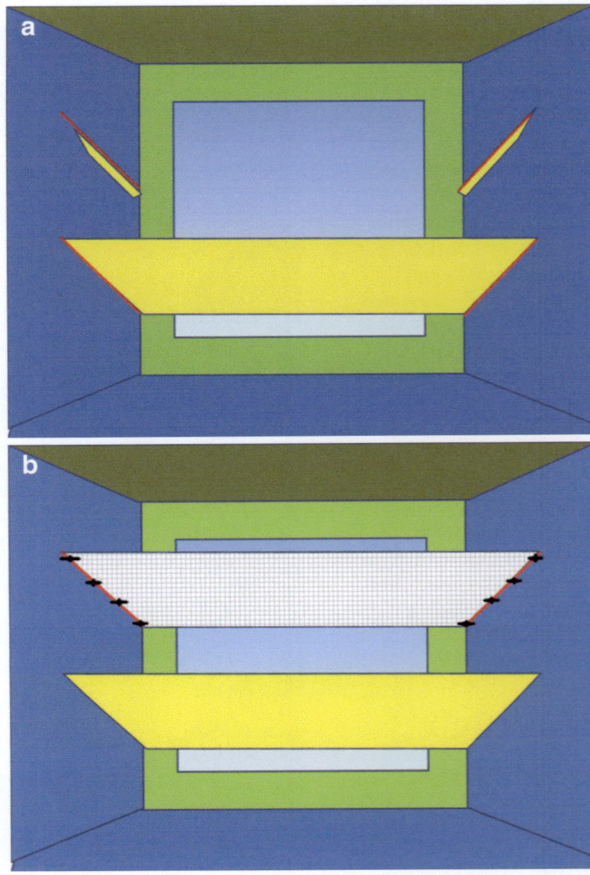

Fig. 7.23 (**a**) Pelvic floor room analogy: absence or severe deficiency of the pubocervical fibromuscularis can result in a cystocele. (**b**) Pelvic floor room analogy: the ideal scenario for synthetic mesh placement when there is total lack of the pubocervical fascia. Anterior mesh replaces the fascia and is sutured to intact lateral walls (arcus tendinous) as shown in red line. (© Shobeiri 2013)

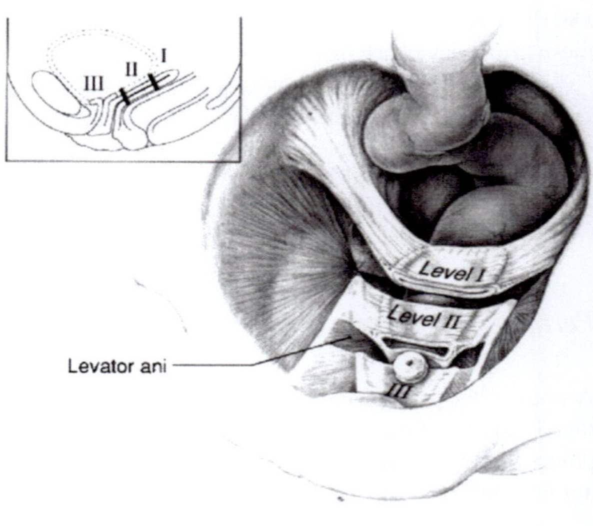

Fig. 7.24 Three levels of support. (From DeLancey [16], with permission Elsevier)

However, this layer is not a single muscle layer with a double layer of fascia ("diaphragm"), but rather a set of connective tissues that surround the urethra; the term perineal membrane has been used more recently to reflect its true nature [24]. The perineal membrane is a single connective tissue membrane, with muscle lying immediately above. The perineal membrane lies at the level of the hymen and attaches the urethra, vagina, and perineal body to the ischiopubic rami.

Posterior Compartment and Perineal Membrane

The use of mesh for the repair of rectoceles has been discredited. As such in this section, we describe the thought process on how the use of mesh may have been plausible from an anatomic perspective.

The posterior compartment is bound to perineal body and the perineal membrane caudad (Level III), paracolpium and the uterosacral ligaments cephalad (Level I), and the posterior arcus connected to the levator ani laterally (Level II). As in the anterior compartment, a simple defect in rectovaginal fibromuscularis (Fig. 7.25) can cause a distention rectocele. This type of disorder (similar to the anterior

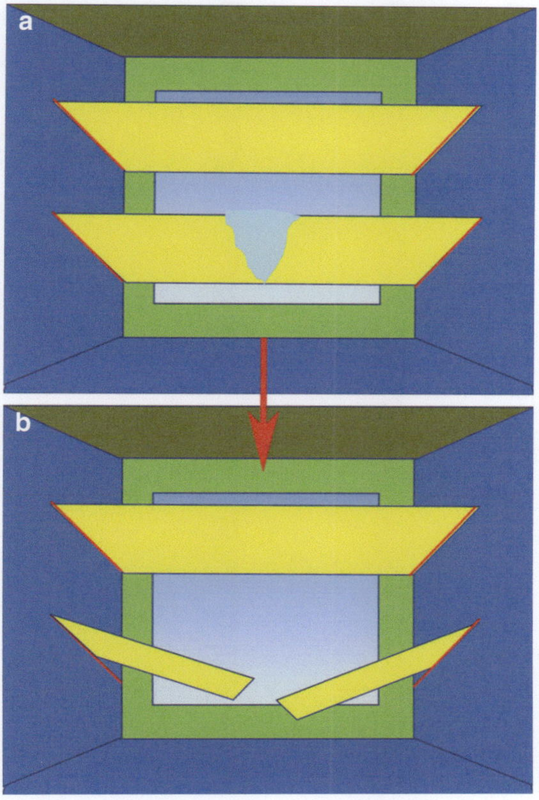

Fig. 7.25 Pelvic floor room analogy: (**a**) an occult rectovaginal defect can result in an overt rectocele (**b**). (© Shobeiri 2013)

distention cystocele) requires a plication and stitching of the rectovaginal fascia, with no need of the use of posterior mesh. A defect in the posterior arcus also called arcus tendineus rectovaginalis (ATRV) is associated with a pararectal defect that can be unilateral (Fig. 7.26) or bilateral (Fig. 7.27). This defect requires a pararectal repair rather than plication of the rectovaginal fascia which might worsen the rectocele stage. Furthermore, in this scenario, the use of posterior mesh is not

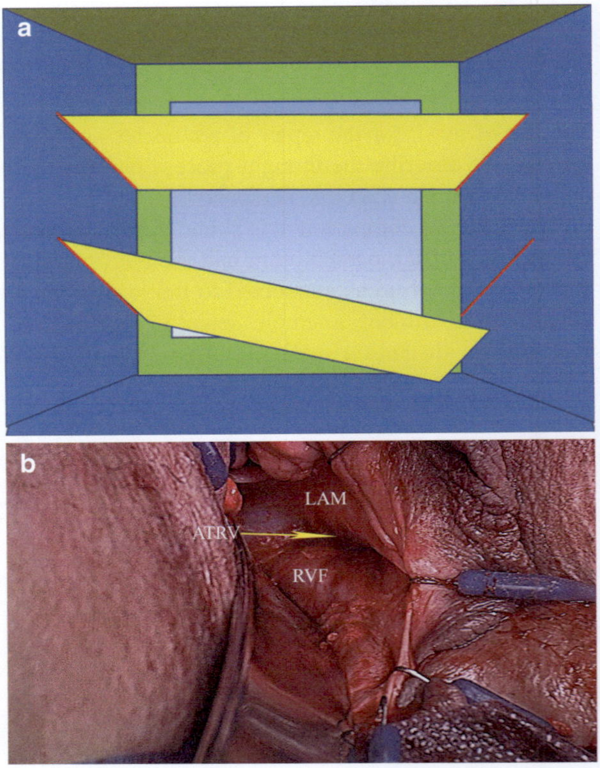

Fig. 7.26 (**a**) Pelvic floor room analogy: right lateral detachment of the rectovaginal septum can result in a rectocele. (**b**) The surgical view of the posterior compartment showing the relationship between the levator ani muscle (LAM), the rectovaginal fibromuscularis (RVF), and the arcus tendineus fasciae rectovaginalis (ATRV). (© Shobeiri 2013)

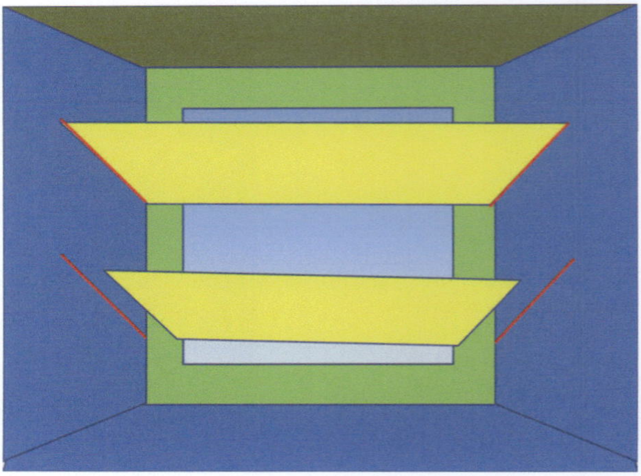

Fig. 7.27 Pelvic floor room analogy: bilateral detachment of the rectovaginal septum can result in a rectocele. (© Shobeiri 2013)

recommended, and since there is no intact lateral wall for the attachment of mesh or for the anchoring of the posterior kits, placing mesh will result in complications as contraction of mesh, pain or erosion. Such defects need to be differentiated from total loss of rectovaginal fibromuscularis (Fig. 7.28a), which was perceived as the ideal scenario in which one should perform an augmentation of the posterior

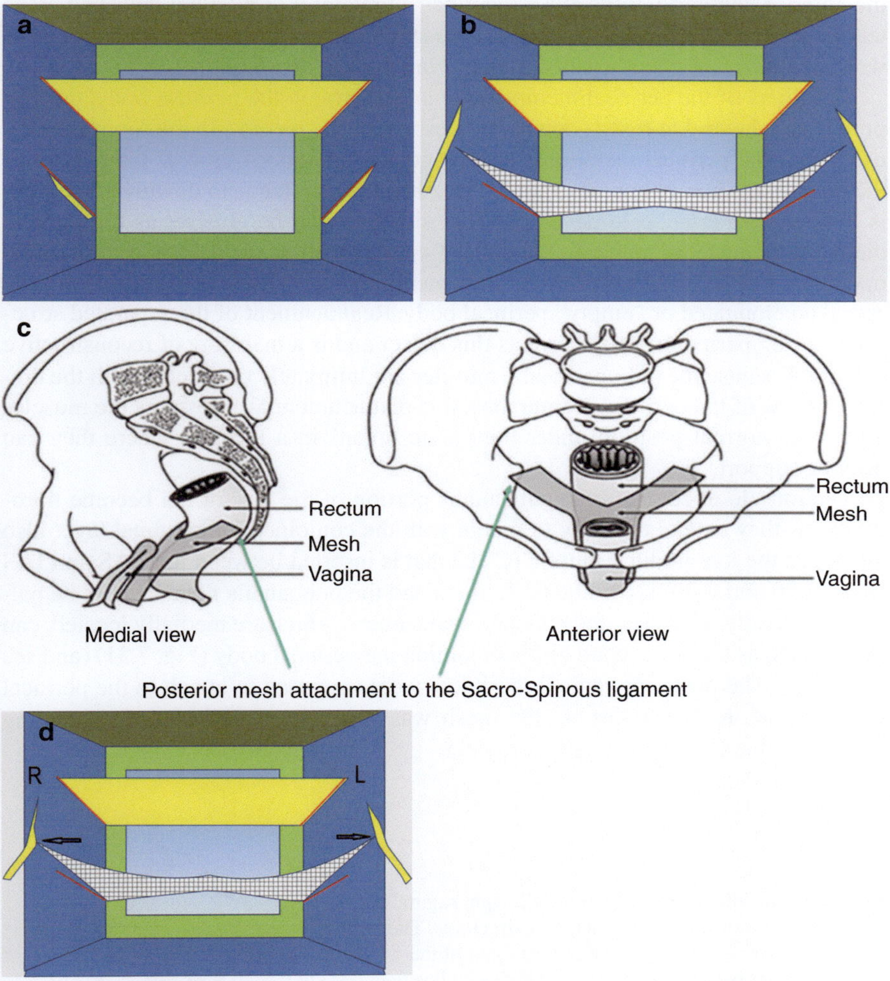

Fig. 7.28 (**a**) Pelvic floor room analogy: absence or severe deficiency of rectovaginal fascia can result in a rectocele. (**b**) Pelvic floor room analogy: This room analogy illustrates a loss of rectovaginal fibromuscularis, which was perceived as the ideal scenario for performing an augmentation of the posterior compartment with mesh. The yellow lines denote the sacrospinous ligaments as the apical attachment point of mesh kit anchors. (**c**) The posterior mesh replaces the rectovaginal fascia. (From Dwyer and O'Reilly [25], with permission John Wiley). (**d**) Pelvic floor room analogy: Bilateral defect of posterior tendinous compartments, a pararectal defect (rectovaginal fascia detachment or levator ani muscle injury), is illustrated in both left and right sides. The first step in this case should be repairing of this detachment by re-approximation of the detached tissues in both sides. Mesh usage without appropriate bilateral repair will lead to contraction of mesh due to the lack of anchoring points. (© Shobeiri 2013)

compartment with autologous, cadaveric tissue, or use posterior mesh/vaginal mesh kits. The posterior compartment mesh kits are mostly designed to be anchored to the sacrospinous ligaments cephalad and go through the perineal membrane and muscles distally (Fig. 7.28b,c) [25]. Most often, the separation of the posterior arcus may be apical and may require reattachment of the posterior arcus to the uterosacral ligament or the iliococcygeal muscle prior to placing posterior mesh. Analogous to the anterior compartment, if the patient has a unilateral or bilateral detached arcus tendinous or doesn't have a levator ani muscle on one or both sides, the mesh arms will not have attachment's walls or anchoring points (Fig. 7.28d).

The fibers of the perineal membrane connect through the perineal body, thereby providing a layer that resists downward descent of the rectum. In the room analogy used here, the perineal membrane is analogous to the door frame. If the bottom of the door frame is missing (see Fig. 7.28a), then the resistance to downward descent is lost, and a perineocele develops. This situation can be elusive, as the clinical diagnosis is made by realizing the patient's need to splint very close to the vaginal opening in order to have a bowel movement, and the physical examination may reveal an elongated or "empty" perineal body. Reattachment of the separated structures during perineorrhaphy corrects this defect and is a mainstay of reconstructive surgery. Because the puboperinealis muscles are intimately connected with the cranial surface of the perineal membranes, this reattachment also restores the muscles to a more normal position under the pelvic organs in a location where they can provide support.

The muscle fibers from the puboanalis portion of the levator ani become fibroelastic as they extend caudally to merge with the conjoined longitudinal layer also known as the longitudinal muscle (CLL) that is inserted between the EAS and IAS (Figs. 7.29 and 7.30) [26]. The CLL fibers and the puboanalis fibers cannot be palpated clinically. However, the puboperinealis fibers, which are medially located, can be palpated as a distinct band of fibers joining the perineal body (Fig. 7.31) (and see Fig. 7.29). The posterior vaginal mesh kits were supposed to attach to the perineal body, but as the mesh shrunk, the mesh was generally pulled cephalad creating either a perineal defect or a low rectocele.

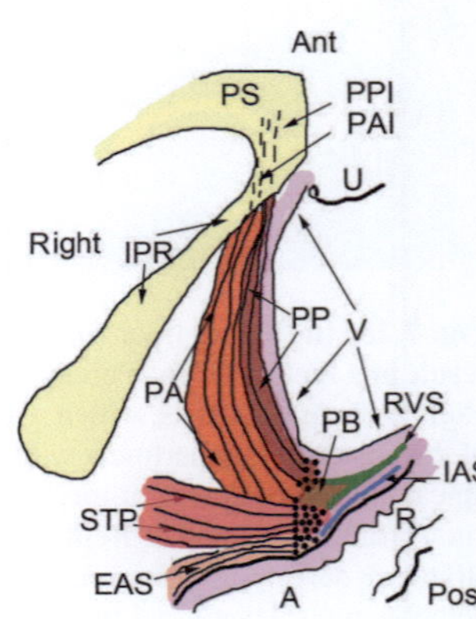

Fig. 7.29 This drawing demonstrates the right sagittal hemipelvis view of the perineal support structures. The perineum, a small seemingly insignificant part of the female body, is packed with muscles and fascial layers that interconnect in an intricate manner. External anal sphincter (EAS), internal anal sphincter (IAS), ischiopubic rami (IPR), puboanalis (PA), puboanalis insertion (PAI), perineal body (PB), puboperinealis (PP), puboperineal insertion (PPI), pubic symphysis (PS), rectum (R), rectovaginal septum, (RVS), superficial transverse perinei (STP), urethra (U), vagina (V). (© Shobeiri 2013)

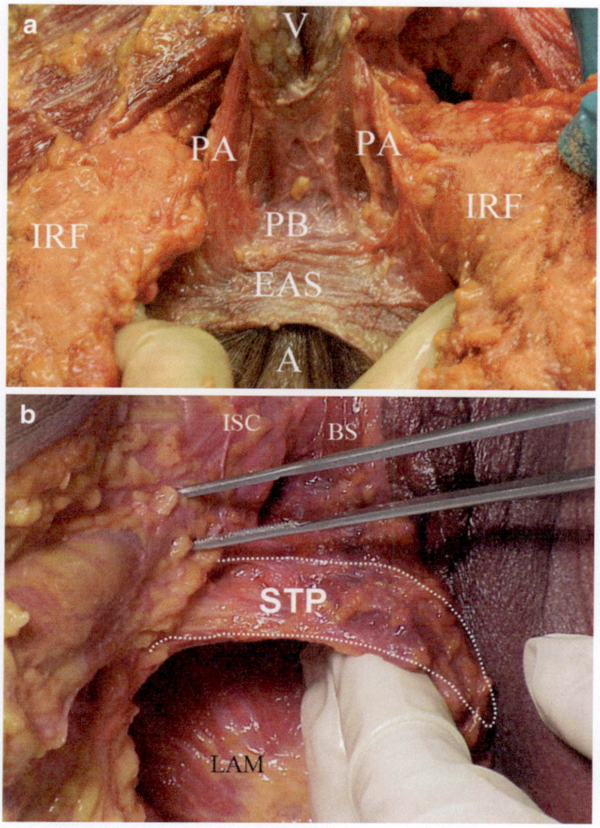

Fig. 7.30 (**a**) Perineal dissection in a fresh frozen pelvis shows the relationship of the external anal sphincter (EAS) to the perineal body (PB) and the puboanalis/puboperinealis complex. Ischiorectal fat (IRF). (**b**) Perineal dissection in a fresh frozen pelvis shows the relationship of the superficial transverse perinei (STP) to the other puboanalis fibers that start inserting at the perineal level at Fig 7.30a and then wrap around the anal canal (LAM). The ischiocavernosus (ISC) and the bulbospongiosus muscle (BS) are depicted here. (© Shobeiri 2013)

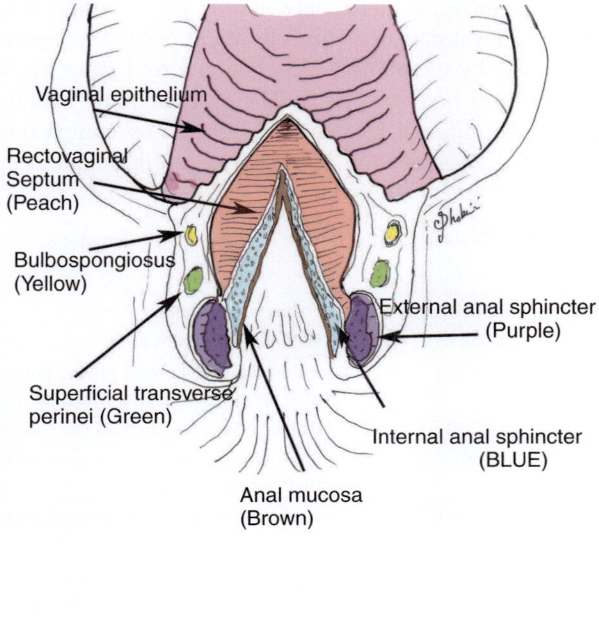

Fig. 7.31 Drawing of perineal region as may be seen after a clean midline episiotomy. The drawing depicts the relationship of muscles to the rectovaginal septum. (© Shobeiri 2013)

Lateral Compartment and the Levator Ani Muscles

It is generally accepted that the levator ani muscles and the associated fascial layer surround pelvic organs like a funnel to form the pelvic diaphragm [27]. Given that we employ concepts such as pelvic floor spasm, levator spasm, and pelvic floor weakness, understanding the basic concepts of pelvic floor musculature is essential to formulate a clinical opinion. The area posterior to the pubic bone is dense with bands of intertwined levator ani muscles; this defies conventional description of the levator ani as comprising the puborectalis, pubococcygeus, and iliococcygeus. The anatomy of distal subdivisions of the levator ani muscle was further described in a study by Kearney et al. [28]. The origins and insertions of these muscles as well as their characteristic anatomical relations are shown in Table 7.1 and Fig. 7.16. Using a nomenclature based on the attachment points, the lesser known subdivisions of the levator ani muscles, the muscles posterior to the pubic bone are identified as pubovaginalis, puboanalis, and puboperinealis. The pubovaginalis is poorly described but may be analogous to the urethrovaginal ligaments. The puboanalis originates from behind the pubic bone as a thin band and inserts around the anus into the longitudinal ligaments. The puboperinealis, which is most often 0.5 cm in diameter, originates from the pubic bone and inserts into the perineal body. The four major components of the levator ani muscle are the iliococcygeus, which forms a thin, relatively flat, horizontal shelf that spans the potential gap from one pelvic sidewall to the other; the pubococcygeus muscle, which travels from the tip of the coccyx to the pubic bone (see Fig. 7.17); the puborectalis muscle, originating from the anterior portion of the perineal membrane and the pubic bone to form a sling behind the rectum; and the puboperinealis and puboanalis, which are thin broad fibromuscular poorly described structures that attach to the perineal body and anus to stabilize the perineal region.

The shortest distance between the pubic symphysis and the levator plate is the minimal levator hiatus. This is different from the urogenital hiatus, which is bounded anteriorly by the pubic bones, laterally by levator ani muscles, and posteriorly by the perineal body and EAS. The baseline tonic activity of the levator ani muscle keeps the minimal levator hiatus closed by compressing the urethra, vagina, and rectum against the pubic bone as they exit through this opening [29]. The levator ani

Table 7.1 Divisions of the levator ani muscles – international standardized terminology

Levator ani muscles	Origin/insertion
Puboperinealis (PP)	Pubis/perineal body
Pubovaginalis (PV)	Pubis/vaginal wall at the level of the mid-urethra
Puboanalis (PA)	Pubis/intersphincteric groove between internal and external anal sphincter to end in the anal skin
Puborectalis (PR)	Pubis/forms sling behind the rectum
Iliococcygeus (IC)	Tendinous arch of the levator ani/the two sides fuse in the iliococcygeal raphe
Pubococcygeus (PC)	Pubic symphysis to superficial part of anococcygeal ligament

fibers converge behind the rectum to form the levator plate. With contraction, the levator plate elevates to form a horizontal shelf over which pelvic organs rest. The deficiency of any portion of the levator ani results in weakening of the levator plate and descensus of pelvic organs [30].

Endopelvic Fascia and Levator Ani Interactions

We mention the levator ani muscle here because although the vaginal mesh kits were designed to replace and support deficient anterior or posterior fascia, they did not take into consideration the levator ani muscle function. The levator ani muscles and the endopelvic fascia work as a unit to provide pelvic organ support. If the muscles maintain normal tone, the ligaments of the endopelvic fascia will have little tension on them even with increases in abdominal pressure (Fig. 7.32). If the muscles are damaged by a tear or complete separation from their attachments, the pelvic floor sags downward over time and the organs are pushed through the urogenital hiatus (Fig. 7.33). In such cases the ligaments and the endopelvic fascia will assume the majority of the pelvic floor load until they fail as well. Different varieties of levator ani injury can cause different interesting types of clinical defects. A partial defect and separation of the pubococcygeus muscles will result in a displacement cystocele (Fig. 7.34). However, the clinician may not be able to distinguish if this is a displacement cystocele due to paravaginal defect and arcus tendineus separation or due to muscle loss. The consequences of this lack of recognition can be that the surgeon may elect to do an anterior repair and, by placating the pubocervical

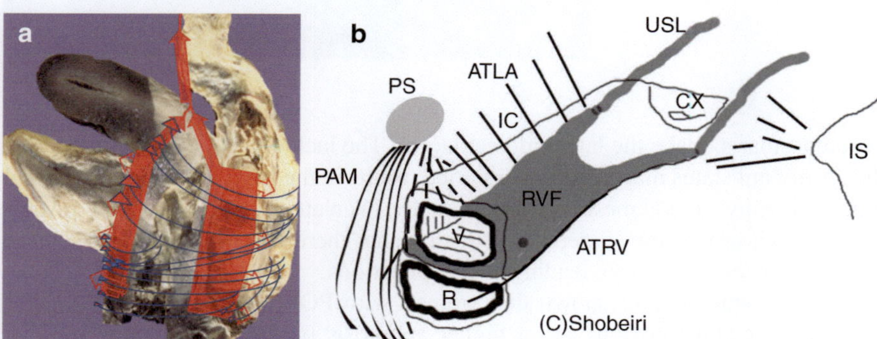

Fig. 7.32 (**a**) Right lateral standing anatomic depiction of the levator ani muscle and uterosacral-cardinal complex interaction. (**b**) Drawing of the interaction between the rectovaginal fibromuscularis and the uterosacral ligaments. The levator ani muscle and uterosacral-cardinal complex give cephalad static support, while the iliococcygeal fibers give lateral support to the posterior compartment. The puboanalis and the puboperinealis muscles stabilize the perineum while the puborectalis closes the levator hiatus. Arcus tendineus levator ani (ATLA), arcus tendineus fascia rectovaginalis (ATRV), cervix (CX), iliococcygeus (IC), ischial spine (IS), pubic symphysis (PS), rectum (R), rectovaginal fibromuscularis (RVF), uterosacral ligament (USL), vagina (V). (© Shobeiri 2013)

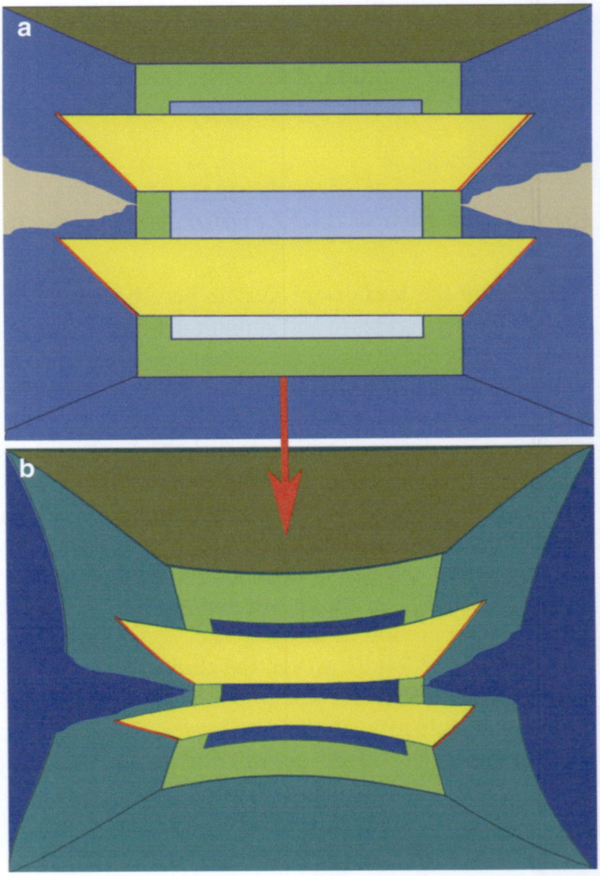

Fig. 7.33 Pelvic floor room analogy: bilateral levator ani tears may or may not result in prolapse or incontinence initially, but over time the other supportive structures will decompensate resulting in pelvic floor laxity. (© Shobeiri 2013)

fibromuscularis, make the lateral defect worse. The lack of basic information about the levator ani status may account for varied results in the anterior repair studies and failure of many vaginal mesh kits. Additionally, in an attempted paravaginal or vaginal mesh kit repair, the surgeon may realize that there is no muscle to attach the arcus tendineus or mesh to, leading to complications.

Previous studies have shown that women with POP have a decreased muscle fiber number and function, and a higher apoptosis pace, and disorganization of smooth muscular fibers. Implanting a mesh into unhealthy muscular tissue may result in a maladaptive remodeling response, which increases the risk for mesh complications, including mesh erosion, extrusion, or contraction. The same is true in implanting anterior vaginal mesh in an individual with unilateral or bilateral levator tear/avulsion (Fig. 7.35) [8, 31, 32].

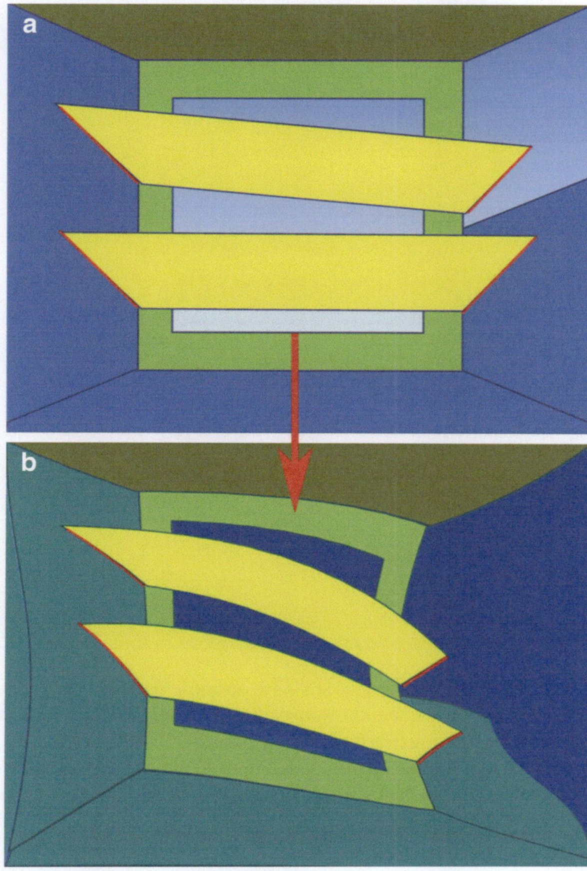

Fig. 7.34 Pelvic floor room analogy: (**a**) unilateral levator ani tears may or may not result in prolapse or incontinence initially, but over time the other supportive structures will decompensate resulting in pelvic floor laxity (**b**). (© Shobeiri 2013)

A partial defect (see Fig. 7.34a) is subjected to excessive forces and may progress over time to involve the apical and posterior compartments as well (see Fig. 7.34b). How fast this occurs depends on the strength of the patient's connective tissue. One woman with injured muscles may have strong connective tissue that compensates and never develops prolapse, while another woman with even less muscle injury but weaker connective tissue may develop prolapse with aging. There are instances of catastrophic injury during childbirth during which complete muscle loss occurs and the patient presents with a displacement cystocele, rectocele, and varied types of incontinence (Fig. 7.35). This scenario is different with patients who have a defect in pubocervical and rectovaginal fibromuscularis (Fig. 7.36), which develops into a distention cystocele and rectocele over time. A cystocele and rectocele repair that can be used for the latter case will worsen the condition of the first patient with levator damage.

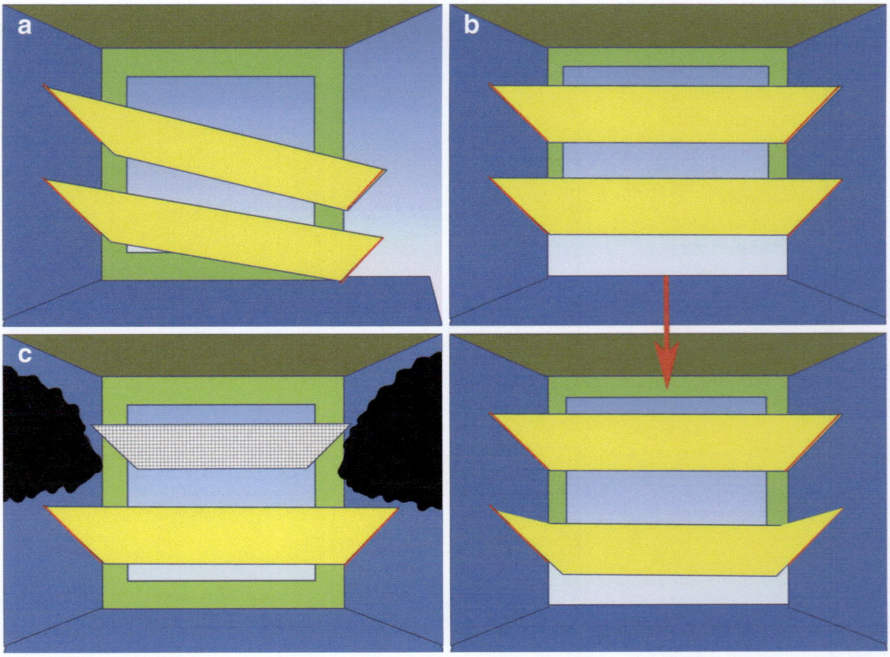

Fig. 7.35 Pelvic floor room analogy: obstetric injuries can be catastrophic or subtle. To the left is a complete right unilateral levator ani detachment (avulsion). To the right is injury to the perineal support (the missing green part of the door frame) (**a**), which may result in sliding of the rectovaginal fascia and a clinical perineocele (**b**). **(c)** Pelvic floor room analogy: anterior mesh displacement /contraction due to the lack of adequate levator ani muscle attachment points. (© Shobeiri 2013)

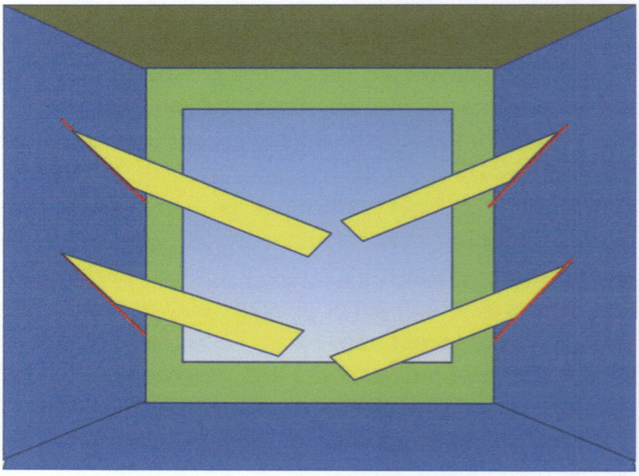

Fig. 7.36 Pelvic floor room analogy: multicompartmental defect – pubocervical fibromuscularis and rectovaginal septum defects. (© Shobeiri 2013)

The Pudendal Nerve

The pudendal nerve is mentioned here because the injury to this nerve caused much irreversible misery for the patients. It supplies the urethral and anal sphincters and the perineal muscles. The pudendal nerve originates from S2 to S4 foramina and runs through the Alcock canal, which is caudal to the levator ani muscles. The pudendal nerve has three branches: the clitoral, perineal, and inferior hemorrhoidal, which innervate the clitoris, the perineal musculature, inner perineal skin, and the EAS, respectively [26]. The blockade of the pudendal nerve decreases resting and squeeze pressures in the vagina and rectum, increases the length of the urogenital hiatus, and decreases electromyography activity of the puborectalis muscle [33]. The pudendal nerve injury due to vaginal mesh kit trocar placement close to or through this nerve is discussed elsewhere, but it is one of the important design flaws of the vaginal mesh kits that resulted in life altering and debilitating pain in many women.

Summary

The knowledge of pelvic floor anatomy, function, and biomechanics is essential for understanding of pelvic floor pathologies and reaching the precise diagnosis and treatment. Moreover, biomechanics studies help to understand part of mesh complications and failures in terms of POP. Models can be used to simulate pelvic floor dysfunction, vaginal childbirth, vaginal meshes, and novel devices for POP treatment and hold significant potential for patient specific diagnostics and surgical planning. The pelvic floor in many ways is a functional unit like the human mouth. Some vaginal mesh kits inhibited vaginal movement and distention because of their stiffness; others inhibited function because their points of attachments were either too firm or too unstable. A good augmentative product takes into account human factors and mechanical properties of pelvic structures and the functionality required for the vaginal tissue.

References

1. NIH state-of-the science conference statement on prevention of fecal and urinary incontinence in adults. NIH Consens State Sci Statements. 2007;24(1):1–37.
2. Nygaard I, Barber MD, Burgio KL, Kenton K, Meikle S, Schaffer J, et al. Prevalence of symptomatic pelvic floor disorders in US women. JAMA. 2008;300(11):1311–6.
3. Olsen AL, Smith VJ, Bergstrom JO, Colling JC, Clark AL. Epidemiology of surgically managed pelvic organ prolapse and urinary incontinence. Obstet Gynecol. 1997;89(4):501–6.

4. Boyles SH, Weber AM, Meyn L. Procedures for pelvic organ prolapse in the United States, 1979–1997. Am J Obstet Gynecol. 2003;188(1):108–15.
5. Smith FJ, Holman CD, Moorin RE, Tsokos N. Lifetime risk of undergoing surgery for pelvic organ prolapse. Obstet Gynecol. 2010;116(5):1096–100.
6. Aigmueller T, Dungl A, Hinterholzer S, Geiss I, Riss P. An estimation of the frequency of surgery for posthysterectomy vault prolapse. Int Urogynecol J. 2010;21(3):299–302.
7. Quiroz LH, Munoz A, Shippey SH, Gutman RE, Handa VL. Vaginal parity and pelvic organ prolapse. J Reprod Med. 2010;55(3–4):93–8.
8. Boreham MK, Wai CY, Miller RT, Schaffer JI, Word RA. Morphometric analysis of smooth muscle in the anterior vaginal wall of women with pelvic organ prolapse. Am J Obstet Gynecol. 2002;187(1):56–63.
9. Morgan DM, Rogers MA, Huebner M, Wei JT, Delancey JO. Heterogeneity in anatomic outcome of sacrospinous ligament fixation for prolapse: a systematic review. Obstet Gynecol. 2007;109(6):1424–33.
10. Jakus SM, Shapiro A, Hall CD. Biologic and synthetic graft use in pelvic surgery: a review. Obstet Gynecol Surv. 2008;63(4):253–66.
11. Burger JW, Luijendijk RW, Hop WC, Halm JA, Verdaasdonk EG, Jeekel J. Long-term follow-up of a randomized controlled trial of suture versus mesh repair of incisional hernia. Ann Surg. 2004;240(4):578–83. discussion 583-5
12. Luijendijk RW, Hop WC, van den Tol MP, de Lange DC, Braaksma MM, Ijzermans JN, et al. A comparison of suture repair with mesh repair for incisional hernia. N Engl J Med. 2000;343(6):392–8.
13. Ricci JV, Thom CH. The myth of a surgically useful fascia in vaginal plastic reconstructions. Q Rev Surg Obstet Gynecol. 1954;11(4):253–61.
14. Gitsch E, Palmrich AH. Operative anatomie. Berlin: De Gruyter; 1977.
15. Albright T, Gehrich A, Davis G, Sabi F, Buller J. Arcus tendineus fascia pelvis: a further understanding. Am J Obstet Gynecol. 2005;193(3):677–81.
16. DeLancey JO. Anatomic aspects of vaginal eversion after hysterectomy. Am J Obstet Gynecol. 1992;166(6 Pt 1):1717–24. discussion 1724-8
17. Shobeiri SA, Leclaire E, Nihira MA, Quiroz LH, O'Donoghue D. Appearance of the levator ani muscle subdivisions in endovaginal three-dimensional ultrasonography. Obstet Gynecol. 2009;114(1):66–72.
18. Campbell RM. The anatomy and histology of the sacrouterine ligaments. Am J Obstet Gynecol. 1950;59(1):1–12.
19. Range RL, Woodburne RT. The gross and microscopic anatomy of the transverse cervical ligaments. Am J Obstet Gynecol. 1964;90:460–7.
20. Richardson AC, Edmonds PB, Williams NL. Treatment of stress urinary incontinence due to paravaginal fascial defect. Obstet Gynecol. 1981;57(3):357–62.
21. DeLancey J. Fascial and muscular abnormalities in women with urethral hypermobility and anterior vaginal wall prolapse. Am J Obstet Gynecol. 2002;187(1):93–8.
22. Chesson RR, Schlossberg SM, Elkins TE, Menefee S, McCammon K, Franco N, et al. The use of fascia lata graft for correction of severe or recurrent anterior vaginal wall defects. J Pelvic Surg. 1999;5(2):96–103.
23. Bump RC, Mattiasson A, Bo K, Brubaker LP, DeLancey JO, Klarskov P, et al. The standardization of terminology of female pelvic organ prolapse and pelvic floor dysfunction. Am J Obstet Gynecol. 1996;175(1):10–7.
24. Oelrich T. The striated urogenital sphincter muscle in the female. Anat Rec. 1983; 205(2):223–32.
25. Dwyer PL, O'Reilly BA. Transvaginal repair of anterior and posterior compartment prolapse with Atrium polypropylene mesh. Br J Obstet Gynaecol. 2004;111(8):831–6.
26. Shobeiri SA, Chesson RR, Gasser RF. The internal innervation and morphology of the human female levator ani muscle. Am J Obstet Gynecol. 2008;199(6):686.e1–6.
27. Lawson JO. Pelvic anatomy. I. Pelvic floor muscles. Ann R Coll Surg Engl. 1974;54(5):244–52.

28. Kearney R, Sawhney R, DeLancey JOL. Levator ani muscle anatomy evaluated by origin-insertion pairs. Obstet Gynecol. 2004;104(1):168–73.
29. Taverner D, Smiddy FG. An electromyographic study of the normal function of the external anal sphincter and pelvic diaphragm. Dis Colon Rectum. 1959;2(2):153–60.
30. Nichols DH, Milley PS, Randall CL. Significance of restoration of normal vaginal depth and axis. Obstet Gynecol. 1970;36(2):251–6.
31. Boreham MK, Wai CY, Miller RT, Schaffer JI, Word RA. Morphometric properties of the posterior vaginal wall in women with pelvic organ prolapse. Am J Obstet Gynecol. 2002;187(6):1501–8; discussion 1508–9.
32. Takac P, Gualtieri M, Nassiri M, Candiotti K, Medina CA. Vaginal smooth muscle cell apoptosis is increased in women with pelvic organ prolapse. Int Urogynecol J Pelvic Floor Dysfunct. 2008;19(11):1559–64.
33. Guaderrama NM, Liu J, Nager CW, Pretorius DH, Sheean G, Kassab G, et al. Evidence for the innervation of pelvic floor muscles by the pudendal nerve. Obstet Gynecol. 2005;106(4):774–81.

Chapter 8
Basic Science of Vaginal Mesh

Katrina Knight, Pamela Moalli, and Rui Liang

Introduction

Following the success of the tension-free vaginal tape (TVT) to repair stress urinary incontinence (SUI) in the 1990s, transvaginal meshes were introduced into the market in the form of kits. These kits were marketed as having shorter operating times and were associated with a procedure that is technically easier to learn than sacrocolpopexy. By 2005, kits were increasingly adopted into prolapse surgery such that by 2010 over 70% of meshes inserted were via the transvaginal approach [1]. As the number of transvaginal mesh implantations increased, so did the awareness of complications associated with polypropylene mesh, prompting the US Food and Drug Administration (FDA) to issue two public health notifications (PHNs) and upregulating prolapse mesh from a Class II to Class III device. These regulatory measures (Section 522 of the Federal Food, Drug, and Cosmetic Act) mandated small clinical postmarket surveillance trials as the FDA continued to assess the safety and effectiveness of prolapse meshes in the market place. Simultaneously, research into the mechanisms of mesh complications accelerated in the direction of elucidating the

K. Knight (✉)
Department of Medicine, School of Medicine, University of Pittsburgh, Pittsburgh, PA, USA
e-mail: kmk144@pitt.edu

P. Moalli
Division of Urogynecology and Pelvic Reconstructive Surgery, Department of Obstetrics, Gynecology and Reproductive Sciences, Magee-Womens Hospital of UPMC, Magee-Womens Research Institute, University of Pittsburgh, Pittsburgh, PA, USA

R. Liang
Department of Obstetrics, Gynecology and Reproductive Sciences, University of Pittsburgh, Pittsburgh, PA, USA

S. A. Shobeiri (ed.), *The Innovation and Evolution of Medical Devices*,
https://doi.org/10.1007/978-3-319-97073-8_8

role of mesh properties and behaviors in the host response and surgical outcomes. The purpose of this chapter is to focus on those *ex vivo* and *in vivo* studies that have shed light on our understanding of mesh mechanics and the host response to mesh. However, given that most current urogynecologic meshes are simply hernia meshes, this chapter will first discuss the biological and mechanical differences between the female pelvis and abdomen and how these differences induce disparate host responses. Next, the impact of mesh textile properties and mesh mechanics on the host response will be explored. This will be followed by a summary of the results from animal and human studies that have aided our understanding of how the body responds to synthetic meshes *in vivo* and how researchers have been able to modulate this response. Finally, this chapter will conclude by discussing the future outlook of basic science research for urogynecologic mesh.

Unique Environments in the Pelvic Floor for Mesh Implantation

To date, most urogynecologic meshes are simply hernia meshes remarketed for the indication of prolapse repair. Consequently, there is not much difference between urogynecologic and hernia meshes in regard to design and construction. However, the biological and mechanical environments in which these meshes are implanted are drastically different. Thus, in the next few sections, the aspects of the biological and mechanical environments within the pelvic floor that distinguish mesh implantation in the pelvis vs. the abdomen will be discussed. Additionally, studies comparing the host response to mesh implanted into the pelvis vs. the abdomen will also be explored.

Biological Environment

Unlike hernia repair meshes, which are positioned in direct contact with the abdominal fascia (consisting of dense connective tissue), vaginal mesh is placed in an environment with heterogeneous soft tissues, consisting of smooth and striated muscle, loose and dense connective tissue, and specialized organs (e.g., the vagina, uterus, rectum, bladder). Additionally, the vagina is metabolically more active than the abdominal fascia, dramatically changing in response to hormone-driven events such as pregnancy, menstrual cycles, and menopause [2, 3]. In women with pelvic organ prolapse (POP), the vagina has been shown to have less compact smooth muscle bundles and altered matrix turnover with higher levels of collagenases and elastases [4–6]. The vagina is also distinct from the abdominal wall in that it is heavily colonized with bacteria and is considered a clean-contaminated surgical field. With these differences, it is not surprising that the host responses to urogynecologic meshes, and consequently the outcome of mesh implantation, are different from the responses to hernia meshes.

Mechanical Environment

The vagina plays a central role in providing support to the pelvic organs. The vagina supports the urethra and bladder anteriorly, the uterus apically, and the rectum posteriorly. Directly supporting the vagina, and indirectly supporting the pelvic organs, is a sophisticated network of striated muscles and connectives tissues. For conceptual purposes, the latter is divided into three levels [7–9]. Apical support to the vagina is provided by the cardinal and uterosacral ligaments (referred to as Level I support), and support to the mid-vagina is provided by the paravaginal attachments, which function to attach the vagina to the pelvic sidewall via the anterior and posterior endopelvic fascia (Level II support). The distal vagina is supported by the perineal body and perineal membrane (Level III support). Striated muscle support, provided by the levator ani (iliococcygeus, pubococcygeus, and pubovisceral muscles), also provides support to the distal vagina and functions to close the hole at the bottom of the bony pelvis [7, 8, 10]. POP is generally understood to occur when there is a loss of support via damage to or abnormalities in the vagina and/or its supportive muscles and connective tissues.

Surgeries to repair prolapse typically involve restoring connective tissue support to the vagina, most commonly at the apex. Since native tissue repairs have high failure rates (40% at 2 years) [11], surgeons have turned to biomaterials, most commonly polypropylene mesh. Mesh can be implanted transabdominally via sacrocolpopexy. By this procedure, two strips of mesh or the arms of a preconfigured Y mesh are placed between the bladder and the vagina and the rectum and the vagina. The two arms (or stem of the Y) are then brought up to the sacrum to restore apical support by attaching the vagina to the sacrum via a mesh bridge. Alternatively, mesh can be implanted transvaginally by which the mesh body is placed in the anterior or posterior compartment, and mesh arms are pulled through the sacrospinous ligaments to restore Level I support bilaterally. For some products, additional arms can be pulled through the arcus tendineous fascia pelvis to restore Level II support. Following both transabdominal and transvaginal insertions, the predominant loading directions are unidirectional or uniaxial. This is in contrast to hernia mesh in which mesh is loaded more uniformly (circumferentially) along the edges of the mesh. These loading configurations ultimately impact the geometry of the mesh pore.

Vaginal Versus Abdominal Host Response to Mesh

Although the abdomen and pelvis are biologically and mechanically distinct in terms of implantation environments, studies involving the implantation of mesh into the abdomen are certainly necessary to validate mesh designs and to test the biocompatibility of mesh at early stages. Given their distinct environments, it is not surprising that the host response to mesh in these two regions differs. Utilizing a rabbit model, Pierce et al. reported that the rate of mesh exposures through the vaginal epithelium as well as the rate of inflammation is higher in the vagina relative to the abdomen [12].

Additionally, Pierce et al. showed that chemically cross-linked porcine dermal mesh degrades faster in the vagina as compared to the abdomen, supporting the finding that the vagina is more biologically active than the abdomen. Moreover, the mechanical behavior of mesh is very different at these two sites, leading to an increased likelihood of mesh contraction or "shrinkage" when implanted in the vagina vs. the abdomen, even though the mesh in both cases may be initially implanted in a flat configuration [13, 14]. Thus, meshes are better suited for the abdomen, and future studies assessing the host response to meshes must consider differences in the host response at these two sites when choosing a model to investigate novel products.

Mesh Textile Properties and Impact on Host Response

Filament Type

The filament structure of mesh can be classified as either mono- or multifilament and has been linked to the host response, specifically in relation to the presence of infection. Particularly, meshes with multifilament fibers, braided or interwoven, are associated with higher bacterial colonization [15]. This finding is believed to be a result of the increased surface area of multifilament fibers, which has been shown to be by a factor of at least 1.57 higher when compared with monofilament fibers [16]. The larger surface is thought to provide more space for bacterial adhesion and increased area for bacterial proliferation. Further, multifilament fibers are thought to have spaces within the fibers themselves, which are less than 10 μm in diameter, allowing for the passage of bacteria, but not macrophages or neutrophils, thus providing a harbor for bacterial proliferation [17]. Consequently, the multifilament design has been avoided for urogynecologic mesh products in the present market.

Knit Pattern

While individual fibers, whether monofilament or multifilament, provide the basic structural element of synthetic mesh implants, the behavior of the entire mesh is governed by the method by which the mesh is constructed, referred to as the knit pattern. Two of the most common knit patterns used to create a mesh are knitting and weaving. Woven meshes are constructed using a simple interlacing technique, with two sets of threads (fibers) running perpendicular to one another. Conversely, knitted meshes are constructed by successive looping of a single fiber in styles of warp-lock, interlock, and circular knit. Comparing the two knit patterns, woven meshes have superior mechanical strength and shape memory relative to knitted meshes. However, woven meshes are usually susceptible to fraying when cut and conform poorly to underlying structures such as the vagina [18]. This is not the case for knitted meshes, which have increased flexibility and high conformity to underlying structures. Additionally, knitted meshes are more porous than woven meshes; thus, the risk of infection is reduced with the larger pore sizes of knitted meshes [19–21]. Therefore knitted meshes are generally preferred relative to woven meshes.

Pore Size and Porosity

Arguably, pore size and porosity are the two most important textile properties that impact both the short- and long-term host immune response to mesh. Overall, the impact of pore size has been well characterized in the abdominal hernia literature. Specifically for polypropylene mesh, large pores are shown to improve tissue ingrowth and the mechanical integrity of the resulting mesh-tissue complex, to increase vascular penetration, and to decrease the risk of bacterial colonization compared to small pores [22]. Additionally, large pore meshes with high porosity yield less inflammation, less fibrous tissue, and decreased potential for adhesion formation relative to meshes with small pores and lower porosity [23–27]. Further, pores with dimensions less than 10 μm provide beds for bacterial proliferation and persistent infection, as macrophages and neutrophils are unable to penetrate these tiny pores [28]. In addition, studies report that the surface of each fiber becomes encased by a granulomatous inflammatory reaction as part of the foreign body response [29–31]. When pore sizes are small or there is a reduction in pore size as a result of pore contraction, the peri-fiber inflammatory reactions become closer together, and once sufficiently close, the fibrous granulation tissue can form a "bridge" with neighboring fibrous granulations. This phenomenon, known as "bridging fibrosis," leads to the formation of a continuous fibrotic response or encapsulation of the mesh. It is believed that the myofibroblasts present in the capsule contract, which creates tension on surrounding tissues and thus increases the risk of pain and contributes to the perception of shrinkage of the mesh [32–36]. Additionally, the thickness of the fibrous capsule likely varies depending on the polymer used, as the amount of fibrous capsule deposition may be dependent on tissue interaction with the fiber surface and may also be related to hydrophobicity of the polymer [37]. Therefore, both the material and pore size play a role in the formation of bridging fibrosis and should be taken into consideration when choosing a mesh. When using polypropylene in hernia repairs, to prevent bridging fibrosis and optimize tissue ingrowth, it is recommended that pore sizes be ≥1 mm [26, 38]. Although the critical pore diameter to prevent bridging fibrosis for urogynecologic meshes has not been identified, it is likely distinct from that found in the abdominal wall studies, given the biologically and mechanically distinct implantation sites in the pelvis vs. the abdomen.

Mesh Weight

Typically, the weight of synthetic meshes is defined by the specific gravity (g/m^2), with heavyweight and lightweight being two of the most commonly used terms to describe urogynecologic meshes. Heavyweight meshes generally have decreased porosity with smaller pores and increased stiffness relative to lightweight meshes, which have high porosity, large pores, and decreased stiffness. Overall, heavier meshes (those with higher specific gravities, typically above 45 g/m^2) tend to induce a more pronounced and prolonged inflammatory response, have more apoptotic cells in the area of the mesh fibers, and increased turnover of tissues surrounding mesh fibers up to 1 year after implantation relative to lightweight meshes as shown in animal abdominal wall and sacrocolpopexy models [39–44]. In addition, lighter-weight meshes (<45 g/m^2) achieved by thinner fibers and larger pore sizes have been shown to have improved biocompatibility compared to heavier-weight meshes [22]. Specifically, lightweight meshes have a reduced potential for adhesion and pain as well as a reduced amount of fibrosis and inflammation with an increased potential for tissue incorporation between the pores of the mesh compared to heavy-weight meshes [23, 26, 39, 45–47]. Although these results strongly suggest that lightweight meshes are clinically more favorable than heavyweight meshes, mesh weight, pore size, and stiffness are all highly interrelated, and, as a result, it is difficult to attribute the impact of a heavier mesh to any single factor. Indeed, while in some studies, the host inflammatory response has been shown to be positively correlated to the amount of material implanted [48], in others, (e.g., Weyhe et al. [49]), pore size rather than mesh weight has been found to be most predictive. For example, the host response to a lightweight microporous mesh was found to provoke a more intense foreign body response with poor tissue integration as compared to a heavyweight mesh with larger pores [49]. This is likely related to a heavier weight mesh having mechanical properties suited to maintaining its pores in an open configuration.

Mesh Mechanics and Impact on the Host Response

Mesh mechanics is a broad term that is used to describe the *ex vivo* and *in vivo* mechanical behaviors of meshes, and it is also used to describe how mesh textile properties impact mesh behavior. Over the past decade, researchers have utilized mechanical testing in order to understand the structural properties and *ex vivo* mechanical behavior of vaginal meshes. These tests have proved to be invaluable in terms of distinguishing one mesh from another and for understanding the mechanical behaviors that may be contributing to complications. In the next few sections, a brief overview of the textile and structural properties of current synthetic meshes will be discussed. Next, the mechanical behaviors of mesh in response to various load (i.e., how deformation or force is applied) and boundary (i.e., boundaries that restrict and/or limit movement in a given direction) conditions will be examined. In addition to discussing the mechanical behaviors of mesh, the clinical implications of these behaviors, if any, will also be discussed.

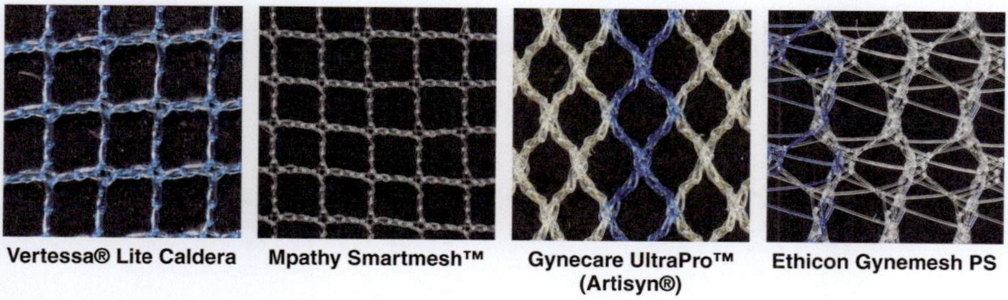

Fig. 8.1 The knit pattern and pore geometry of urogynecologic meshes are unique. Each mesh depicted is 10 mm × 10 mm

Textile and Structural Properties

Current synthetic meshes are all knitted, lightweight (<45 g/m^2), wide-pore (>1 mm, porosity >55%), type I (pore sizes exceed 75 μm) polypropylene meshes. Despite the similarities in the manufacturing of synthetic meshes, the knit pattern, pore geometries, and pore diameters are all distinct (Fig. 8.1). Some meshes, such as Vertessa® Lite (Caldera Medical, Agoura Hills CA, USA) and Restorelle™ (Coloplast, Minneapolis, MN, USA), have a square-shaped pore, whereas the pores of other meshes, such as UltraPro™ (a.k.a. Artisyn®) and Gynemesh PS™ (both manufactured by Gynecare, Ethicon, Somerville NJ, USA), are diamond and hexagon shaped, respectively. Ultimately, the pore geometry impacts the mechanics of mesh, and this will be explored further below under *Tensile Loading*.

To determine the structural properties of mesh, researchers have primarily utilized uniaxial tensile and ball-burst tests. Uniaxial tensile testing involves clamping a rectangular-shaped sample of mesh on opposing ends and elongating (or loading) the mesh to a specific load or until failure. Similar to uniaxial tensile testing, ball-burst testing also involves clamping the mesh; however, instead of clamping the ends of a rectangular piece of mesh, a square piece is clamped circumferentially (between two clamps) and a steel ball head is pushed through the mesh until failure. From these two tests, a load-elongation curve is generated (Fig. 8.2), and the following structural properties for synthetic meshes are commonly reported: ultimate load (N), ultimate elongation or displacement (mm), relative elongation (mm/mm), stiffness (N/mm), and energy absorbed (N mm). In the event that the load-elongation curve is bilinear, stiffness is typically reported as low and high stiffness (N/mm).

The ultimate load refers to the maximum amount of force that a mesh can withstand prior to failure, and the ultimate elongation (or ultimate displacement) refers to the amount that the mesh elongated (or displaced) at failure. Relative elongation is the normalized version of elongation, and it is calculated by dividing the amount of elongation by the initial length of the mesh. Stiffness is a parameter that describes the ability of the mesh to resist deformation, and it can be reported as two different

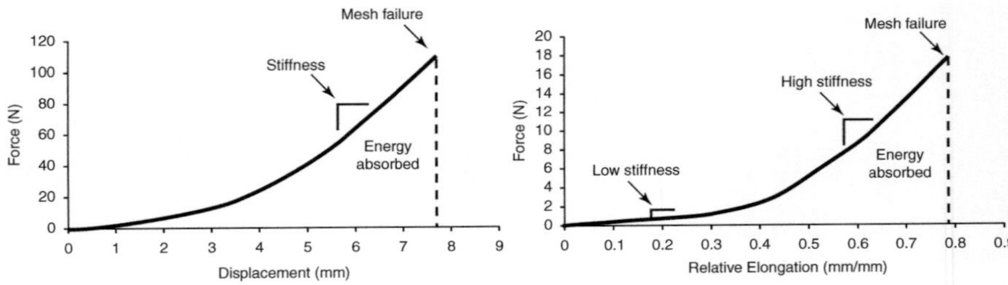

Fig. 8.2 Characteristic load-elongation curves generated after load to failure tests of synthetic mesh via ball-burst (*left graph*) and uniaxial tensile (*right graph*) tests. A single stiffness is typically reported for ball-burst testing, whereas low and high stiffness are reported for uniaxial tensile tests, which generally have a bilinear-shaped curve

values: low and high stiffness. Low stiffness, which is typically used to characterize the behavior of mesh in the physiologic range, is defined as the minimum stiffness over a defined interval of elongation. High stiffness describes the highest stiffness value over a defined interval of elongation and typically occurs with elongations in the supraphysiologic ranges. Energy absorbed refers to the toughness of the mesh. It is important for readers to note that the structural properties reported from uniaxial tensile and ball-burst tests are similar (e.g., stiffness, load at failure, and elongation at failure); however, the values of these structural properties are not the same (Tables 8.1 and 8.2) [50, 51]. This is a result of the differences in the boundary and loading conditions between the uniaxial tensile test and the ball-burst test. For more detailed information regarding the mechanical testing of synthetic meshes (including specific protocols, assumptions, and the calculation of structural properties), the interested reader should refer to Knight et al. [52].

In addition to having distinct textile properties, the structural properties of vaginal meshes also vary among products (see Tables 8.1 and 8.2) [50, 51, 53–56]. However, it is important to note that mesh textile and structural properties are not mutually exclusive. Utilizing ball-burst mechanical testing, Feola et al. in 2013 found that specific weight (also referred to as mesh weight and typically represented as g/m^2) and porosity positively correlate with stiffness, ultimate load, and energy absorbed [51].

Currently, no optimal stiffness has been defined for urogynecologic meshes. The uniaxial stiffness of vaginal meshes ranges from 0.009 N/mm to 1.66 N/mm [50, 53]. Interestingly, a single vaginal mesh can have a different stiffness depending on the direction in which it is tested – a phenomenon referred to as anisotropy. For example, the stiffness of UltraPro™ (aka Artisyn®) in the direction perpendicular to the blue orientation lines is 0.009 ± 0.002 N/mm, whereas the stiffness in the direction parallel to the blue orientation lines is 0.258 ± 0.085 N/mm [57]. This anisotropic behavior of vaginal meshes has also been observed with abdominal hernia meshes [58]. Clinically, understanding the anisotropic behavior of mesh is important information for a surgeon to have prior to implanting mesh, as it will alert surgeons to the direction in which a mesh should be implanted.

Table 8.1 Uniaxial structural properties of synthetic meshes. Data represented as mean ± standard deviation

Synthetic mesh	Low stiffness (N/mm)	High stiffness (N/mm)	Load at mesh failure (N)	Relative elongation at failure (%)
Boston Scientific Polyform™	0.130 ± 0.01	1.42 ± 0.11	53.8 ± 4.8	86.5 ± 2.4
Coloplast NovaSilk™	0.072 ± 0.05	0.508 ± 0.09	19.6 ± 4.5	89.4 ± 21.4
Gynecare, Ethicon Gynemesh PS™	0.286 ± 0.02	1.37 ± 0.09	46.3 ± 2.6	66.7 ± 4.6
Gynecare, Ethicon UltraPro™ (Artisyn®)	0.009 ± 0.00	0.236 ± 0.02	7.83 ± 0.7	87.9 ± 5.6
Coloplast Restorelle™	0.178 ± 0.03	0.592 ± 0.04	22.7 ± 1.8	68.5 ± 2.5

Adapted from Shepherd et al. [50], with permission

Table 8.2 Structural properties of synthetic meshes obtained via ball-burst testing. Data represented as mean ± standard deviation

Synthetic mesh	Stiffness (N/mm)	Load at mesh failure (N)	Extension at mesh failure (mm)	Energy absorbed (J)
Boston Scientific Polyform™	28 ± 0.43	108 ± 5.7	7.8 ± 0.05	261 ± 27
Coloplast NovaSilk™	16 ± 5.5	54 ± 19	6.3 ± 0.56	113 ± 43
Gynecare, Ethicon Gynemesh PS™	28 ± 2.7	108 ± 8.6	7.3 ± 0.31	288 ± 37
Gynecare, Ethicon UltraPro™ (aka Artisyn®)	22 ± 2.8	76 ± 12	7.3 ± 0.21	170 ± 11
Coloplast Restorelle™	11 ± 0.89	45 ± 3.8	6.7 ± 0.45	109 ± 11

From Feola et al. [51], with permission

Stiffness is an important parameter mechanically and biologically given that a mesh that is not stiff enough can result in recurrent prolapse, whereas a mesh that is too stiff can result in stress shielding. Stress shielding is a phenomenon that occurs when two neighboring materials with differing stiffnesses are in contact with each other; the stiffer material bears the majority of the load, thereby shielding the less stiff material [59, 60]. This phenomenon can ultimately lead to degeneration and atrophy of the less stiff material [61, 62]. In studies conducted by Liang et al. in 2013 and 2015, Feola et al. in 2013, and Jallah et al. in 2016, stress shielding was shown to be a likely mechanism by which stiffer prolapse meshes exerted a negative impact on the vagina when implanted by sacrocolpopexy in the rhesus macaque [40, 63–65]. Increased apoptosis surrounding mesh fibers, thinning of the smooth muscle layer, and decreases in collagen and elastin content were all negative responses to prolapse meshes with the greatest negative response observed with the stiffest mesh (Fig. 8.3) [40]. Concomitant with a decrease in collagen and elastin content, there was also an associated increase in active matrix metalloproteinases MMP-1, MMP-8, and MMP-13, and total MMP-2 and MMP-9 which is indicative of ongoing tissue degradation [65].

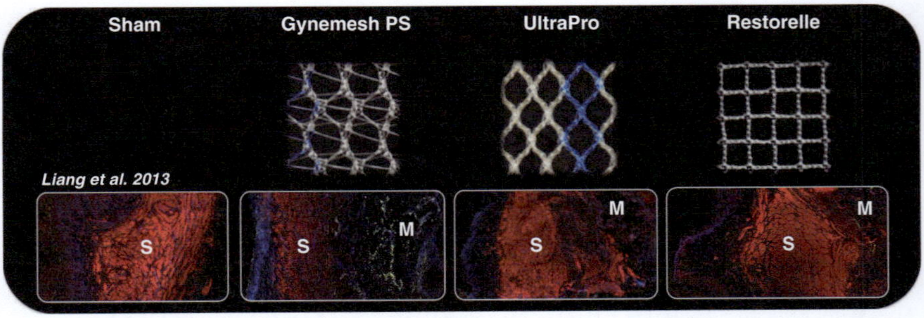

Fig. 8.3 Immunofluorescent labeling (bottom) demonstrates the effect of various synthetic mesh products (top) on vaginal tissue [40]. Here the red signal represents positive staining of alpha-smooth muscle actin, the green signal represents apoptotic cells, and the blue signal represents nuclei. Gynemesh PS™, the stiffest of all meshes, was found to significantly reduce the thickness of the smooth muscle layer (*layer designated by S*). Further, increased apoptosis was observed surrounding the mesh fibers (mesh designated by M) (Magnification 100×)

Similarly, the greatest deterioration in the mechanical properties of the vagina, particularly the functional capacity of the smooth muscle, was observed with the stiffest mesh [63, 64].

Tensile Loading

Uniaxial tensile tests have not only played a crucial role in defining the structural properties of mesh, but they have also aided the understanding of how the geometry of the mesh pores impacts the mechanical response of mesh to loading. The majority of current synthetic meshes have pore geometries that are either square, diamond, or hexagon shaped. In general, studies have shown that the pores of synthetic meshes tend to collapse in response to uniaxial loading, and this behavior is observed for both transvaginal and abdominal meshes [29, 66]. However, the degree of pore collapse is dependent on the geometry of the pore [57, 67]. In a study conducted by Barone et al. in 2016, initially the pores of Restorelle™, square-shaped pores; UltraPro™ (aka Artisyn®), diamond-shaped pores; and Gynemesh PS™, hexagon-shaped pores are all open at 0.1 N (Fig. 8.4) [66]. However, at 10 N, the pores of Restorelle™ remained relatively open compared to UltraPro™ (aka Artisyn®) and Gynemesh PS™, in which the pores of these meshes significantly collapsed (see Fig. 8.4). Specifically for Restorelle™, nearly 89% of the pores had diameters that were greater than 1 mm, resulting in only a 2% reduction in the mesh porosity (defined as the percent of open space relative to mesh area). Conversely, all of the pores of Gynemesh PS™ collapsed, resulting in a porosity of only 15.5%, and none of the pores had a diameter that was greater than 1 mm. Similar results were observed for UltraPro™ (aka Artisyn®). At 10 N, none of the pore diameters were greater than 1 mm for UltraPro™ (aka Artisyn®). Interestingly, uniaxially loading Restorelle™

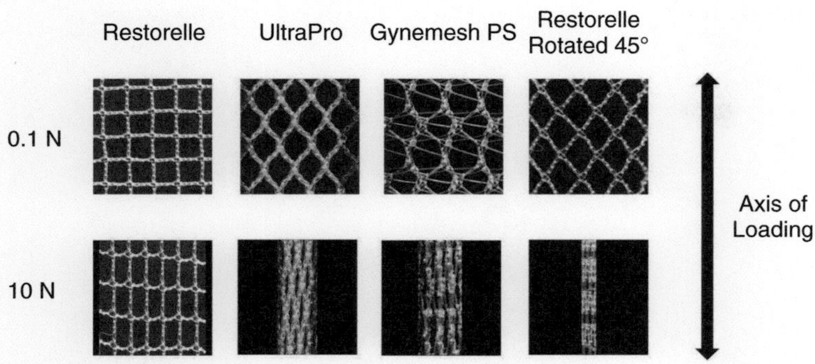

Fig. 8.4 The geometry of the mesh pores impacts the mechanics of polypropylene meshes. For example, meshes with square-shaped pores, such as Restorelle™, maintain their geometry in response to uniaxial loading, whereas meshes with diamond UltraPro™ (aka Artisyn®) or hexagon pores (Gynemesh PS™) do not. In the latter two meshes, the pores collapse with uniaxial loading. However, rotating a square-shaped pore by 45° (Restorelle™ rotated 45° pictured) to an unstable diamond configuration results in pore collapse. The dimensions of each image is 10 mm × 10 mm

with the pores rotated 45° (referred to as Restorelle™ 45°), such that the pores were in the diamond configuration, resulted in pore collapse similar to Gynemesh PS™ and UltraPro™ (aka Artisyn®) (see Fig. 8.4). The observed collapse of pores was also associated with a 91% decrease in the porosity of Restorelle™ 45°, and none of the pores had a diameter that was greater than 1 mm. Collectively, these results suggest that the geometry of the pore ultimately dictates the behavior of the mesh, with square-shaped pores being more stable in terms of maintaining their pore shape in response to uniaxial loading relative to diamond- and hexagon-shaped pores.

In a study conducted by Barone et al. in 2016, pore collapse was demonstrated for meshes intended for abdominal sacral colpopexy [66]. Pore collapse is also observed with transvaginal meshes. In transvaginal meshes, the construction is more complicated, with pores oriented in multiple varied directions along a single device due to complicated shapes with a body and mesh arms. Otto et al. in 2014 observed a loss of porosity in both the body and mesh arms of Prolift and Prolift+M (Gynecare, Ethicon) (also known as UltraPro™) (a.k.a. Artisyn®) transvaginal meshes after exposing these meshes to relatively small loads [29]. Barone et al. in 2015 observed pore collapse with Direct Fix (Coloplast), a transvaginal mesh product, and a computational model of this product [68]. This mesh is identical to Restorelle™, but while the proximal arms are loaded on the square, those in the body of the mesh and in the distal arms are loaded on the diamond. The results of this study revealed that with minimal loading of the proximal and distal arms, the pores across the proximal body and distal arms collapsed. Interestingly, altering the angle in which the model arms were loaded (analogous to the insertion site direction of the proximal arms) from a directly horizontal position (insertion into the arcus tendineous) to a more vertical position (sacrospinous ligament toward the sacrum) reduced the amount of pore collapse in the body of the mesh and model.

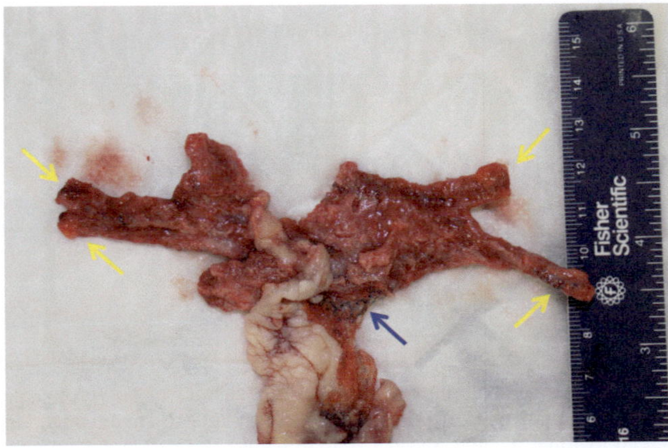

Fig. 8.5 Mesh removed from a patient with an exposure. The arms of the mesh (*yellow arrows*) have contracted into thin bands and are encapsulated with dense tissue, which is consistent with pore collapse. In the area of exposure, which occurred at the apex (*blue arrow*), the vagina is thinned

In the abdominal hernia literature, the impact of pore size and porosity on the host response to mesh has been widely characterized. Studies have shown that large pore, high porosity meshes are associated with decreased inflammation and less fibrous tissue relative to small pore, low porosity meshes [26, 27]. Additionally, meshes with larger pores yield better tissue integration with increased collagen deposition and decreased adhesion formation relative to smaller pore meshes [23, 24]. To allow for optimal tissue ingrowth and to decrease bridging fibrosis, 1 mm has been identified as the minimal pore diameter for polypropylene meshes [26]. When mesh pore sizes decrease, especially below 1 mm, bridging fibrosis increases (i.e., pore size and bridging fibrosis are inversely related) [26, 27]. Interestingly, mesh complications are often located in areas where the pores of the mesh have collapsed (Fig. 8.5). Thus from a biocompatibility standpoint, it is important that mesh pores remain open (with diameters >1 mm for polypropylene meshes) at the time of implantation and throughout the time period in which the mesh will be implanted.

Given the importance of pore size and porosity, the reduction in pore size (less than 1 mm), porosity, and effective porosity (percentage of pores with dimensions that are greater than 1 mm in all directions) with loading are factors that likely decrease the biocompatibility of urogynecologic meshes. Indeed collapsed pores that are less than 1 mm could be expected to be associated with an unfavorable host response characterized by an increased risk of bridging fibrosis, inflammation, poor tissue integration, and fibrosis, resulting in poor patient outcomes and corresponding to the clinical observation of mesh "shrinkage" or "contraction" after implantation [14, 69–72]. While mesh shrinkage may involve in part tissue contraction associated with wound healing, this phenomenon is thought to contribute only to 10–15% of the loss of mesh size [71, 72]. The remaining 20–30% observed with prolapse meshes is likely due to placement of the mesh at the time of implantation, unstable mesh geometry with loading, and subsequent encapsulation and fibrosis. Therefore, the type of mesh, the *in vivo* tensile forces to which the mesh is exposed, and the amount of tension applied are all important factors to consider when placing a mesh.

Cyclic Loading

Cyclically loading mesh from 0.5 N to 15 N, Jones et al. in 2009 and Shepherd et al. in 2012 found that mesh permanently deforms (i.e., the mesh elongates beyond the point of repair) [50, 53]. Clinically, permanent deformation of mesh can be problematic during the initial stages of mesh implantation, prior to the incorporation of tissue within the mesh pores. It is during this time that the mesh is allowed to elongate freely without any restrictions.

Boundary Conditions

During the implantation of vaginal mesh, sutures are used to attach the mesh to the vagina and the pelvic side wall (e.g., arcus tendineous or sacrospinous ligament) or sacrum. From a mechanical perspective, sutures function as boundaries, and studies have shown that the boundary conditions to which vaginal meshes are subjected can impact the mechanical behavior of these devices [50, 51, 67]. For example, during a uniaxial tensile test, the mesh is clamped on opposing ends, which allows the mesh to contract in the perpendicular direction, whereas circumferentially constraining the entire border of the mesh, as is done with ball-burst testing, prevents the pores from collapsing. This not only affects how the mesh deforms, but it ultimately results in differing structural properties for a single mesh (e.g., the uniaxial stiffness of Gynemesh PS™ is 0.286 ± 0.02 N/mm, whereas the ball-burst stiffness is 28 ± 2.7 N/mm) (see Tables 8.1 and 8.2 in *Textile and Structural Properties*) [50, 51]. Similarly, Barone et al. in 2015 found that the boundary conditions also impact surface curvature of mesh [67]. Specifically, clamping mesh by completely constraining both ends of the mesh (analogous to implanting mesh with a continuous suture), as is done with traditional uniaxial tensile tests, results in less out-of-plane deformation (observed in the form of mesh bunching/wrinkling/buckling) relative to constraining mesh using point loads (analogous to implanting mesh with interrupted sutures). Specifically, increasing the number of sutures – for example, from 0 to 4 as demonstrated by Barone et al. in 2015 – significantly increased the amount of out-of-plane deformation (Fig. 8.6) [67]. However, it is important to note that after a certain point, increasing the number of point loads (i.e., adding a lot of sutures) will act to distribute the load more uniformly, resulting in a similar effect as constraining the entire border of the mesh. From a clinical perspective, however, out-of-plane deformation of a mesh likely results in regional increases in the concentration of mesh on the vagina (increased mesh burden), which ultimately may

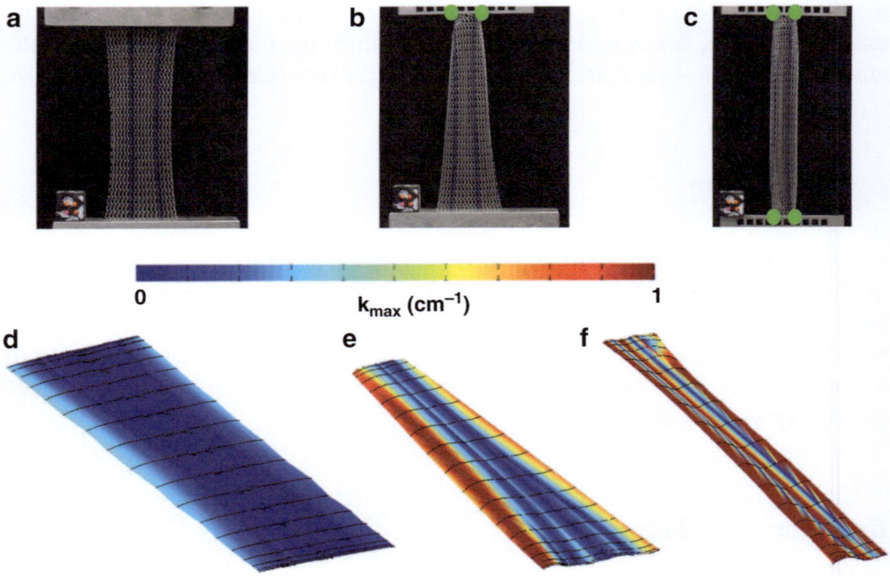

Fig. 8.6 Increasing the number of point loads (suture attachments) from 2 to 4 resulted in increasing out-of-plane deformation observed as mesh wrinkling k_{max}. (**a**) Standard uniaxial tensile loading (**d** corresponding computational model); (**b**) two-point loading (**e** corresponding computational model); and (**c**) four-point loading (**f** corresponding computational model). *Green dots* represent suture attachments

increase the foreign body response to mesh, thus leading to mesh complications such as pain. Alternatively, buckling can lead to stress mismatches with the underlying tissue, resulting in degeneration and atrophy, thereby increasing the risk of mesh exposure. It is therefore important for surgeons to understand how sutures impact the mechanics of mesh, specifically the ability of the mesh to remain flat when implanted.

In Vivo Studies Assessing the Host Response to Mesh

Similar to any synthetic material, polypropylene mesh behaves as a foreign body when implanted, inducing a robust inflammatory response to each individual mesh fiber with the inflammatory reaction positively correlated to the amount of material implanted [22, 48, 73]. Multiple immune cell types are involved in the inflammatory response, each releasing numerous cytokines and chemokines to orchestrate this process and direct a final response of resolution of inflammation or transition into a chronic inflammatory response. While early on in the healing process, mild to moderate inflammation may be beneficial for tissue incorporation, persistent or chronic inflammation is thought to increase the risk of complications such as pain, exposure, and erosion. To date, much of the information regarding the host response to mesh was obtained via animal-abdominal studies, and this is largely due to the limitations and ethical dilemmas surrounding the use and procurement of human subjects and human tissues in research. Nevertheless, recent human and animal studies have collectively aided our understanding of the host response to mesh and have begun to elucidate potential mechanisms for mesh complications. Thus, the findings of these studies will be discussed as follows, with an emphasis placed on those studies investigating the host response to mesh implanted in the vagina. This section will then conclude by discussing efforts that researchers have made to attenuate the host response to synthetic mesh.

Animal and Human Studies

As one of the primary cell types responding to mesh implants, macrophages have been indicated as a critical component in determining the downstream long-term functional outcomes of mesh [74, 75]. Emerging early in the area of foreign antigens, macrophages can differentiate into different phenotypes that exist along a continuum ranging from M1 (classically activated, pro-inflammatory) to M2 (anti-inflammatory, homeostatic, wound healing) with differential functional properties and patterns of gene expression in response to microenvironmental cues [76–78]. An M1 dominant reaction tends to be pro-inflammatory, associated with an increased release of high levels of inducible nitric oxide synthase (iNOS), toxic reactive oxygen species, and pro-inflammatory cytokines such as IL-1β, IL-6, and TNF-α affording removal of pathogens and tissue debris but in the process also inducing damage to host tissues. In contrast, an M2-polarized reaction (subpopulations M2a, M2b, and M2c) is associated with the production of remodeling/reconstruction cytokines such as low molecular weight IL-12 and IL-23, high molecular weight IL-10, and other molecules that favor constructive remodeling [76, 78–80]. However, a prolonged M2 macrophage response can result in excessive tissue deposition and fibrosis [81].

For prolapse meshes, M1 macrophages are the predominant macrophage at the mesh-tissue interface (Fig. 8.7) [43, 44]. However, Brown et al. in 2015 observed that implanting a lighter-weight, higher-porosity mesh can attenuate the M1 macrophage response [43]. In addition to a predominantly M1 pro-inflammatory response, a concomitant increase of inflammatory cytokines and chemokines such as tumor necrosis factor-α, IL-12p40p70, IL-12p70, CXCL10, and CCL17 was observed by Nolfi et al. in 2016 when examining mesh-vaginal tissue complexes excised from women with complications of pain and mesh exposure months to years after implantation [44].

Additionally, mesh-vaginal tissue complexes removed for the indication of exposure were associated with increased levels of MMP-9 relative to mesh removed for the indication of pain, which is suggestive of ongoing tissue degradation in tissues associated with mesh exposure. In this same study, there was also a positive

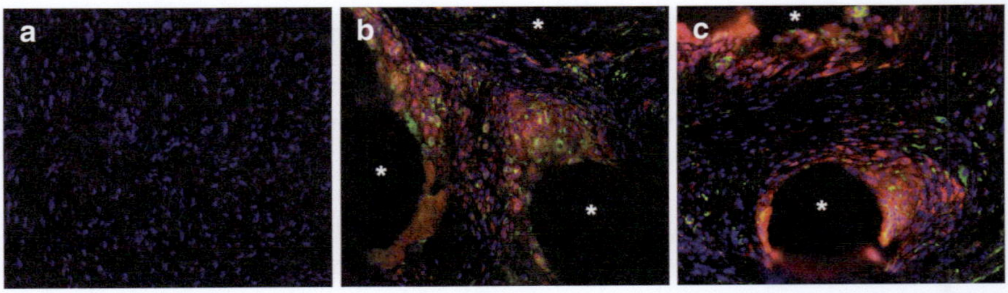

Fig. 8.7 Immunofluorescent labeling of pan-macrophage marker CD68 (*red*), M1 pro-inflammatory marker CD86 (*orange*), M2 pro-remodeling macrophage marker CD206 (*green*), and DAPI (*blue*). (**a**) Control tissue from patients without mesh; (**b**) a mesh-tissue section from a patient presenting with pain and implanted with the Gynecare TVT Secur™ (Ethicon, Somerville NJ, USA) for 6 months; (**c**) a mesh-tissue section from a patient presenting with an exposure after implantation with transvaginal mesh Perigee™ (American Medical Systems, Minnetonka MN, USA) for 93 months. A predominance of pro-inflammatory M1 macrophages surround mesh fibers (*) consistent with a prolonged immune response was observed in both (**b**) and (**c**); however, this response was limited to the area immediately adjacent to mesh fibers. Control tissue contained few or no macrophages as compared to mesh patient tissue (Magnification 200×). (Adapted from Nolfi et al. [44], with permission)

correlation between the percentage of M2-polarized macrophages and IL-10 (a pro-fibrotic cytokine) with the mesh explants removed from women for pain, which is consistent with fibrosis. The data suggest two distinct pathways lead to these two mesh complications.

Modifying the Host Response to Mesh

As a way to prevent mesh complications, researchers have coated mesh with various biological and chemical agents such as collagen, S-nitrosoglutathione (GSNO), and extracellular matrix (ECM) in order to mitigate the host response to mesh with limited success [82–90]. Hachim et al. in 2017 utilized a more targeted approach to mitigate the host response to mesh in which a polypropylene mesh was designed to release IL-4 early following implantation. The released IL-4 modified the host immune response to polypropylene, altering the macrophage phenotype at the mesh-tissue interface from a predominant M1 to an M2 phenotype. Additionally, the IL-4 slow eluting coating resulted in a decrease in capsule area and thickness, and this capsule consisted of an increased amount of thin collagen fibers compared to a mesh without IL-4. Collectively, these findings are promising; however, they should be interpreted with caution as they have been evaluated solely in an abdominal wall model. Given the differences in the host response to mesh implanted in the abdomen vs. the vagina, future studies assessing the impact of this coating on the host response in a vaginal model are warranted.

Future Outlook for Urogynecologic Basic Science Research

Over the past 10 years, basic science studies have afforded an improved understanding of urogynecologic mesh based on investigations of mesh materials, properties, mechanical behaviors, and the host responses to mesh. With this knowledge, surgeons are able to identify and appreciate differences between the various polypropylene meshes available on the market, and they are also able to select the most appropriate mesh for their patients. However, there is still more to be learned, particularly in the area of mesh complications. To date, the exact etiology of mesh complications is unclear. However, with basic science research, researchers and clinicians now understand that the pathogenesis of mesh complications likely involves multiple factors including the patient's general health condition when the mesh is placed, the quality of the host tissue, the route of implantation (vaginal vs. abdominal), the technique of the surgeon, the host immune response, the mesh textile properties, and the mechanical behavior of the mesh. It is anticipated that over the next decade, there will be an increase in the number of mechanistic studies that will aim to determine the exact etiology of mesh complications. Such studies would not only aid in preventing mesh complications but would also play an integral role in the development of the next generation of urogynecologic meshes. In addition to mechanistic studies, it is anticipated that studies investigating mesh coatings to mitigate the host response to mesh, and hence decrease the risk of mesh complications, will also increase.

Although synthetic mesh was the main focus of this chapter, exploration of augmentation with biological materials for the purpose of reversing the adverse impact of synthetic meshes on host responses has long been and continues to be investigated. In a recent nonhuman primate (NHP) study, a non-cross-linked degradable acellular porcine urinary bladder matrix, MatriStem® Surgical Matrix RS (ACell, Columbia MD, USA), was able to attenuate the negative impact of polypropylene mesh on the vagina when used with Gynemesh PS™ as a composite mesh [91]. Compared to Gynemesh PS™, the host inflammatory response and presence of apoptotic cells surrounding mesh fibers were reduced with the Gynemesh PS™–MatriStem® composite mesh relative to Gynemesh PS™ implanted alone. Additionally, the contractile function of the vaginal smooth muscle as well as the thickness of the smooth muscle layer was similar to sham animals for the composite mesh, whereas these parameters were reduced for Gynemesh PS™. As a standalone material, MatriStem® was also utilized in another NHP study to investigate the potential use of this bioscaffold to restore disrupted vaginal support (i.e., disrupted Level I and Level II support) [92]. Newly formed tissue bands were present in the location where Level I and Level II supports were disrupted. The locations of the newly formed tissue coincided with the locations where MatriStem® was implanted. This is one of the first studies that utilized a bioscaffold to specifically regenerate Level I and II support, and given the increased popularity of using regenerative medicine strategies to treat medical diseases and disorders, this study will likely not be the last. Over the next 10 years, it is expected that there will be an increase in the number of basic science studies using regenerative medicine and tissue engineering approaches to improve treatment of POP.

Ultimately, improving patient outcomes with mesh augmentation is not only limited by our knowledge of the pathogenesis of mesh complications but is also limited by our knowledge of the pathogenesis of POP. As our knowledge increases in these two areas, so will our ability to develop a mesh treatment that has minimal risk for complications. Complete understanding of the etiology of mesh complications and POP will require a collaborative effort between clinicians, scientists, and engineers. The basic science studies presented in this chapter utilized primarily animal implantation studies that evaluated the host response to mesh and *ex vivo* mechanical testing to characterize the mechanical behavior of mesh. Although these techniques have yielded invaluable information, advanced imaging techniques, such as ultrasound and magnetic resonance imaging, and computational modeling are also useful tools that will aid with elucidating the etiology of mesh complications and POP. Researchers within the urogynecology field have already begun to utilize these tools, and it is anticipated that over the next 10–15 years, new discoveries and advances will be made in vaginal mesh research and in the treatment of POP.

References

1. Funk MJ, Edenfield AL, Pate V, Visco AG, Weidner AC, Wu JM. Trends in use of surgical mesh for pelvic organ prolapse. Am J Obstet Gynecol. 2013;208(1):79.e1–e7.
2. Moalli PA, Talarico LC, Sung VW, Klingensmith WL, Shand SH, Meyn LA, Watkins SC. Impact of menopause on collagen subtypes in the arcus tendineous fasciae pelvis. Am J Obstet Gynecol. 2004;90(3):620–7.
3. Moalli PA, Shand SH, Zyczynski HM, Gordy SC, Meyn LA. Remodeling of vaginal connective tissue in patients with prolapse. Obstet Gynecol. 2005;106(5 I):953–63.
4. Boreham MK, Wai CY, Miller RT, Schaffer JI, Word RA. Morphometric analysis of smooth muscle in the anterior vaginal wall of women with pelvic organ prolapse. Am J Obstet Gynecol. 2002;187(1):56–63.
5. Boreham MK, Wai CY, Miller RT, Schaffer JI, Word RA, Weber AA. Morphometric properties of the posterior vaginal wall in women with pelvic organ prolapse. Am J Obstet Gynecol. 2002;187(6):1501–9.
6. Zong W, Stein SE, Starcher B, Meyn LA, Moalli PA. Alteration of vaginal elastin metabolism in women with pelvic organ prolapse. Obstet Gynecol. 2010;115(5):953–61.
7. DeLancey JO. Anatomy and biomechanics of genital prolapse. Clin Obstet Gynecol. 1993;36(4):897–909.
8. DeLancey JO. The anatomy of the pelvic floor. Curr Opin Obstet Gynecol. 1994;6(4):313–6.
9. Norton PA. Pelvic floor disorders: the role of fascia and ligaments. Clin Obstet Gynecol. 1993;36(4):926–38.
10. Wei JT, De Lancey JO. Functional anatomy of the pelvic floor and lower urinary tract. Clin Obstet Gynecol. 2004;47(1):3–17.
11. Barber MD, Brubaker L, Burgio KL, Richter HE, Nygaard I, Weidner AC, et al. Comparison of 2 transvaginal surgical approaches and perioperative behavioral therapy for apical vaginal prolapse: the OPTIMAL randomized trial. JAMA. 2014;311(10):1023–34.
12. Pierce LM, Rao A, Baumann SS, Glassberg JE, Kuehl TJ, Muir TW. Long-term histologic response to synthetic and biologic graft materials implanted in the vagina and abdomen of a rabbit model. Am J Obstet Gynecol. 2009;200(5):546.e1–e8.

13. Feola A, Endo M, Urbankova I, Vlacil J, Deprest T, Bettin S, et al. Host reaction to vaginally inserted collagen containing polypropylene implants in sheep. Am J Obstet Gynecol. 2015;212(4):474.e1–474.e8.
14. Manodoro S, Endo M, Uvin P, Albersen M, Vláčil J, Engels A, et al. Graft-related complications and biaxial tensiometry following experimental vaginal implantation of flat mesh of variable dimensions. BJOG. 2013;120(2):244–50.
15. Engelsman AF, Van Dam GM, Van Der Mei HC, Busscher HJ, Ploeg RJ. In vivo evaluation of bacterial infection involving morphologically different surgical meshes. Ann Surg. 2010;251(1):133–7.
16. Klinge U, Junge K, Spellerberg B, Piroth C, Klosterhalfen B, Schumpelick V. Do multifilament alloplastic meshes increase the infection rate? Analysis of the polymeric surface, the bacteria adherence, and the in vivo consequences in a rat model. J Biomed Mater Res. 2002;63(6):765–71.
17. Iglesia CB, Fenner DE, Brubaker L. The use of mesh in gynecologic surgery. Int Urogynecol J Pelvic Floor Dysfunct. 1997;8(2):105–15.
18. Cosson M, Debodinance P, Boukerrou M, Chauvet MP, Lobry P, Crépin G, Ego A. Mechanical properties of synthetic implants used in the repair of prolapse and urinary incontinence in women: which is the ideal material? Int Urogynecol J Pelvic Floor Dysfunct. 2003;14(3):169–78.
19. Chen CC, Ridgeway B, Paraiso MF. Biologic grafts and synthetic meshes in pelvic reconstructive surgery. Clin Obstet Gynecol. 2007;50(2):383–411.
20. Wohlrab KJ, Erekson EA, Myers DL. Postoperative erosions of the Mersilene® suburethral sling mesh for antiincontinence surgery. Int Urogynecol J Pelvic Floor Dysfunct. 2009;20(4):417–20.
21. Cobb WS, Peindl RM, Zerey M, Carbonell AM, Heniford BT. Mesh terminology 101. Hernia. 2009;13(1):1–6.
22. Patel H, Ostergard DR, Sternschuss G. Polypropylene mesh and the host response. Int Urogynecol J Pelvic Floor Dysfunct. 2012;23(6):669–79.
23. Conze J, Rosch R, Klinge U, Weiss C, Anurov M, Titkowa S, et al. Polypropylene in the intraabdominal position: influence of pore size and surface area. Hernia. 2004;8(4):365–72.
24. Greca FH, De Paula JB, Biondo-Simões MLP, Da Costa FD, Da Silva APG, Time S, Mansur A. The influence of differing pore sizes on the biocompatibility of two polypropylene meshes in the repair of abdominal defects: experimental study in dogs. Hernia. 2001;5(2):59–64.
25. Greca FH, Souza-Filho ZA, Giovanini A, Rubin MR, Kuenzer RF, Reese FB, Araujo LM. The influence of porosity on the integration histology of two polypropylene meshes for the treatment of abdominal wall defects in dogs. Hernia. 2008;12(1):45–9.
26. Klinge U, Klosterhalfen B, Birkenhauer V, Junge K, Conze J, Schumpelick V. Impact of polymer pore size on the interface scar formation in a rat model. J Surg Res. 2002;103(2):208–14.
27. Orenstein SB, Saberski ER, Kreutzer DL, Novitsky YW. Comparative analysis of histopathologic effects of synthetic meshes based on material, weight, and pore size in mice. J Surg Res. 2012;176(2):423–9.
28. Amid PK. Classification of biomaterials and their related complications in abdominal wall hernia surgery. Hernia. 1997;1(1):15–21.
29. Otto J, Kaldenhoff E, Kirschner-Hermanns R, Mühl T, Klinge U. Elongation of textile pelvic floor implants under load is related to complete loss of effective porosity, thereby favoring incorporation in scar plates. J Biomed Mater Res A. 2014;102(4):1079–84.
30. Junge K, Binnebösel M, Von Trotha KT, Rosch R, Klinge U, Neumann UP, Jansen PL. Mesh biocompatibility: effects of cellular inflammation and tissue remodelling. Langenbeck's Arch Surg. 2012;397(2):255–70.
31. Mühl T, Binnebösel M, Klinge U, Goedderz T. New objective measurement to characterize the porosity of textile implants. J Biomed Mater Res B Appl Biomater. 2008;84((1):176–83.
32. Desmouliere A, Chaponnier C, Gabbiani G. Tissue repair, contraction, and the myofibroblast. Wound Repair Regen. 2005;13(1):7–12.
33. Duffield JS, Lupher M, Thannickal VJ, Wynn TA. Host responses in tissue repair and fibrosis. Ann Rev Pathol. 2013;8:241–76.

34. Hinz B. Formation and function of the myofibroblast during tissue repair. J Invest Dermatol. 2007;127(3):526–37.
35. Rudolph R, Utley JR, Woodward M. Contractile fibroblasts (myofibroblasts) in a painful pacemaker pocket. Ann Thorac Surg. 1981;31(4):373–6.
36. Tomasek JJ, Gabbiani G, Hinz B, Chaponnier C, Brown RA. Myofibroblasts and mechano-regulation of connective tissue remodelling. Nat Rev Mol Cell Biol. 2002;3(5):349–63.
37. Klinge U, Klosterhalfen B, Öttinger AP, Junge K, Schumpelick V. PVDF as a new polymer for the construction of surgical meshes. Biomaterials. 2002;23(16):3487–93.
38. Klinge U, Klosterhalfen B. Modified classification of surgical meshes for hernia repair based on the analyses of 1,000 explanted meshes. Hernia. 2012;16(3):251–8.
39. Klinge U, Junge K, Stumpf M, Öttinger AP, Klosterhalfen B. Functional and morphological evaluation of a low-weight, monofilament polypropylene mesh for hernia repair. J Biomed Mater Res. 2002;63(2):129–36.
40. Liang R, Abramowitch S, Knight K, Palcsey S, Nolfi A, Feola A, et al. Vaginal degeneration following implantation of synthetic mesh with increased stiffness. BJOG. 2013;120(2):233–43.
41. Novitsky YW, Cristiano JA, Harrell AG, Newcomb W, Norton JH, Kercher KW, Heniford BT. Immunohistochemical analysis of host reaction to heavyweight-, reduced-weight-, and expanded polytetrafluoroethylene (ePTFE)-based meshes after short- and long-term intraabdominal implantations. Surg Endosc. 2008;22(4):1070–6.
42. Costello CR, Bachman SL, Grant SA, Cleveland DS, Loy TS, Ramshaw BJ. Characterization of heavyweight and lightweight polypropylene prosthetic mesh explants from a single patient. Surg Innov. 2007;14(3):168–76.
43. Brown BN, Mani D, Nolfi AL, Liang R, Abramowitch SD, Moalli PA. Characterization of the host inflammatory response following implantation of prolapse mesh in rhesus macaque. Am J Obstet Gynecol. 2015;213(5):668.e1–668e.10.
44. Nolfi AL, Brown BN, Liang R, Palcsey SL, Bonidie MJ, Abramowitch SD, Moalli PA. Host response to synthetic mesh in women with mesh complications. Am J Obstet Gynecol. 2016;215(2):206.e1–206.e8.
45. Klinge U, Klosterhalfen B, Conze J, Limberg W, Obolenski B, Öttinger AP, Schumpelick V. Modified mesh for hernia repair that is adapted to the physiology of the abdominal wall. Eur J Surg. 1998;64(12):951–60.
46. Klinge U, Klosterhalfen B, Muller M, Ottinger AP, Schumpelick V. Shrinking of polypropylene mesh in vivo: an experimental study in dogs. Eur J Surg. 1998;164(12):965–9.
47. O'Dwyer PJ, Kingsnorth AN, Molloy RG, Small PK, Lammers B, Horeyseck G. Randomized clinical trial assessing impact of a lightweight or heavyweight mesh on chronic pain after inguinal hernia repair. Br J Surg. 2005;92(2):166–70.
48. Rosch R, Junge K, Schachtrupp A, Klinge U, Klosterhalfen B, Schumpelick V. Mesh implants in hernia repair: inflammatory cell response in a rat model. Eur Surg Res. 2003;35(3):161–6.
49. Weyhe D, Schmitz I, Belyaev O, Grabs R, Muller KM, Uhl W, Zumtobel V. Experimental comparison of monofile light and heavy polypropylene meshes: less weight does not mean less biological response. World J Surg. 2006;30(8):1586–91.
50. Shepherd JP, Feola AJ, Abramowitch SD, Moalli PA. Uniaxial biomechanical properties of seven different vaginally implanted meshes for pelvic organ prolapse. Int Urogynecol J Pelvic Floor Dysfunct. 2012;23(5):613–20.
51. Feola A, Barone W, Moalli P, Abramowitch S. Characterizing the ex vivo textile and structural properties of synthetic prolapse mesh products. Int Urogynecol J Pelvic Floor Dysfunct. 2013;24(4):559–64.
52. Knight K, Moalli PA. Mechanics of pelvic floor prosthetic devices. In: Hoyte L, Damaser M, editors. Biomechanics of the female pelvic floor. 2nd ed. London: Academic Press/Elsevier; 2016. p. 149–78.
53. Jones KA, Feola A, Meyn L, Abramowitch SD, Moalli PA. Tensile properties of commonly used prolapse meshes. Int Urogynecol J Pelvic Floor Dysfunct. 2009;20(7):847–53.

54. Moalli PA, Papas N, Menefee S, Albo M, Meyn L, Abramowitch SD. Tensile properties of five commonly used mid-urethral slings relative to the TVT™. Int Urogynecol J Pelvic Floor Dysfunct. 2008;19(5):655–63.
55. Afonso JS, Martins PA, Girao MJ, Natal Jorge RM, Ferreira AJM, Mascarenhas T, et al. Mechanical properties of polypropylene mesh used in pelvic floor repair. Int Urogynecol J Pelvic Floor Dysfunct. 2008;19(3):375–80.
56. Dietz HP, Vancaillie P, Svehla M, Walsh W, Steensma AB, Vancaillie TG. Mechanical properties of urogynecologic implant materials. Int Urogynecol J Pelvic Floor Dysfunct. 2003;14(4):239–43.
57. Feola A, Pal S, Moalli P, Maiti S, Abramowitch S. Varying degrees of nonlinear mechanical behavior arising from geometric differences of urogynecological meshes. J Biomech. 2014;47(11):2584–9.
58. Saberski ER, Orenstein SB, Novitsky YW. Anisotropic evaluation of synthetic surgical meshes. Hernia. 2011;15(1):47–52.
59. Goel VK, Lim TH, Gwon J, Chen JY, Winterbottom JM, Park JB, et al. Effects of rigidity of an internal fixation device. A comprehensive biomechanical investigation. Spine. 1991;16(3 Suppl):S155–61.
60. Huiskes R, Weinans H, Grootenboer HJ, Dalstra M, Fudala B, Slooff TJ. Adaptive bone-remodeling theory applied to prosthetic-design analysis. J Biomech. 1987;20(11–12):1135–50.
61. Rumian AP, Draper ER, Wallace AL, Goodship AE. The influence of the mechanical environment on remodelling of the patellar tendon. J Bone Joint Surg Br. 2009;91(4):557–64.
62. Yamamoto N, Ohno K, Hayashi K, Kuriyama H, Yasuda K, Kaneda K. Effects of stress shielding on the mechanical properties of rabbit patellar tendon. J Biomech Eng. 1993;115(1):23–8.
63. Feola A, Abramowitch S, Jallah Z, Stein S, Barone W, Palcsey S, Moalli P. Deterioration in biomechanical properties of the vagina following implantation of a high-stiffness prolapse mesh. BJOG. 2013;120(2):224–32.
64. Jallah Z, Liang R, Feola A, Barone W, Palcsey S, Abramowitch S, et al. The impact of prolapse mesh on vaginal smooth muscle structure and function. BJOG. 2016;123(7):1076–85.
65. Liang R, Zong W, Palcsey S, Abramowitch S, Moalli PA. Impact of prolapse meshes on the metabolism of vaginal extracellular matrix in rhesus macaque. Am J Obstet Gynecol. 2015;212(2):174.e1–174.e7.
66. Barone WR, Moalli PA, Abramowitch SD. Textile properties of synthetic prolapse mesh in response to uniaxial loading. Am J Obstet Gynecol. 2016;215(3):326.e1–326.e9.
67. Barone WR, Amini R, Maiti S, Moalli PA, Abramowitch SD. The impact of boundary conditions on surface curvature of polypropylene mesh in response to uniaxial loading. J Biomech. 2015;48(9):1566–74.
68. Barone WR. Mechanical characterization of synthetic mesh for pelvic organ prolapse repair [dissertation]. Pittsburgh: University of Pittsburgh; 2015. http://d-scholarship.pitt.edu/25620/. Accessed 8 Sept 2017.
69. Caquant F, Collinet P, Debodinance P, Berrocal J, Garbin O, Rosenthal C, et al. Safety of trans vaginal mesh procedure: retrospective study of 684 patients. J Obstet Gynaecol Res. 2008;34(4):449–56.
70. Feiner B, Maher C. Vaginal mesh contraction: definition, clinical presentation, and management. Obstet Gynecol. 2010;115(2 Part 1):325–30.
71. Rogowski A, Bienkowski P, Tosiak A, Jerzak M, Mierzejewski P, Baranowski W. Mesh retraction correlates with vaginal pain and overactive bladder symptoms after anterior vaginal mesh repair. Int Urogynecol J Pelvic Floor Dysfunct. 2013;24(12):2087–92.
72. Svabik K, Martan A, Masata J, El-Haddad R, Hubka P, Pavlikova M. Ultrasound appearances after mesh implantation—evidence of mesh contraction or folding? Int Urogynecol J. 2011;22(5):529–33.
73. Clavé A, Yahi H, Hammou J-C, Montanari S, Gounon P, Clavé H. Polypropylene as a reinforcement in pelvic surgery is not inert: comparative analysis of 100 explants. Int Urogynecol J. 2010;21(3):261–70.

74. Brown BN, Londono R, Tottey S, Zhang L, Kukla KA, Wolf MT, et al. Macrophage phenotype as a predictor of constructive remodeling following the implantation of biologically derived surgical mesh materials. Acta Biomater. 2012;8(3):978–87.
75. Brown BN, Ratner BD, Goodman SB, Amar S, Badylak SF. Macrophage polarization: an opportunity for improved outcomes in biomaterials and regenerative medicine. Biomaterials. 2012;33(15):3792–802.
76. Mantovani A, Sica A, Sozzani S, Allavena P, Vecchi A, Locati M. The chemokine system in diverse forms of macrophage activation and polarization. Trends Immunol. 2004;25(12): 677–86.
77. Mills CD, Kincaid K, Alt JM, Heilman MJ, Hill AM. M-1/M-2 macrophages and the Th1/Th2 paradigm. J Immunol. 2000;164(12):6166–73.
78. Mosser DM, Edwards JP. Exploring the full spectrum of macrophage activation. Nat Rev Immunol. 2008;8(12):958–69.
79. Brown BN, Badylak SF. Expanded applications, shifting paradigms and an improved understanding of host-biomaterial interactions. Acta Biomater. 2013;9(2):4948–55.
80. Gundra UM, Girgis NM, Ruckerl D, Jenkins S, Ward LN, Kurtz ZD, et al. Alternatively activated macrophages derived from monocytes and tissue macrophages are phenotypically and functionally distinct. Blood. 2014;123(20):e110–22.
81. Murray PJ, Wynn TA. Protective and pathogenic functions of macrophage subsets. Nat Rev Immunol. 2011;11(11):723–37.
82. Dias FG, Prudente A, Siniscalchi RT, de Vidal BC, Riccetto CL. Can highly purified collagen coating modulate polypropylene mesh immune-inflammatory and fibroblastic reactions? Immunohistochemical analysis in a rat model. Int Urogynecol J Pelvic Floor Dysfunct. 2015;26(4):569–76.
83. Huffaker RK, Muir TW, Rao A, Baumann SS, Kuehl TJ, Pierce LM. Histologic response of porcine collagen-coated and uncoated polypropylene grafts in a rabbit agina model. Am J Obstet Gynecol. 2008;198(5):582.e1–582.e7.
84. Pierce LM, Asarias JR, Nguyen PT, Mings JR, Gehrich AP. Inflammatory cytokine and matrix metalloproteinase expression induced by collagen-coated and uncoated polypropylene meshes in a rat model. Am J Obstet Gynecol. 2011;205(1):82.e1–82.e9.
85. Tayrac R, Alves A, Thérin M. Collagen-coated vs noncoated low-weight polypropylene meshes in a sheep model for vaginal surgery. A pilot study. Int Urogynecol J. 2007;18(5):513–20.
86. Siniscalchi RT, Melo M, Palma PC, Fabbro IM, De Campos Vidal B, Riccetto CL. Highly purified collagen coating enhances tissue adherence and integration properties of monofilament polypropylene meshes. Int l Urogynecol J. 2013;24(10):1747–54.
87. Prudente A, Favaro WJ, Reis LO, Riccetto CL. Nitric oxide coating polypropylene mesh increases angiogenesis and reduces inflammatory response and apoptosis. Int Int Urol Nephrol. 2017;49(4):597–605.
88. Faulk DM, Londono R, Wolf MT, Ranallo CA, Carruthers CA, Wildemann JD, et al. ECM hydrogel coating mitigates the chronic inflammatory response to polypropylene mesh. Biomaterials. 2014;35(30):8585–95.
89. Wolf MT, Carruthers CA, Dearth CL, Crapo PM, Huber A, Burnsed OA, et al. Polypropylene surgical mesh coated with extracellular matrix mitigates the host foreign body response. J Biomed Mater Res A. 2014;102(1):234–46.
90. Wolf MT, Dearth CL, Ranallo CA, LoPresti ST, Carey LE, Daly KA, et al. Macrophage polarization in response to ECM coated polypropylene mesh. Biomaterials. 2014;35(25):6838–49.
91. Liang R, Knight K, Barone W, Powers RW, Nolfi A, Palcsey S, et al. Extracellular matrix regenerative graft attenuates the negative impact of polypropylene prolapse mesh on vagina in rhesus macaque. Am J Obstet Gynecol. 2017;216(2):153.e1–153.e9.
92. Liang R, Knight K, Easley D, Palcsey S, Abramowitch S, Moalli PA. Towards rebuilding vaginal support utilizing an extracellular matrix bioscaffold. Acta Biomater. 2017;57:324–33.

Chapter 9
Vaginal Mesh for Prolapse: An Epidemiologic and Historical Perspective

Cheryl B. Iglesia and Pakeeza A. Alam

History of Vaginal Mesh Use for Prolapse and FDA Clearance

Following the well-documented, long-term subjective and objective success of synthetic midurethral slings in the late 1990s, and the ensuing randomized comparative trials showing increased benefits of synthetic slings over retropubic urethropexies [1], pelvic reconstructive surgeons felt more comfortable using synthetic polypropylene mesh in the vagina. In 2004, the first transvaginal mesh "kits" for treatment of pelvic organ prolapse (which included the surgical mesh material plus the tools and introducers used for mesh delivery in the vesicovaginal and rectovaginal spaces) were cleared by the US Food and Drug Administration (FDA) with the Perigee™ and Apogee™ devices (American Medical Systems, AMS, Minnetonka, MN, USA) followed by Prolift™ (Ethicon, Somerville, NJ, USA), Elevate™ (AMS), and Uphold™ (Boston Scientific, Marlborough, MA, USA) in 2008 [2]. Figure 9.1 shows the number of surgical mesh devices cleared for urogynecologic use between 1992 and 2010, representing 168 submissions under 510(k)s for which 49 were related to surgical mesh for pelvic organ prolapse (POP) and the majority of the other mesh devices for stress urinary incontinence (SUI) [2]. The 510(k) review is a comparative process, wherein devices have been determined by the FDA to be "substantially equivalent" to a previously cleared predicate device. In the case of transvaginal mesh for prolapse, the predicate device was both the ProteGen™ sling (Boston Scientific), initially cleared in 1996, and also surgical polypropylene hernia mesh. Of note, the ProteGen™ sling was later recalled by the manufacturer in 1999 due to a higher-than-anticipated mesh complication (particularly urethral erosion)

C. B. Iglesia · P. A. Alam (✉)
Section of Female Pelvic Medicine and Reconstructive Surgery, MedStar Washington Hospital Center, Departments of Obstetrics/Gynecology and Urology, Georgetown University School of Medicine, Washington, DC, USA

S. A. Shobeiri (ed.), *The Innovation and Evolution of Medical Devices*,
https://doi.org/10.1007/978-3-319-97073-8_9

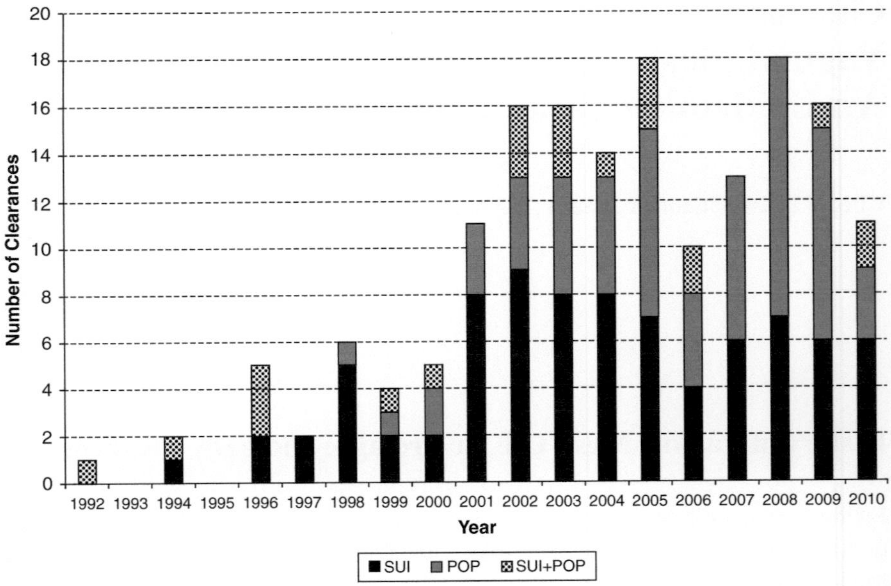

Fig. 9.1 FDA surgical mesh 510(k) clearance by year. Stacked columns show number of devices cleared each year for SUI (stress urinary incontinence), POP (pelvic organ prolapse), and SUI + POP (both). (From Surgical Mesh for Treatment of Women with Pelvic Organ Prolapse and Stress Urinary Incontinence, FDA Executive Summary, ObGyn Devices Advisory Committee, Sept 8–9, 2011 [2])

rate. Over 300 adverse events had been reported after the first year of ProteGen™ use, and the product was no longer manufactured after January 1999.

Littman and Culligan demonstrated the predicate devices for transvaginal mesh kits and their evolution (Fig. 9.2) [3]. The two main predicates cleared by the Office of Device Evaluation (ODE), Division of General, Restorative and Neurological Devices, Plastic and Reconstructive Surgery Devices Branch, were the ProteGen™ sling and Prolene™ soft mesh used for hernia repair. Subsequent to the public health notifications, vaginal mesh was evaluated by urology and gynecology reviewers in a different division of ODE (Division of Reproductive, Abdominal and Radiological Devices, DRARD). The clearance process for medical devices by the FDA has come under increased public scrutiny with many calling for a more evidence-based approach prior to device clearance and increased post-marketing surveillance once devices have been cleared [4, 5].

Training for Surgical Implantation of Vaginal Mesh

After initial clearance, surgeons (gynecologists, urologists, and urogynecologists) often received training through industry and manufacturer-sponsored hands-on and didactic courses as well as preceptorships. Since many surgeons already felt very comfortable with placement of retropubic and transobturator slings, training

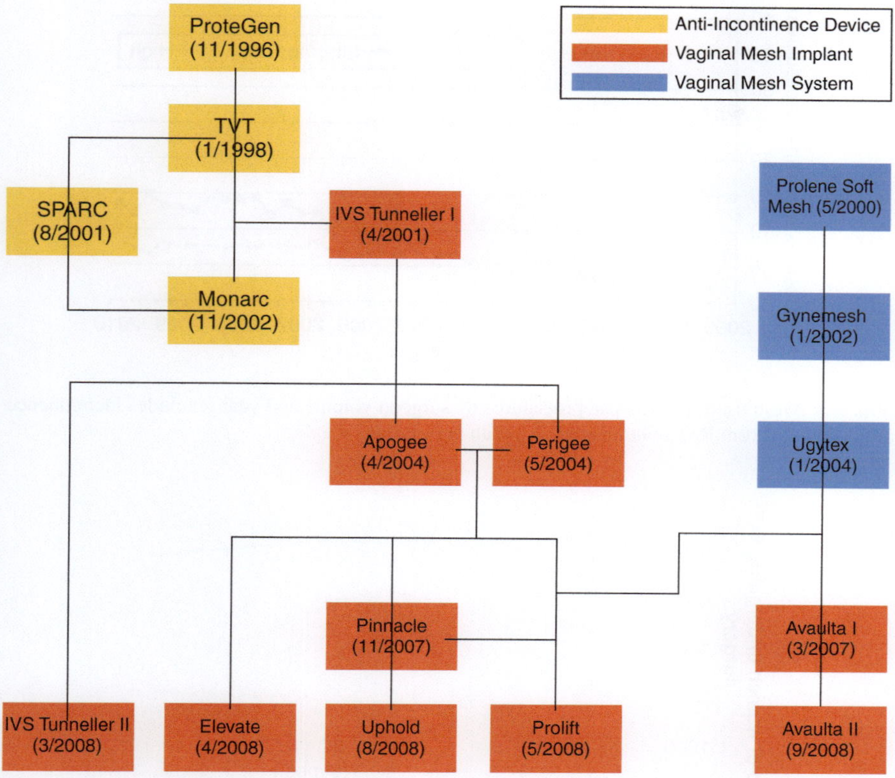

Fig. 9.2 Origin of predicate devices for transvaginal mesh kits (adapted from Littman and Culligan [3])

for vaginal mesh for prolapse was a progression for those who had performed midurethral slings. By 2006, among patients undergoing surgery for prolapse, nearly one-third involved surgical mesh placement. Figure 9.3 shows use of mesh for prolapse repair by year, with peak at year 2005–2007, and mirrored by high-volume surgeons, compared to low- and intermediate-volume surgeons [6].

In this review, Rogo-Gupta et al. analyzed the Perspective database (a healthcare quality database) representing approximately 15% of all hospitalizations in the United States for women who underwent prolapse repair between 2000 and 2010 [6]. During this time period, mesh was used in 7.9% of patients undergoing prolapse repair in 2000 and increased to a peak of 32.1% in 2006 and then declined to 27.5% in 2010. The investigators found that high-volume surgeons used mesh for prolapse repairs more frequently than low-volume surgeons.

Findings from the New York Statewide Planning and Research Cooperative System showed that use of mesh for pelvic organ prolapse increased from 21% to 31% from 2008 to 2010; however, after the second FDA PHN warning in 2011, mesh use significantly decreased from 30% in 2011 to 23% in 2013, perhaps in part due to the stronger language about mesh-related complications [7] (Fig. 9.4), with most of the decline in use being among low- and medium-volume surgeons [8] (Fig. 9.5).

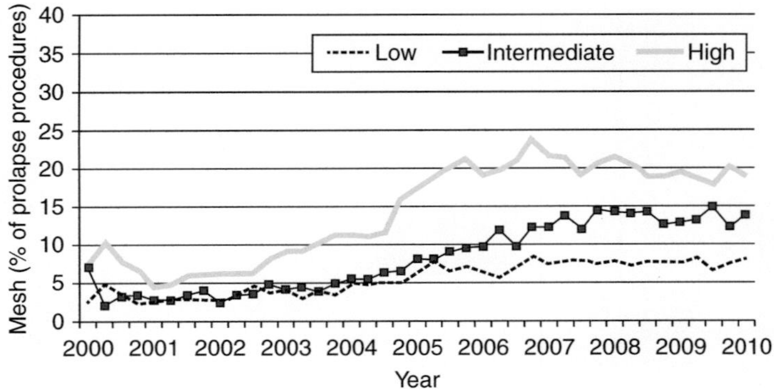

Fig. 9.3 Mesh used for prolapse procedures by surgeon volume and year (excludes incontinence procedures) (From Rogo-Gupta et al. [6], with permission)

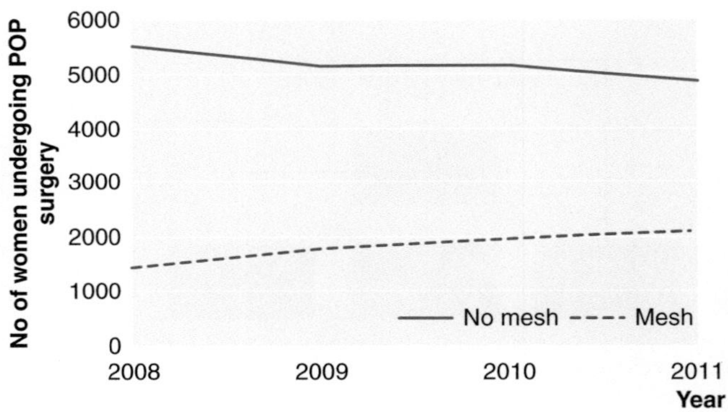

Fig. 9.4 Prolapse repair with no mesh and with mesh from 2008 to 2011 in New York State (From Chughtai et al. [7], with permission)

Standard US FDA Regulatory Process and Vaginal Mesh Up-Classification

The FDA medical device regulation is categorized into three classes:

I. Class I devices represent low-risk products such as bandages, gloves, and surgical instruments and are regulated under a general controls process, including product labeling and good manufacturing practices.

II. Class II devices generally include moderate-risk devices, such as catheters, X-ray machines, urodynamic equipment, wheelchairs, infusion pumps, and (initially) surgical mesh implants for prolapse and incontinence, and are regulated by general and special controls and cleared through the 510(k) process, meaning the device has substantial equivalence to a predicate (previously approved) device.

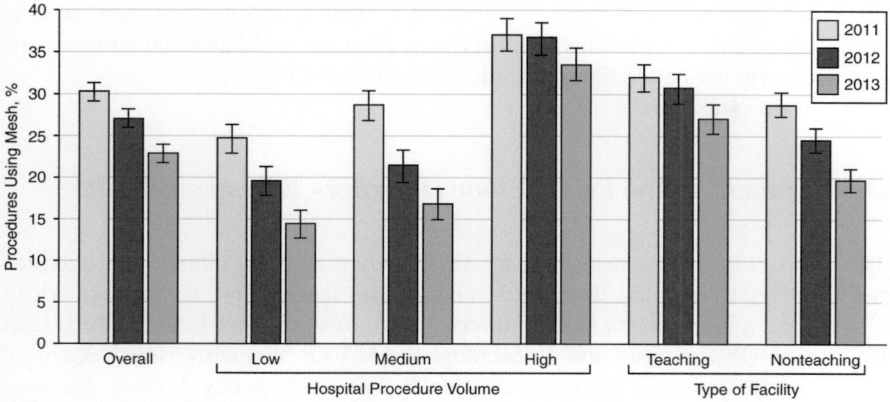

Fig. 9.5 Percent of prolapse procedures using mesh in New York from 2011 to 2014 and categorized by low-, medium-, and high-volume centers and academic versus nonacademic centers (From Sedrakyan et al. [8], with permission)

Table 9.1 Timeline of events surrounding vaginal mesh kits 2008–2016 [9]

Oct 2008 and Jul 2011	The US Food and Drug Administration (FDA) issued two safety communications warning doctors and consumers about an increase in adverse event reports related to urogynecologic mesh. The July 2011 public health notification questioned the safety and effectiveness of vaginal repair with mesh
Sept 2011	The FDA convened an advisory panel to solicit recommendations on surgical mesh for transvaginal pelvic organ prolapse (POP) repairs
Jan 2012	The FDA issued 522 orders to manufacturers to conduct post-market surveillance studies to address safety and effectiveness concerns surrounding transvaginal mesh for POP and mini-slings
May 2014	The FDA proposed orders to reclassify the devices from class II to class III and to require manufacturers to submit a premarket approval (PMA) application
Jan 2016	The FDA issued the order to reclassify these medical devices from class II to class III, requiring manufacturers to submit a PMA application to support the safety and effectiveness of surgical mesh for the transvaginal repair of POP

III. Class III devices generally include high-risk devices and are regulated through a premarket approval (PMA) process and require studies demonstrating efficacy and safety. Examples include cardiac pacemakers, defibrillators, direct sacral stimulation devices, heart valves, and endometrial ablation devices.

Originally, in 2004, vaginal mesh kits were considered class II devices and approved through the 510(k) process. In 2006, an increase in adverse event and safety reports prompted an initial review of the Manufacturer and User Facility Device Experience (MAUDE) database. A timeline of the events surrounding vaginal mesh kit review by the FDA is summarized in Table 9.1 [9].

After the 522 orders were issued on January 3, 2012, to 33 manufacturers of urogynecologic surgical mesh for prolapse, many companies ceased manufacturing of vaginal mesh kits or withdrew from the market. Multidistrict litigation lawsuits were filed against several mesh manufacturers. Other companies invested millions to meet the FDA requirements to satisfy the 522 orders and partnered with investigators to form the Pelvic Floor Disorders Registry (PFDR).

Development of the Pelvic Floor Disorders Registry (PFDR)

The Pelvic Floor Disorders Registry (https://www.augs.org/clinical-practice/pfd-research-registry/) was developed under the leadership of the American Urogynecologic Society (AUGS) in collaboration with the FDA, the American College of Obstetricians and Gynecologists (ACOG) Women's Health Registry Alliance, the National Institutes of Health Eunice Kennedy Shriver National Institute of Child Health and Human Development (NICHD), medical device and industry manufacturers, and other professional societies (AUA, SUFU). The stakeholders advocated for a registry to scientifically study and track the safety and effectiveness outcomes for a variety of treatment options for pelvic floor disorders including (1) pessary, (2) native tissue repair, (3) transvaginal mesh (biologic and synthetic) for prolapse repair, (4) sacrocolpopexy, and (5) obliterative procedures. The PFDR will allow for tracking of surgeon volume, patient demographics, and treatment effectiveness, incorporating composite outcomes (anatomic, patient-centered, and need for repeat treatment) [10]. The registry emphasizes both short- and long-term anatomic outcomes, patient-centered outcomes (including symptoms of prolapse, sexual function, and quality-of-life outcomes), and complications and safety for the surgical and medical management of prolapse [11]. Another major role of the PFDR, in addition to facilitation of post-market FDA 522 studies sponsored by vaginal mesh device manufacturers, is the opportunity for participants to report quality metrics to agencies such as the Centers for Medicare and Medicaid Services (CMS) and other agencies involved in physician payment incentive and penalty programs.

New Guidelines for Vaginal Mesh Use and Training

In addition to more robust post-market surveillance programs for transvaginal mesh devices, recommendations for training and guidelines for use have been published to assist surgeons. In December 2011, ACOG and AUGS published a joint document on vaginal placement of synthetic mesh for pelvic organ prolapse [12]. Recommendations include the following:

> "Pelvic organ prolapse vaginal mesh repair should be reserved for high-risk individuals in whom the benefit of mesh placement may justify the risk, such as individuals with recurrent prolapse (particularly of the anterior compartment) or with medical comorbidities that preclude more invasive and lengthier open and endoscopic procedures."

ACOG and AUGS support the PFDR for post-market surveillance and recommend training specific to each device. In 2012 AUGS published guidelines for credentialing for transvaginal mesh procedures [13], including general knowledge through fellowship or continuing medical education (CME) training, specific procedural knowledge (including device-specific training) through fellowship training or proctoring, significant experience in treating pelvic floor disorders incorporating fellowship training or a minimum 50% surgical practice dedicated to pelvic floor disorders, and annual internal audit.

Indeed, multiple studies confirm a tenet that high-volume surgeons and hospitals have better outcomes and lower complication rates, compared to low-volume surgeons and centers. In a recent study by Eilber et al., a 2007–2008 audit of the CMS of all transvaginal mesh for prolapse repairs showed that the majority of cases were performed by low-volume surgeons (one case annually) who had significantly higher reoperation rates compared to higher-volume surgeons [14]. Clearly, transvaginal mesh should be reserved for the right patient at the right time by the right surgeon, preferably a fellowship-trained or board-certified high-volume specialist who will track outcomes through the Pelvic Floor Disorders Registry.

Conclusion

Over the past decade, there has been a rapid cycling of transvaginal mesh products on and off the US market. Many lessons have been learned, resulting in significant improvement in mesh design and delivery, as well as improved understanding of the basic science of mesh, and new guidelines for mesh use and potential benefit in the treatment of pelvic organ prolapse. Transvaginal mesh for prolapse should be performed by a trained, high-volume surgeon able to track objective and subjective short- and long-term outcomes with the full consent of the patient, who has been informed of potential benefits, risks, and treatment alternatives. Provider and patient participation in the PFDR will enable improved comparative effectiveness data of transvaginal mesh procedures to native tissue and nonsurgical (pessary) treatment options, which will ultimately aid in patient counseling and provide opportunities for surgeons to review their own outcome data.

References

1. Ward K, Hilton P. Prospective multicentre randomized trial of tension-free vaginal tape and colposuspension as primary treatment for stress incontinence. BMJ. 2002 Jul 13;325 (7355):67.
2. Surgical mesh for treatment of women with pelvic organ prolapse and stress urinary incontinence. FDA Executive Summary, ObGyn Devices Advisory Committee, Sept 8–9, 2011. https://wayback.archive-it.org/7993/20170404140406/https://www.fda.gov/downloads/AdvisoryCommittees/CommitteesMeetingMaterials/MedicalDevices/MedicalDevicesAdvisoryCommittee/ObstetricsandGynecologyDevices/UCM270402.pdf. Accessed 7 Sept 2017.

3. Littman PM, Culligan PJ. The rapid evolution of vaginal mesh delivery systems for the correction of pelvic organ prolapse, Part 1: clinical data. The Female Patient. 2009;34:32–8.
4. Challoner DR, Vodra WW. Medical devices and health—creating a new regulatory framework for moderate-risk devices. N Engl J Med. 2011;365:977–9.
5. Curfman GD, Redberg RF. Medical devices—balancing regulation and innovation. N Engl J Med. 2011;365:975–7.
6. Rogo-Gupta L, Rodriguez LV, Litwin MS, Herzog TJ, Neugut AI, Lu Y, et al. Trends in surgical mesh use for pelvic organ prolapse from 2000 to 2010. Obstet Gynecol. 2012;120(5):1105–15.
7. Chughtai B, Mao J, Buck J, Kalan S, Sedrakyan A. Use and risks of surgical mesh for pelvic organ prolapse surgery in women in New York state: population based cohort study. BMJ. 2015;350:h2685. Correction: BMJ 2015;350:h3060.
8. Sedrakyan A, Chughtai B, Mao J. Regulatory warnings and use of surgical mesh in pelvic organ prolapse. JAMA Intern Med. 2016;176(2):275–7.
9. FDA strengthens requirements for surgical mesh for the transvaginal repair of pelvic organ prolapse to address safety risks. FDA News Release, 4 Jan 2016. http://www.fda.gov/NewsEvents/Newsroom/PressAnnouncements/ucm479732.htm. Accessed 7 Sept 2017.
10. Bradley CS, Visco AG, Weber LeBrun EE, Barber MD. The pelvic floor disorders registry: purpose and development. Female Pelvic Med Reconstr Surg. 2016;22(2):77–82.
11. Weber LeBrun EE, Adam RA, Barber MD, Boyles SH, Iglesia CB, Lukacz ES, et al. Pelvic floor disorders registry: study design and outcome measures. Female Pelvic Med Reconstr Surg. 2016;22:70–6.
12. Vaginal placement of synthetic mesh for pelvic organ prolapse. Committee Opinion No. 513. American College of Obstetricians and Gynecologists. Obstet Gynecol 2011;118:1459–64.
13. Guideline for providing privileges and credentials to physicians for transvaginal placement of surgical mesh for pelvic organ prolapse. Female Pelvic Med Reconstr Surg. 2012;18:194–6.
14. Eilber KS, Alperin M, Khan A, Wu N, Pashos CL, Clemens JQ, Anger JT. The role of the surgeon on the outcomes of vaginal prolapse surgery with mesh. Female Pelvic Med Reconstr Surg. 2017;23(5):293–6.

Chapter 10
Innovation Breeds Innovation: How Pelvic Floor Ultrasound Filled the Diagnostic Gap for Vaginal Mesh Kit Complications

Jonia Alshiek and S. Abbas Shobeiri

Introduction

Vaginal mesh kit complications created dilemmas that the physicians, the patients, or the industry had not encountered before. As the patients suffered, the manufacturers did not offer innovative solutions for diagnosis, evaluation or management of defective products. The innovative gap in all these areas were offered by the physicians. This has been a recurrent theme in the story of medical device innovations. When bad things happen, the physician has to create new tools to solve the problem or adapt the existing tools to the needs at hand. In this chapter we discuss the adaptive innovative role that ultrasound played in diagnois and management of mesh complications.

The use of vaginal mesh kits in urogynecologic and urologic practices has increased rapidly in the past two decades. The pelvic floor is a multifaceted structure functionally and anatomically. Muscles, nerves, and connective tissue all play a role in its adequate functioning. Many factors, including birth-related trauma and age, play a role in pelvic floor dysfunctions. Much progress has been made in the diagnosis of pelvic floor dysfunction, and pelvic floor ultrasonography is becoming mainstream in the academic and major medical centers. Traditionally, physical examination, cystoscopy, and urodynamics have been the bases of pelvic floor diagnosis. Now,

J. Alshiek
Department of Obstetrics and Gynecology, Inova Women's Hospital, Virginia Commonwealth University, Falls Church, VA, USA

Tel Aviv Sourasky Medical Center, Sackler Faculty of Medicine, Tel Aviv University, Tel Aviv, Israel

S. A. Shobeiri (✉)
INOVA Health System, Falls Church, VA, USA
e-mail: Abbas.shobeiri@inova.org

S. A. Shobeiri (ed.), *The Innovation and Evolution of Medical Devices*,
https://doi.org/10.1007/978-3-319-97073-8_10

cheap, simple, noninvasive two-dimensional (2D), three-dimensional (3D), or four-dimensional (4D) office ultrasound is in widespread use. Physicians have learned to view all compartments of the pelvic floor in order (1) to find the causes of dysfunction, (2) to plan treatment, and (3) to evaluate outcomes. More and more clinical studies are illustrating the value of a thorough pelvic floor ultrasound examination that includes endovaginal and endoanal as well as transperineal imaging.

Polypropylene mesh, which is difficult to visualize clearly with radiography, computed tomography (CT), or magnetic resonance imaging (MRI), is hyperechogenic [1] on pelvic floor ultrasound [2]. With the emergence of vaginal mesh complications, physicians soon learned that ultrasound was the only modality to reliably visualize the course of vaginal mesh. The use of these diverse techniques and approaches of ultrasound imaging became highly helpful in assessing the presence of transvaginal mesh (TVM), its locations, and its complications [3–8]. Ultrasound allowed fast, multicompartmental assessment, facilitating optimal patient throughput. It allowed for high-resolution assessment of the morphology and function of the different parts of the pelvic floor. It facilitated observation of the entire pelvic floor with minimal disruption to the natural condition of the structures. Moreover, ultrasound findings have aided in surgical planning for correction in patients involved with vaginal mesh complications or reoperations. Ultrasound has proven useful in understanding the etiology of dyspareunia and pelvic pain associated with mesh. It has also been helpful in patients with a previous mesh surgery in whom the exact nature of the surgery or the location of mesh is unknown. The information derived from pelvic floor ultrasonography has affected the success and failure of surgical procedures and the rate of mesh complications [9–11].

This chapter will focus on the history and types of mesh used in pelvic organ prolapse (POP) operations and on the ultrasound imaging of mesh complications gained from different imaging approaches.

Historical Perspective on How Ultrasound Became Important for Mesh Imaging and Type of Vaginal Meshes

Increasing life expectancy produces a growing number of older women looking for gynecological care; POP is the most common gynecological pathology leading to hysterectomy in women older than 55 years of age [12]. Pelvic organ prolapse has significant unfavorable effects on women's health and quality of life. The lifetime risk for POP surgery has been approximated to be around 11.1% [13], and 30% of these women will undergo at least one reoperation for recurrent prolapse [14]. Studies regarding the etiology and genetic influence that are targeted at explicating this problem are still ongoing. The need for POP surgery rises with age [15], and it has been anticipated that the surgical workload associated with POP will increase by 46% over the next three decades as our population ages [16]. As stated by the 2010 Census population report, the female population in the United States has reached more than 157 million (50.8%); as many as 9,420,000 of these women could be vulnerable for POP surgery [17].

Pelvic reconstructive surgery for genital prolapse, with or without mesh, is accompanied by a considerable improvement in quality of life and prolapse-related symptoms [18]. Sacrocolpopexy has become the standard abdominal procedure to correct POP; in the past century, the Amreich-Richter sacrospinous fixation had been used widely as a vaginal surgical approach. However, the simple design of vaginal mesh kits, combined with the forceful marketing of these products to general obstetrician/gynecologists and urologists, resulted in prompt adoption of these techniques in clinical practice without well designed long-term trials or scientific evidence.

In the past decade, various heterologous meshes for POP treatments were introduced to the market in order to popularize vaginal POP surgery. The use of artificial meshes has a long tradition in abdominal wall surgery. Since the 1950s, surgical mesh has been used to repair abdominal hernias. Abdominal hernia repair has been plagued with complications, including pain, mesh shrinkage, and recurrence. In the 1970s, gynecologists started using abdominal hernia mesh products for abdominal POP repair, and in the 1990s urogynecologists began using surgical mesh for surgical treatment of stress urinary incontinence (SUI). In selective cases, skilled surgeons would cut the mesh to the required shape for POP or SUI repair and then implant the mesh through a corresponding incision. Medical device representatives often insisted on being in the operating rooms to capture these observations and to report up to the chain of command. This observation motivated manufacturers to create vaginal mesh products targeted for SUI and POP repair marketed to a wider audience of gynecologists and urologists [19].

In 1996, the surgical fabrics device (ProteGen Sling) (Boston Scientific, Marlborough, Massachusetts, USA) was the first pre-configured surgical mesh product designed for surgical treatment of SUI. The ProteGen was soon removed from the market because of its complications, and to this day patients still present with its complications. In 2002, Gynemesh® PS (Ethicon/Gynecare, Somerville, New Jersey, USA) became the first surgical mesh product designed for POP repair, which surgeons could cut and use for either abdominal or vaginal repair. Again, this observation prompted the manufacturers to create vaginal mesh products that metamorphosed into "kits" that included tools helping in the delivery and insertion of the vaginal mesh. The industry's rationale behind the creation of vaginal mesh kits was that the mesh for sacrocolpopexies had minimal profit margin and could be used only by more skilled or fellowship-trained physicians. The industry was looking for a disruptive technology to disseminate POP repair among the less trained general obstetrician/gynecologists and urologists.

Because of the precedence for mesh use for abdominal hernia repair and trocar use in sling procedures, the industry made the gigantic leap of putting the meshes and trocars together and introducing them into the POP market via the US Food and Drug Administration (FDA) 510(k) process. A 510(k) is a premarket submission made to the FDA to demonstrate that the device to be marketed is at least as safe and effective – that is, substantially equivalent to – a legally marketed device (21 Code of Federal Regulations [CFR] 807.92[a] [3]), and it is not subject to premarket approval. Meanwhile Tyco (Australia) introduced IVS Tunneller, which was a dual-purpose incontinence sling or POP repair sling that could be inserted into the apex of the vagina via two perirectal incisions. The first kits for POP repair, the AMS Apogee™ System and the AMS Perigee™ System (American Medical Systems, Minnetonka, Minnesota, USA), were cleared in 2004. Surgical mesh kits continued to differ in regard to introducer instrumentation, tissue fixation anchors, surgical technique, and incorporation of absorbable materials into the mesh, features intended to differentiate one company's kit from another's as the companies rushed to enter the POP market [19]. The FDA then approved the Prolift (Ethicon/Gynecare) among many other kits. The Prolift required inserting trocars into the pudendal nerve space between the sacrospinous and sacrotuberous ligaments. This is a sacred space to pelvic surgeons, as the pudendal nerve is responsible for the clitoral, urethral, vaginal, perineal, and anal selection. Injury to the main branch of the pudendal nerve results in pain in all branches, and selective injury to single branches can result in anything from pain to spasm or voiding and defecatory dysfunction. Pudendal neuralgia in the presence of mesh and scarring was a new area of diagnostic and therapeutic challenge. Based on the update released by the FDA in 2010, "at least 100,000 POP repairs that used surgical mesh" were performed and "about 75,000 of these were transvaginal procedures" [19]. This statement suggested that at least 225,000 TVM procedures were done in a 3-year period (2008–2010) [20].

During the past decade, gynecologists have been introduced to a variety of graft materials placed in the vagina as an alternative or augmentation to the traditional native tissue surgical repairs of POP. This was attributed to the assumption that use of mesh improves the outcome of the surgical correction while reducing the recurrence rate of POP. This hypothesis has since been disproven for the posterior compartment. Nonetheless, several "mesh kits" were introduced onto the surgical market, promoting a minimally invasive alternative to the conventional methods of surgical repairs of rectocele and posterior POP. The purpose of developing mesh kits was to raise the longevity of POP repairs. In general, mesh products for POP repair were designed to match the anatomical defect they are targeted to correct. The majority of the meshes are used for anterior prolapse repair, followed by posterior and apical vaginal repair. The main goal of using grafts in reconstructive surgery was reconstructing the deformed anatomy with a material that was apparently safe and offered an anatomically proper result. The ideal graft desired was believed to be inert, non-carcinogenic, with high tensile strength and flexibility, nonallergenic, noninflammatory, able to be sterilized, non-modifiable by body tissue, convenient, and cheap. However, except for the patient's native tissues, there has never been an obtainable graft that has all of these features.

Synthetic meshes are classified into four types based on filament number and pore size:

- Type 1 meshes are polypropylene, monofilament, and microporous (75 m) (e.g., Marlex; Atrium™ [American Medical Systems, Minnetonka, Minnesota, USA], Gynecare Gynemesh™ [Ethicon, Somerville, New Jersey, USA], Pelvitex™ [C. R. Bard, Murray Hill, New Jersey, USA]).
- Type 2 meshes are microporous (10 m) and multifilamentous (e.g., Gore-Tex™ [W. L. Gore Associates, Newark, Delaware, USA]).
- Type 3 meshes are multifilamentous, although having both microporous and microporous components (e.g., Teflon™ [DuPont de Nemours, Wilmington, Delaware, USA], Mersilene [Ethicon], IVS™ [Tyco Healthcare/US Surgical, Norwalk, Connecticut, USA]).

- Type 4 meshes, also known as polypropylene sheets, have a pore size of 1 micrometer (e.g., Silastic™ [C. R. Bard], Celgard™ [Celgard, Charlotte, North Carolina, USA]) [21].

The first FDA formal public alert regarding complications related to the use of mesh for POP repair was in 2008. Despite this warning, interest in mesh kits continued between 2008 and 2010 [20]. Complications reported to the MAUDE (Manufacturer and User Facility Device Experience) database following the initial warning ultimately led the FDA to issue an updated public health notification in 2011 that included a significantly stronger warning for transvaginal POP meshes [20]. In 2014, the FDA suggested that surgical mesh for transvaginal POP repair be reclassified from class II devices to class III, thus necessitating better safety and efficacy data for mesh kits prior to FDA approval. This reclassification was based on the tentative determination that the previously used mechanisms of approval were not sufficient to provide reasonable assurance of safety and effectiveness for this device. In addition, the FDA proposed to reclassify urogynecologic surgical mesh instrumentation (e.g., manual gastroenterology-urology surgical instrument and accessories or manual surgical instrument for general use) from class I to class II. On its own initiative based on new information [20], the FDA is reclassifying both the surgical mesh for transvaginal repair and the urogynecologic surgical mesh instrumentation. A fivefold increase in the number of adverse medical device reports associated with mesh for POP in the years after the initial warning also prompted the FDA to release a safety communication in 2011 [22]. The updated FDA warning stated that vaginal mesh was not consistently found to be more efficient than native tissue repair and may expose patients to higher risks [19]. Although the FDA communication was written to prompt understanding of the risks associated with vaginal mesh and to encourage informed decision-making by patients and healthcare providers, it caused in a lot of confusion, controversy, and concern regarding the role of vaginal mesh [22]. At the present time, most urogynecologists are trained mostly with vaginal mesh kits, thus missing the benefit of training to perform traditional pelvic reconstructive surgery. Against this historical background, we review mesh complications, with specific emphasis on vaginally placed mesh and ultrasound findings.

2D Transperineal, 2D/3D Endovaginal, and Endoanal Instrumentation and Techniques for Pelvic Floor Imaging

A fair amount of information can be obtained with an abdominal 2D concave probe that is placed on the perineum [23]. Additional information can be obtained by endovaginal and endoanal imaging. For 2D imaging any available 2–8-MHz abdominal probe can be used for scanning of the pelvic floor. The images in this chapter are from a BK abdominal probe used for transperineal imaging, unless specified otherwise (Fig. 10.1). In skilled hands, much can be accomplished even with this simple probe. Endocavitary or introital high-resolution 3D allows the automatic acquisition and construction of high-resolution data volumes by synthesis of a high

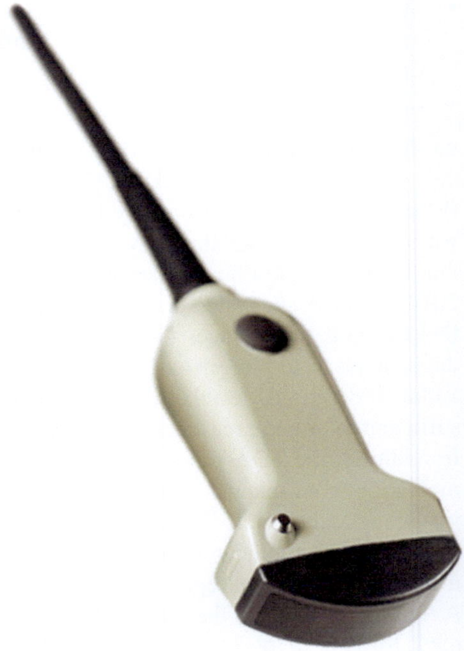

Fig. 10.1 BK abdominal probe used for transperineal imaging (BK Ultrasound, Analogic, Peabody, MA, USA)

number of parallel transaxial or radial 2D images, ensuring that true dimensions in all three *x*, *y*, and *z* planes are equivalent. The constructed data cube technique provides accurate distance, area, angle, and volume measurements. The volume-rendering technique resulting from high-resolution 3D provides accurate visualization of the deeper structures. High-resolution endovaginal or endoanal anatomy can be obtained in 30–60 s. The scanned data set is also highly reproducible, with limited operator dependency. The probe can visualize all rectal wall layers; evaluate the radial, longitudinal extension of sphincter tears; and measure detailed pelvic floor architecture in all *x*, *y*, and *z* planes accurately (Fig. 10.2). The 3D probes allow for acquisition of radial or axial 2D images without any movement of the probe within the cavity. The set of 2D images is instantaneously reconstructed into a high-resolution 3D image for real-time manipulation and volume rendering. The 3D volume can also be archived for offline analysis.

Multicompartmental Ultrasonographic Techniques

During examination, the patient may be placed in the dorsal lithotomy, the left lateral, or the prone position. The patient's positioning depends on cultural factors, local acceptable practices, physician's specialty, and equipment availability. In the United States, urogynecologists perform pelvic examination in dorsal lithotomy

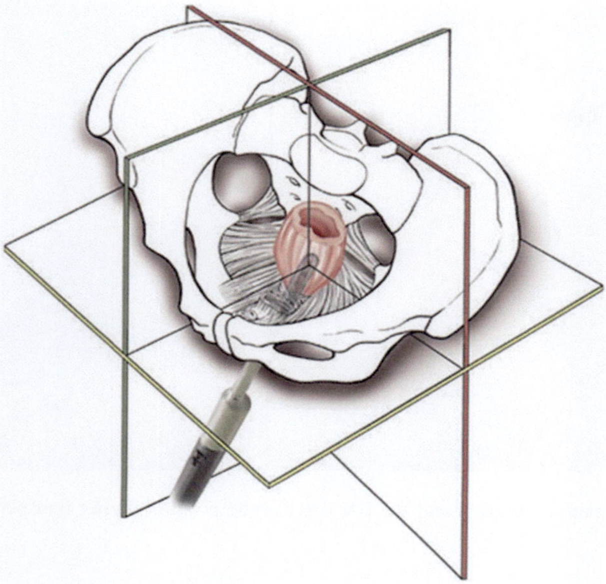

Fig. 10.2 *x*, *y*, *z* planes in relation to an endocavitary probe

position. At our institution, the pelvic floor ultrasound, including endoanal examinations, is performed in dorsal lithotomy position. This position allows symmetrical acquisition of ultrasound volumes regardless of their being done endovaginally or endoanally [24, 25]. Transperineal ultrasound is most useful for indirect assessment of pelvic floor function. Measuring the distance from the symphysis pubis to the levator plate gives the anterior posterior (AP) measurement of the minimal levator hiatus, which can be measured at rest and in Valsalva (Fig. 10.3).

2D endovaginal or introital anterior compartment imaging is indicated for voiding dysfunction, enterocele, cystocele, location of mesh and slings, anterior vaginal masses and cysts, and fistulas. The probe is gently placed at the introitus or in the vagina (Fig. 10.4). Measurements of the urethral structures or any visible mesh or sling can be obtained (Fig. 10.5) [26].

2D endovaginal posterior compartment imaging is indicated for defecatory dysfunction, constipation, intussusception, sigmoidocele, enterocele, rectocele, perineocele, mesh, posterior vaginal masses and cysts, and fistulas. 2D dynamic view of the anal canal and the levator plate comes to view (Fig. 10.6). Measurements of the external anal sphincter (EAS), internal anal sphincter (IAS), and any visible mesh can be obtained. Even in 2D posterior imaging, an EAS that is intact at the 12 o'clock position can be visualized. Ask the patient to squeeze and Valsalva to visualize any high rectocele, enterocele, sigmoidocele, or intussusception.

3D 360° endovaginal imaging is indicated for mesh, vaginal masses and cysts, levator ani muscle subdivisions, and defects. During endocavitary imaging the

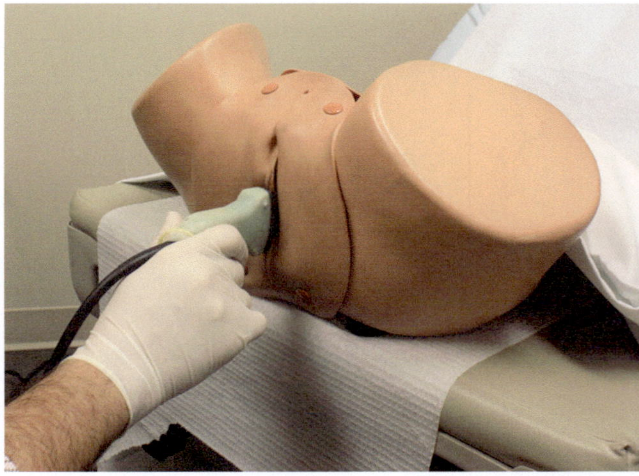

Fig. 10.3 The patient position and the BK 8802 probe position during transperineal scanning. (© Shobeiri)

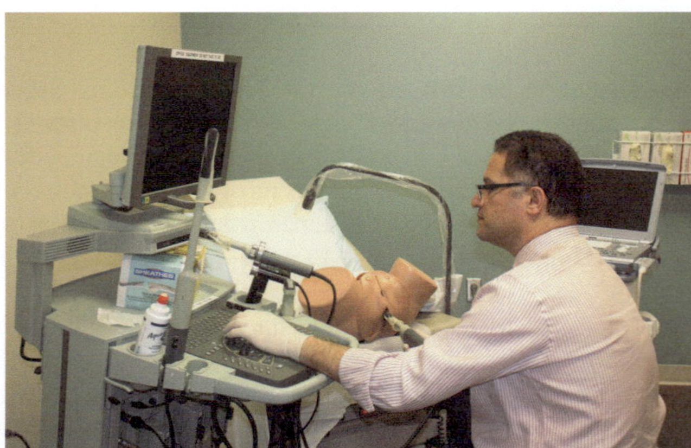

Fig. 10.4 Correct two-handed operation of the probe and the machine. (© Shobeiri 2013)

patient may be tempted to talk to alleviate her anxiety. It is important to calm the patients, let them know what is happening, and share with them that during scanning their talking and body movements may distort the desired image acquisition [27–29]. Once the probe is in position, the 3D button is pushed and 3D volume acquisition is started (Fig. 10.7).

3D 360 endoanal imaging is indicated for perianal masses and cysts, perianal fistulas, and anal sphincter injury. This modality is used only if anal sphincter injury is suspected or in cases where the vagina is short, such as in cases of vaginal agenesis or vaginal collapse and scarring due to implanted mesh. This modality is excellent for getting close to the sacrospinous ligaments to view the mesh arms.

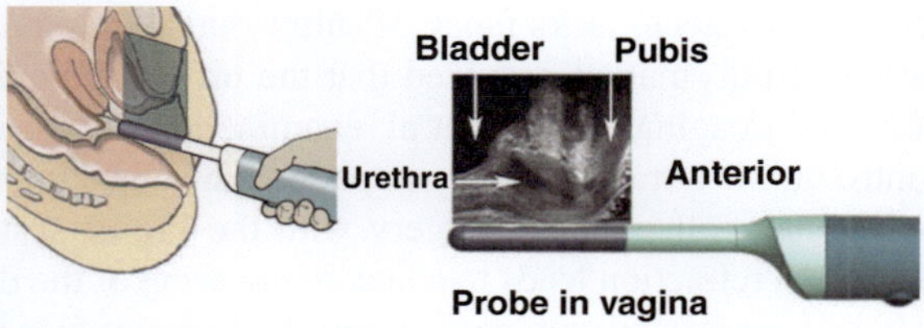

Fig. 10.5 Composite of anterior compartment imaging with BK 8838 probe. To the *right* the image as seen on the screen is demonstrated. The probe is advanced to the vesicourethral junction to visualize the full length of the urethra. (© Shobeiri 2013)

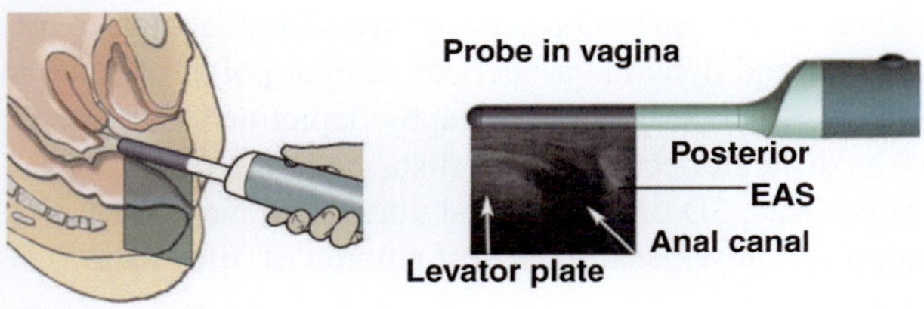

Fig. 10.6 Composite of posterior compartment imaging with 8838 probe. To the *right* the image as seen on the screen is demonstrated. The probe is advanced until the perineal body/EAS complex is visualized to the *right* of the screen. (© Shobeiri 2013)

Fig. 10.7 8838 probe vaginal placement. The probe is generally advanced until the vesicourethral junction is viewed. Pressing the 3D button will obtain radial images of the pelvic floor that will be packaged as a 3D volume

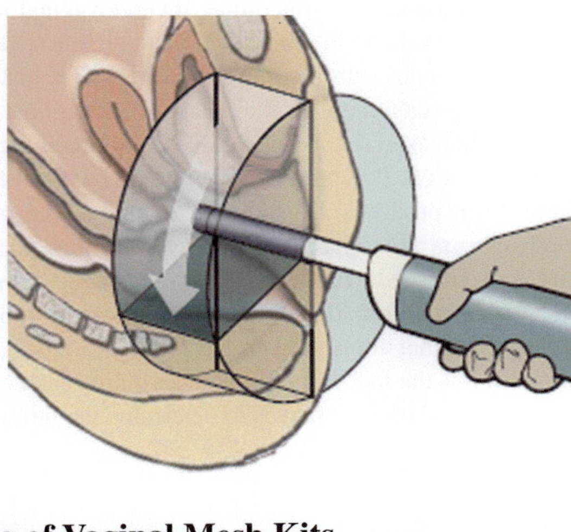

Ultrasonographic Imaging of Vaginal Mesh Kits

Perineal/Introital Approach

Tunn et al. reported polypropylene mesh identification postoperatively using the introital approach. A 5-MHz vaginal sector probe was used to identify the implants in midsagittal view to measure the distal-to-proximal length and thickness [4]. The study demonstrated that much could be accomplished with a simple 2D perineal ultrasound probe. If a physician lacks fancy 3D ultrasound equipment, 2D imaging may provide sufficient information provided that the urogynecologist is trained in pelvic floor ultrasound imaging. Velemir et al. examined mesh appearance postoperatively using introital 2D ultrasonography in patients who had undergone anterior and/or posterior vaginal wall prolapse surgery with the Prolift system. They concluded that severe mesh retraction leads to a lack of covering of the distal part of the vaginal walls, which is associated with posterior prolapse recurrence [6]. In addition, in a previous study aimed at exploring the correlation between mesh appearance and success after 6 months of anterior vaginal mesh repair, the introital ultrasound approach was used and demonstrated that mesh retraction was significantly greater in patients who reported de novo overactive bladder and vaginal pain [30].

In the literature 2D, 3D, and 4D perineal/introital techniques are widely reported to identify anatomic and dynamic aspects of vaginal polypropylene mesh implants [7, 23, 31]. However, 2D perineal sonography depiction of the location of vaginal mesh kits may be difficult because of the distance to the mesh arms. Therefore, for these groups of patients, 3D or 4D perineal ultrasound may be helpful [32], and the endovaginal approach provides the greatest amount of information.

Endovaginal Approach

A recent study demonstrated that 3D endovaginal ultrasound (EVUS) imaging is the best tool to evaluate the presence, location, and extent of polypropylene mesh, especially in patients with a complicated treatment history [3]. 3D EVUS has proven to have a high sensitivity for the detection of vaginal mesh or slings. As a result, it can explain the reason for complications or failure and aid in the planning of further surgical intervention. Polypropylene mesh can be clearly identified with 3D EVUS sonography, as it produces a distinct echogenic signal on sonography [5]. Polypropylene mesh appears as a thin echogenic wavy structure adjacent to the vaginal wall with minimal acoustic shadowing. The anterior mesh is demonstrated under the bladder neck and proximal urethra (Fig. 10.8), and the posterior mesh is demonstrated under vaginal and transvaginal ultrasound probe (Fig. 10.9). The advantage of multicompartment 3D ultrasound is the fact that the 3D data volume can be manipulated using a combination of straight and oblique planes to determine the intrapelvic course of mesh implants.

Endoanal Approach

Endoanal ultrasonography (EAUS) and endorectal ultrasonography (ERUS) are also useful in determining the location and extent of mesh implants. EAUS is especially useful in evaluating vaginal mesh kits when the upper vagina has collapsed. By using the endoanal approach, one can get past the short vagina and image the

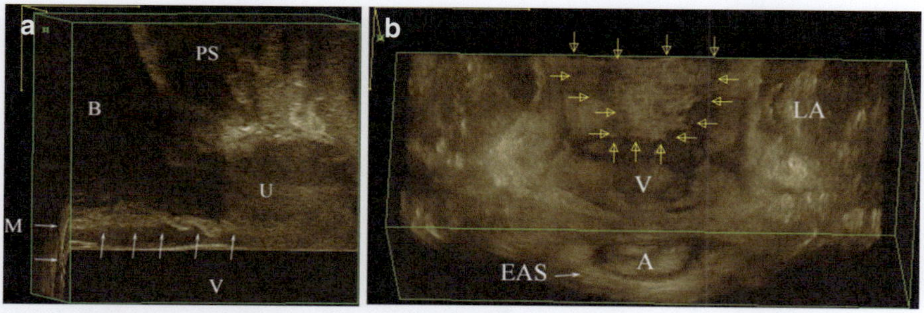

Fig. 10.8 (**a**) 3D endovaginal ultrasound image (anterior compartment) in sagittal plane showing the anterior vaginal wall mesh (M). Bladder (B), urethra (U), vagina (V), pubic symphysis (PS). (**b**) 3D coronal tilted view of the posterior compartment obtained using an endovaginal probe. *Arrows* point to the edges of the posterior mesh. External anal sphincter (EAS), vagina (V), levator ani (LA), anus (A). (© Shobeiri)

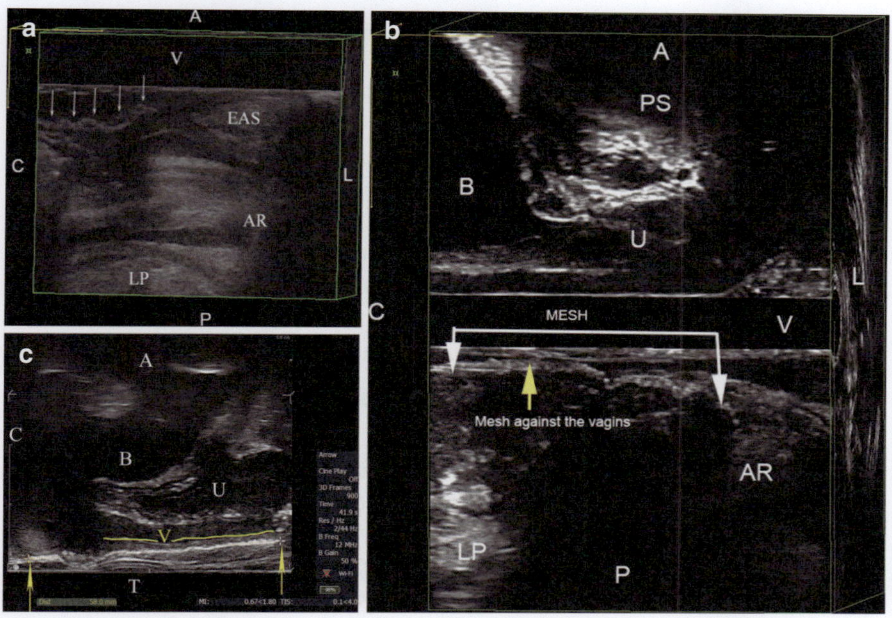

Fig. 10.9 (**a**) 3D endovaginal ultrasound image (posterior compartment) in sagittal plane showing the posterior vaginal wall mesh (*white arrows*). Vagina (V), anorectum (AR), external anal sphincter (EAS), levator plate (LP); anterior (A), posterior (P), cephalad (C), left (L). (**b**) 3D endovaginal ultrasound image in midsagittal plane showing the posterior vaginal wall mesh prominence (*white arrows*). Vagina (V), anorectum (AR), levator plate (LP), anterior (A), posterior (P), cephalad (C), left (L), urethra (U). (**c**) 3D endoanal ultrasound image in midsagittal plane showing the posterior vaginal wall mesh in full length (*yellow arrows* point to the 58-mm cursors) past the apex of the vagina (V) (*yellow line*). Transducer (T) in the anorectum, anterior (A), bladder (B), cephalad (C), urethra (U). (© Shobeiri)

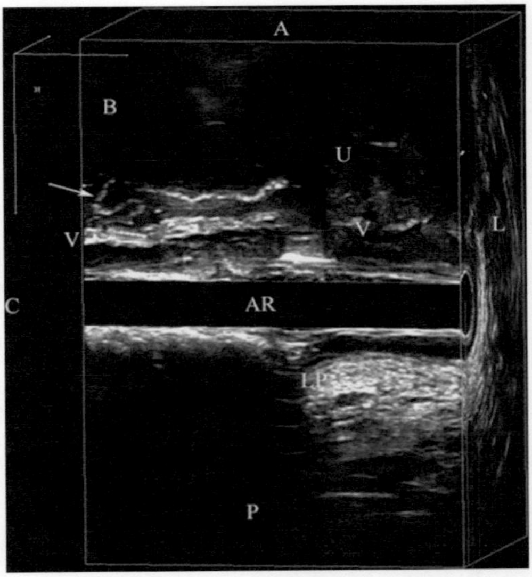

Fig. 10.10 360° 3D endoanal ultrasound image in sagittal plane showing the folding anterior vaginal wall mesh (*yellow arrow*). Bladder (V), urethra (U), vagina (V), anorectum (AR), levator plate (LP), anterior (A), posterior (P), cephalad (C), left (L). © Shobeiri

sacrospinous-sacrospinous mesh bridge created by the mesh (see Fig. 10.9c). When a tight bridge exists, the operator must be careful while advancing the probe, should there be any resistance. Additionally, sometimes the endoanal approach may be better tolerated in patients with levator ani muscle spasm or myalgia. The folded anterior vaginal mesh is demonstrated in Fig. 10.10. Figure 10.11 shows posterior vaginal mesh located at the perineum. A useful modality for visualization of mesh is the rendered view of the mesh (see Fig. 10.11b, c).

Mesh Complications and Ultrasonographic Findings

Transvaginal mesh has been used for POP repair for many years, and complications related to mesh have been widely reported. A Cochrane review reported an erosion rate of 10.3% after anterior vaginal wall repair with polypropylene mesh [33]. A systematic review from 2014 concluded that the mean total complication rates in anterior, posterior, and combined mesh repair are 8–27%, 3.5–20%, and 13–40%, respectively [34]. Complications related to mesh in female pelvic floor surgery are classified according to the International Urogynecological Association (IUGA)/International Continence Society (ICS) into (1) local complications, (2) complications to surrounding organs, and (3) systemic complications [35]. A recent retrospective multicenter chart review stated that the affected site of mesh complications could occur at the area or away from the suture line in 250 patients with TVM complications after POP surgery [36]. Ultrasound findings related to complications of TVM will be discussed according to the IUGA/ICS classification.

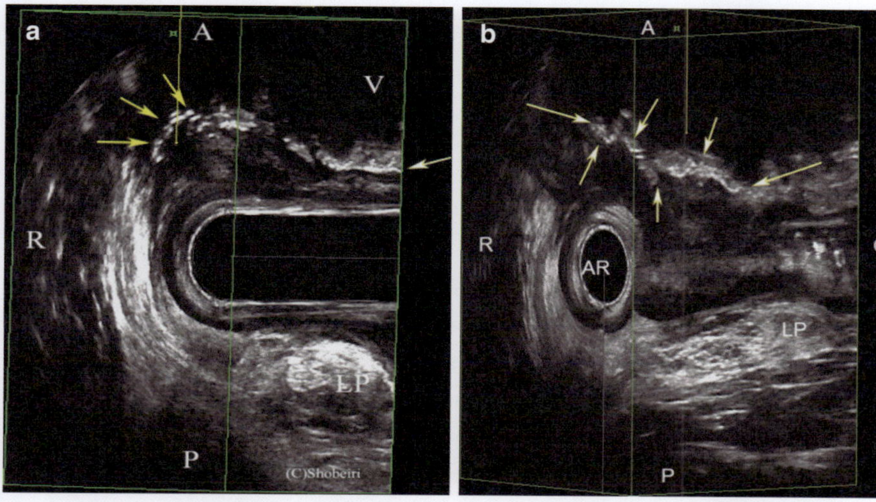

Fig. 10.11 (**a**) 360° 3D endoanal ultrasound image in midsagittal plane showing the posterior vaginal wall mesh (*yellow arrows*) at the perineum. Vagina (V), levator plate (LP), anterior (A), posterior (P), right (R). (**b**) 360° 3D endoanal ultrasound image in left parasagittal plane showing the posterior vaginal wall mesh (*yellow arrows*) with anterior extrusion. Levator plate (LP), anterior (A), posterior (P), right (R), cephalad (C), anterior (A). (**c**) 360° 3D endoanal ultrasound rendered image in left parasagittal plane showing the posterior vaginal wall mesh (*yellow arrows*) with anterior extrusion. The mesh is enhanced in the rendered post-processing. Levator plate (LP), anterior (A), posterior (P), right (R), cephalad (C). (**d**) Unprocessed view of a 3D endovaginal ultrasound volume cut in coronal plane showing the posterior vaginal wall mesh (*outlined* is the pathognomonic mesh lattice). In this view the vagina cannot be seen, as the image is looking posteriorly from inside the vagina. Anorectum (AR), levator ani muscle (levator M), anterior (A), cephalad (C), left (L), posterior (P), right (R). (**e**) Post-processed rendered view of a 3D endovaginal ultrasound volume cut in coronal plane showing the posterior vaginal wall mesh (*outlined* is the pathognomonic mesh lattice); the arrows point to the left mesh arm. In this view the vagina cannot be seen, as the image is looking posteriorly from inside the vagina. Note that the posterior mesh generally pulls away from the anal sphincter complex. Here a *line* is drawn to denote where the detached mesh is shrunken and coiled compared to the more superior aspect of the mesh. Anorectum (A), puborectalis (PR), iliococcygeus (IC), ischiorectal fat (IRF), cephalad (C), left (L), posterior (P), right (R). (**f**) 360° 3D endovaginal ultrasound volume midsagittal plane showing the left side of the pelvis with anterior and posterior vaginal wall mesh. In this view the mesh in the anterior vagina is 1 mm, and the posterior mesh is 2 mm (*large arrows*) from the vaginal epithelium. Vagina (V), anorectum (AR), anterior (A), cephalad (C), left (L), posterior (P), urethra (U), bladder (B). (**g**) 360° 3D endovaginal ultrasound volume midsagittal plane showing the left side of the pelvis with posterior sacrocolpoperineopexy mesh (SCP) and a sling (S). In this view the SCP mesh is deeper than what is typically seen with vaginal mesh. Note that both the SCP and the sling mesh create acoustic shadowing that obscures underlying structures. Transducer (T), sling (S), bladder (B), anorectum (AR), anterior (A), cephalad (C), left (L), posterior (P). (**h**) 360° 3D endovaginal ultrasound volume midsagittal plane showing the bladder with an implanted mesh (*arrows*) and a growth at the trigone (*denoted with Ca)*. The growth proved to be a neoplasm. Transducer (T), bladder (B), anterior (A), cephalad (C), bladder (B), urethra (U). (© Shobeiri)

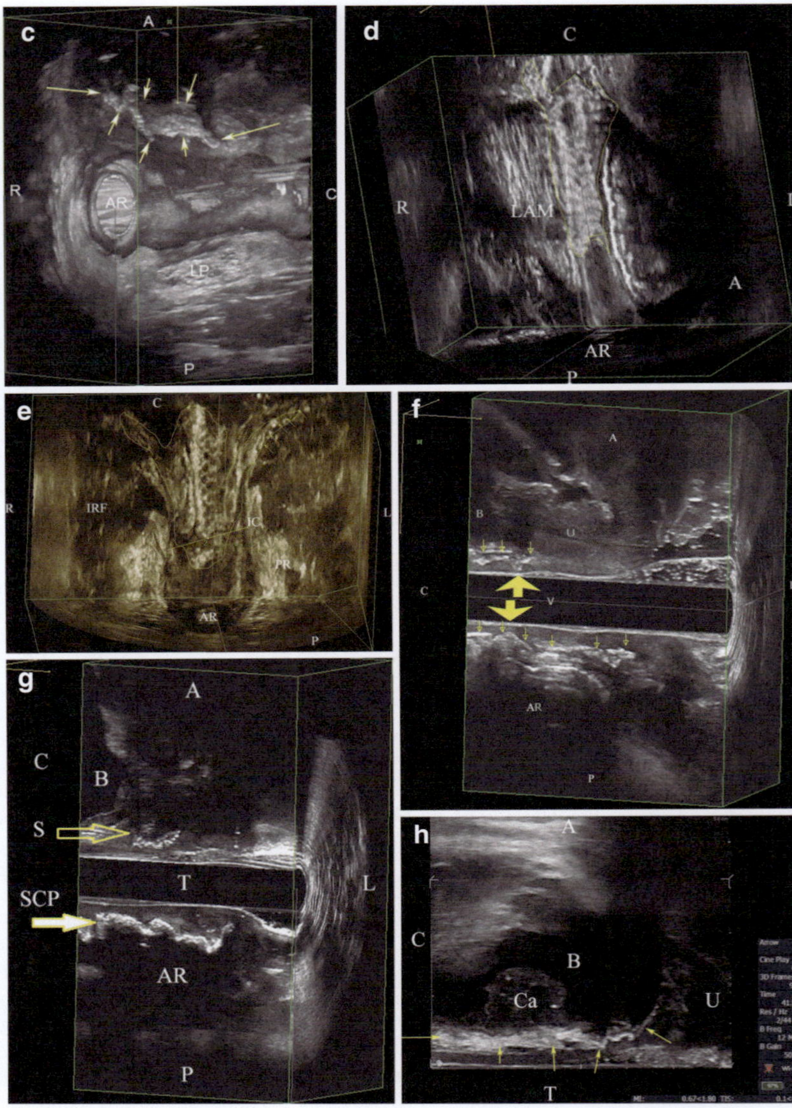

Fig. 10.11 (continued)

Mesh Contraction (Shrinkage)

One of the more disappointing aspects of vaginal mesh was the fact that it sometimes failed, especially in the anterior compartment. The anterior mesh kits such as the AMS Perigee did not have secure anterior anchoring points and bunched up (Fig. 10.12). Mesh contraction can be associated with the development of focally painful segments of hardened mesh. This phenomenon likely underlies the

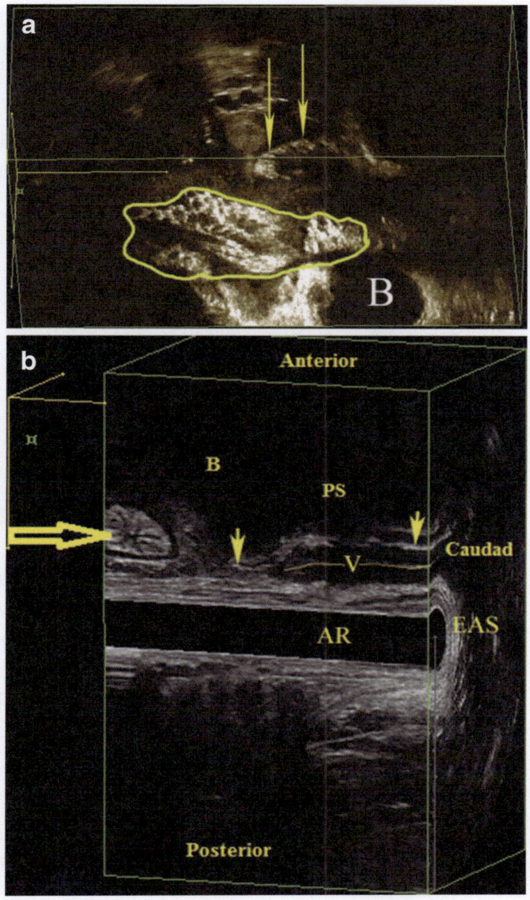

Fig. 10.12 (**a**) 360° 3D endovaginal ultrasound rendered image showing the apical shrunken mesh and one arm of the mesh. Bladder (B). (**b**) 360° 3D endoanal ultrasound midsagittal image showing an anterior mesh that is flat (*two yellow arrows*). The patient has an apical symptomatic enterocele (*hollow arrow*). The physical exam is not significant. An apical sacrocolpopexy relieved patient of her symptoms. Bladder (B), transducer in anorectum (AR), pubic symphysis (PS), vagina (V), external anal sphincter (EAS). (© Shobeiri)

development of primary vaginal pain syndromes and dyspareunia following vaginal mesh use. Pain can usually be reproduced by palpation of the contracted mesh segment, typically along the apical mesh arms. Collagen deposition and contraction within the mesh pores may be responsible for mesh hardening and nerve fiber entrapment; a more plausible cause of this finding is over-tensioning of the mesh arms during implantation. The main clinical features include severe vaginal pain with movement, dyspareunia, and focal tenderness over contracted portions of the mesh on vaginal examination. Exact etiology of shrinkage of synthetic mesh after implantation is most likely inflammation and tissue ingrowth, but different theories have been suggested. Graft shrinkage could be due to physical consequence of the inflammatory response to the mesh or the result of inadequate tissue ingrowth into the mesh. There is growing evidence to suggest that synthetic mesh shrinks significantly once incorporated in the biological tissues.

There has been controversy as to whether or not mesh shrinkage and folding are continuous processes or are limited to the immediate postoperative period [4, 6, 37, 38].

The current consensus is that mesh folding and shrinkage are associated with complications and pain [9]. Based on this assumption, it has been proposed that, together with investing in the development of new materials, the focus should be on improving surgical technique and quality control in order to allow the mesh to be implanted flat and well spread out, anchored to underlying tissues, thus preventing immediate postoperative folding [9]. Ultrasound imaging is used to evaluate the appearance of polypropylene meshes on the significance of mesh shrinkage and folding. Moreover, 3D EVUS can also be helpful in mapping meshes placed in multiple compartments when physical examination cannot exactly locate the existence of contraction. 3D EVUS also nicely demonstrates the mesh arms to the sacrospinous ligaments. An arm under tension may be harder to see as it ropes (see Fig. 10.11d, e).

Mesh Extrusion

One of the more recognized complications related to vaginally placed mesh is mesh extrusion. Mesh extrusion is considered to be mesh visualized through the vaginal epithelium. Although standardized terminology now exists to describe complications such as mesh erosion or extrusion [35], the variability of the use of the term in the literature makes it difficult to identify exact exposure rates.

Mesh extrusion rates vary from 0% to 25% in different studies [39–41]. A Cochrane review by Maher et al. [33] suggested that use of vaginal mesh was associated with an 11.4% rate of mesh extrusion and a 6.8% rate of surgical re-intervention. A nonsignificant increase in rates of vaginal mesh exposure and reoperation for vaginal mesh exposure after vaginal mesh surgery in comparison with laparoscopic sacrocolpopexy has also been recognized (13% vs. 2%, $P = 0.07$ and 9% vs. 2%, $P = 0.11$, respectively). Symptoms associated with mesh extrusion are not insignificant; they include pelvic pain, infection, de novo dyspareunia (painful sex for patient or partner), de novo vaginal bleeding, atypical vaginal discharge, and the need for additional corrective surgeries [42, 43].

A number of risk factors for mesh extrusion have been identified. Patient factors such as smoking status and vaginal atrophy can affect both the tissue integrity and surgical site healing, making exposure in these individuals more likely [42]. Some studies have recognized older age as a risk factor for exposure, but it is unclear if this association is due strictly to age or to the more advanced vaginal atrophy often seen in older women, especially since a number of studies have not found a difference in extrusion rates between younger and older women [44].

It was recognized early on in the adoption of vaginal meshes that factors related to the mesh itself were capable of increasing the risk of mesh exposure. The majority of studies evaluate the effect of mesh type on extrusion; however, it is reasonable to extrapolate from the effects to their use in prolapse mesh kits. These factors are primarily related to pore size and mesh materials. Polypropylene meshes with large pore size (type 4 meshes) are associated with a lower exposure rate than many of their predecessors, which were designed to be tightly woven or nonporous. Another risk factor for mesh exposure that is now recognized is the depth of the vaginal dissection prior to mesh placement. As evidenced by the recognized risk factors for mesh exposure, prevention of exposure is the optimal "management" strategy for these (and other) complications. Preventative measures include avoiding the above-mentioned risk factors wherever possible, such as the use of lighter-weight polypropylene materials with larger pore sizes, use of transverse vaginal incisions for vaginal dissection (rather than vertical or t-shaped vaginal incisions), avoidance of folding the mesh, appropriate thickness of dissection, and deferring mesh placement to a time remote from hysterectomy. That said, there are no long-term studies showing how long mesh extrusion can be prevented, given the fact that it is implanted in the vesicovaginal or rectovaginal tissue that has an average thickness of 5 mm. Endovaginal ultrasound imaging has the added benefit of placing the probe adjacent to the area of interest. Ultrasound is the only imaging modality that can visualize mesh easily. It has higher sensitivity for detection of mesh presence when physical examination fails to visualize or palpate the mesh in the vaginal canal. The mesh implanted via sacrocolpoperineopexy looks different, as it is deep and anterior to the rectum (see Fig. 10.11f, g).

Urinary Tract or Lower Gastrointestinal Tract Compromise or Perforation

Urinary tract and gastrointestinal tract complications after vaginal mesh surgery are less common than after surgery for the anti-incontinence sling [45]. The violation of the genitourinary system or the gastrointestinal tract by mesh is called erosion. Mesh complications involving the bladder and rectum represent the minority of cases reported [46–49]. Recently, there was increased interest regarding the association between the polypropylene mesh/slings and bladder cancer. Ostergard et al. suggested that since oncogenesis is related to the presence of a foreign body that causes the chronic inflammatory reaction, implantation of the polypropylene mesh may cause carcinogenesis many years later [50]. The possibility of such association has been raised and needs further surveillance. However, based on current evidence, the risk of carcinogenesis related to polypropylene mesh is low [51–53]. Regardless, if a focus of cancer that needs to be resected or removed is close to the underlying mesh, the intervention may be complicated. 3D EVUS can easily demonstrate uroepithelial masses on the trigonal area (see Fig. 10.11h).

In patients with a history of TVM for POP repair or slings for SUI, vaginal, urinary, or bowel problems should be carefully investigated [42]. A detailed clinical history taking and thorough physical examination are essential. Symptoms of abnormal vaginal discharge or bleeding, dyspareunia, pelvic or groin pain, urinary tract infections, voiding dysfunction, urinary incontinence, as well as vaginal bulge and bowel complaints should be documented. Information regarding previous pelvic surgeries, type of mesh used, complications, and treatments is crucial. A careful and gentle pelvic examination is necessary to assess mesh exposure in the relevant compartments, taking account of scar tissue, prolapse, recurrence, SUI, vaginal discharge/bleeding, and areas of tenderness or discomfort. Valsalva maneuver should be performed to investigate prolapse recurrence and SUI. Ultrasound imaging is useful to identify the location of mesh or sling in patients with complications. 3D EVUS of the anterior pelvic compartment shows polypropylene mesh eroding into the bladder in Fig. 10.13.

Musculoskeletal: Pain, Lump, Decreased Elasticity, and Sinus Formation

Pelvic pain, including dyspareunia, is a widely acknowledged complication of mesh exposure. The incidence of mesh-related pelvic pain is as high as 30%. Pelvic pain may be groin pain related to the passage of the mesh arms through the muscle tissue, ligament, or nerve entrapment. In some cases mesh designed to be anchored in the sacrospinous ligament can lead to pudendal and sciatic neuropathies, while mesh passing through the obturator space can cause obturator neuropathies. In our practice, we have seen many patients with pain originating after a mesh procedure develop pelvic floor myalgias, which in turn cause pelvic pain and dyspareunia. A focally painful segment of hardened mesh due to shrinkage of the vaginal mesh implant may lead to primary vaginal pain syndromes and dyspareunia following vaginal mesh use. A recent case series reported high incidence of pain along contracted mesh sites. Severe vaginal pain and focal tenderness are

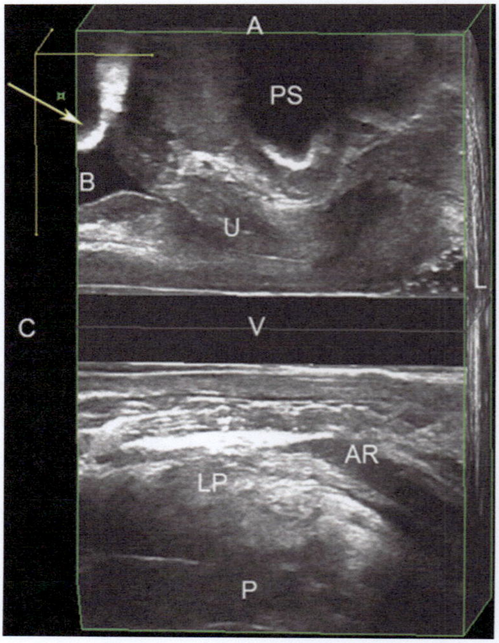

Fig. 10.13 360° 3D endovaginal ultrasound image in sagittal plane showing the sling mesh (*yellow arrow*) in the bladder (B). Vagina (V), pubic symphysis (P), external anal sphincter (EAS), anorectum (AR), levator plate (LP), anterior (A), posterior (P), cephalad (C), left (L). (© Shobeiri)

reported, which can be confirmed by palpation of the mesh segment [54]. To do so, a long cotton swab is introduced in front of the ultrasound probe and the area is probed under ultrasound visualization. It is best to touch the area away from the area of pain in a random fashion and subsequently touch the mesh (Fig. 10.14). In a patient with pudendal neuralgia, all the nerve branch territory is painful. Pressing on the ischial spine may produce pain, and because of nerve entrapment and scarring, the patient may have constant rather than positional pain. Removal of the mesh arms needs to be done via a transgluteal approach, which requires expertise and specialized training. The sacrotuberous ligament is divided or cut to access the pudendal nerve, and then the nerve itself is freed up by removing the underlying sacrospinous ligament. In the presence of mesh and scar tissue, it is almost impossible to remove the mesh arms; even if mesh removal is achieved, the pudendal pain will persist (Fig. 10.15).

The main clinical features of mesh pain can include groin pain, suprapubic pain, dyspareunia, vaginal tightness, severe vaginal pain with movement, and vaginal shortening on vaginal examination. Over-tensioning of the mesh arms during implantation and collagen deposition and contraction within the mesh pores are reported to be responsible for mesh hardening and nerve fiber entrapment. It is always necessary to characterize pain symptoms related to mesh complications vs. chronic pain syndromes or myalgias. The worst cases are patients with chronic pain whose pain is exacerbated due to new mesh pain. Pelvic sonography has the fundamental role in the evaluation of pelvic pain. Transvaginal sonography (TVS) and endovaginal sonography (EVS) with higher resolution of anatomic detail are always the first option in patients with history of mesh placement, especially in the cases

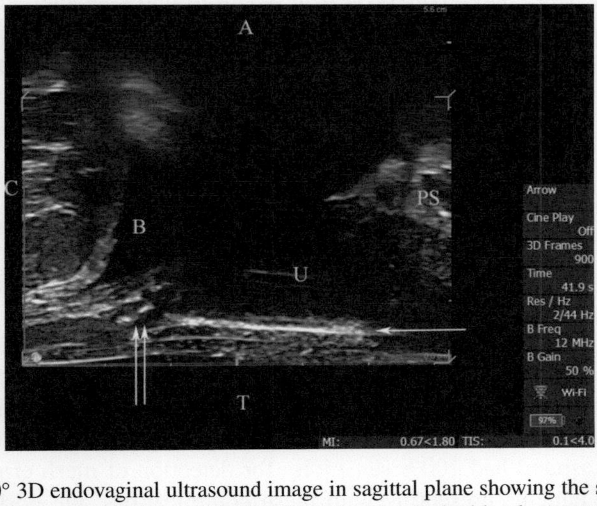

Fig. 10.14 360° 3D endovaginal ultrasound image in sagittal plane showing the sling mesh remnant (*double yellow arrow*) under the bladder (B) being touched with a long cotton swab (*single arrow*) for sensitivity testing with ultrasound guidance. Transducer (T) in vagina, pubic symphysis (PS), anterior (A), cephalad (C), urethra (U). (© Shobeiri)

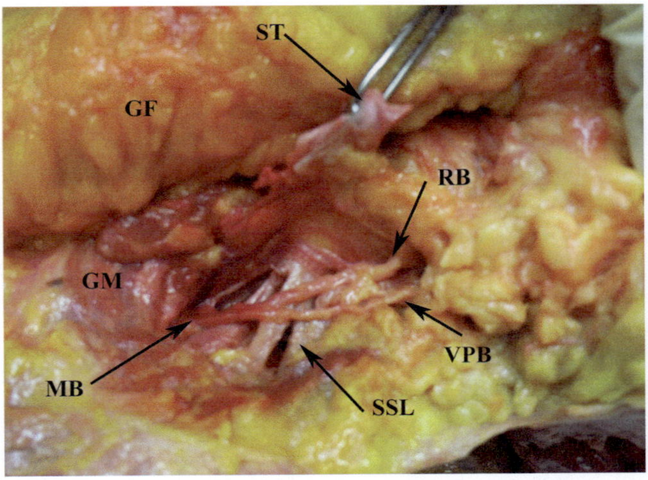

Fig. 10.15 Cadaveric dissection demonstrating the course of the pudendal nerve in relation to the sacrospinous ligament. The pudendal nerve through a space in between the sacrospinous (SSL) and sacrotuberous (ST) ligaments. Here the ST is cut and lifted with an Allis clamp. To get to this space via a posterior approach, the skin is cut, the gluteal fat (GF) is traversed, the glutinous maximus (GM) fascia and fibers are divided, and the ST is located, divided, or cut. The main body of the pudendal nerve (MB) divides and forms the rectal branch (RB) and the vaginoperineal branch (VPB). The RB-VPB division is variable even from one side to the other side of the same patient. Depending on the placement of trocar and mesh, the patient's presentation can be variable. (© Shobeiri)

that involve patients that have had polypropylene mesh inserted into their vaginal wall to treat SUI of POP.

In a recent paper, we reported on in vivo ultrasound characteristics of vaginal mesh kit complications [55]. Comparing mesh length between posterior and anterior compartments, the posterior meshes were significantly longer than the anterior (42.1 mm ± 11.9 vs. 25.8 mm ± 9, $P < 0.0001$) and more often associated with pain. In the posterior compartment, the mean mesh length seen on ultrasound was significantly longer in women with pain than women without pain (46.5 ± 9 mm vs. 31.8 ± 12.1 mm, $P = 0.0001$). There was also a higher proportion of a "flat" mesh pattern 14/25 (58.3%) in the posterior compartment associated with the presence of pain ($P = 0.013$). In the posterior compartment, a smaller distance between the distal edge of the mesh and the anal sphincter was significantly associated with the presence of pain (8 mm (0, 37)) vs. 21 mm (8, 35), ($P = 0.024$). In the anterior compartment, there was no significant association between ultrasound appearance of the mesh and the presence of pain. However, there were a higher number of mesh erosions (6/26) in the anterior compartment, most of which had an abnormal pattern on ultrasound (three had a folding pattern and one was convoluted). In both compartments the ultrasound had 100% sensitivity for detection of mesh erosions. In this population of patients presenting with mesh complications, the posterior meshes were more often visualized as a "flat" pattern with a higher frequency of pain. Mesh complications of the anterior compartment had a higher frequency of folding and shrinkage (Table 10.1) [56].

Table 10.1 Pain in a population of patients presenting with mesh complications – posterior vs. anterior compartments

	Patients with pain *n* (%)	Patients without pain *n* (%)	*P* Value
Posterior	(*n* = 25)	(*n* = 10)	
Folding	6 (24)	8 (80)	0.002
Prominence	4 (16.6)	0	0.23
Flat	14 (58.3)	1 (10)	0.013
Convoluted	0	1 (10)	0.42
Anterior	(*n* = 17)	(*n* = 9)	
Folding	7 (41.1)	6 (66.6)	0.45
Prominence	2 (11.7)	0	0.23
Flat	7 (41.1)	2 (22)	0.34
Convoluted	1 (5.6)	1 (11)	0.72

From Javadian and Shobeiri [56], with permission

Ultrasound Imaging of Slings

Although ultrasound imaging of slings has changed management of sling complications significantly, we limit this chapter to vaginal mesh kit complications. (A more detailed description of the ultrasonography of slings can be found in *Practical Pelvic Floor Ultrasonography: A Multicompartmental Approach to 2D/3D/4D Ultrasonography of the Pelvic Floor,* 2nd ed., Shobeiri SA, editor, Springer International.)

Intraoperative Ultrasound for Management of Mesh Complications

The question that frequently arises is how ultrasound can change management in the operating room or the examination room. This section showcases some advanced ultrasound techniques to augment physical examination, techniques that can be used intraoperatively for vaginal mesh kit complications. Evaluation and assessment of the value of intraoperative ultrasound in urogynecological procedures are essentially nonexistent.

Pelvic pain, including dyspareunia, is a widely acknowledged complication of vaginal mesh procedures. Although dyspareunia can be associated with restrictive anterior and posterior repairs, the etiology of pain is different from mesh, which causes chronic inflammation. The incidence of mesh-related pelvic pain is as high as 30% [57]. Pelvic pain may present as groin pain related to the passage of the mesh arms through muscle tissue. Meshes designed to be anchored in the sacrospinous ligament can lead to pudendal and sciatic neuropathies; meshes passing through the obturator space can cause obturator neuropathies. Visualization of the sacrospinous ligament and the mesh within it can be very useful for both intraoperative management and, in cases were pudendal nerve block is required, for diagnostic or therapeutic management of pudendal neuralgia (Fig. 10.16).

In our practice, we have seen many patients with pain originating after a mesh procedure develop pelvic floor myalgias, pelvic pain, and dyspareunia. A focally painful segment of hardened mesh due to shrinkage of the vaginal mesh implant may lead to primary vaginal pain syndromes and dyspareunia following vaginal mesh use [37]. A recent case series reported high incidence of pain along contracted mesh sites. Severe vaginal pain and focal tenderness are reported which can be reproduced by palpation of the mesh segment. The main clinical features include groin pain, suprapubic pain, dyspareunia, vaginal tightness, severe vaginal pain with movement, and vaginal shortening on vaginal examination. Over-tensioning of the mesh arms during implantation and collagen deposition and contraction within the mesh pores are reported to be responsible for mesh hardening and nerve fiber entrapment [37]. This complication needs to be more robustly characterized and addressed in all studies reporting outcomes with synthetic TVM-augmented prolapse repairs. However, it is difficult to characterize this complication, as the symptoms are often similar to other mesh-related complications or are compounded by chronic pain syndromes or myalgias. The pain syndromes related to mesh, like other pain syndromes, can be debilitating and have a profound adverse psychosocial effect in patients who suffer from it. Thus, treatment of pain related to mesh is typically multimodal and should be promptly recognized and instituted. Muscle relaxants and analgesics may improve pain in some individuals and are frequently first-line therapies. Physical therapy has been shown to improve some myalgias, as well as some neuropathies, and should be attempted prior to more aggressive

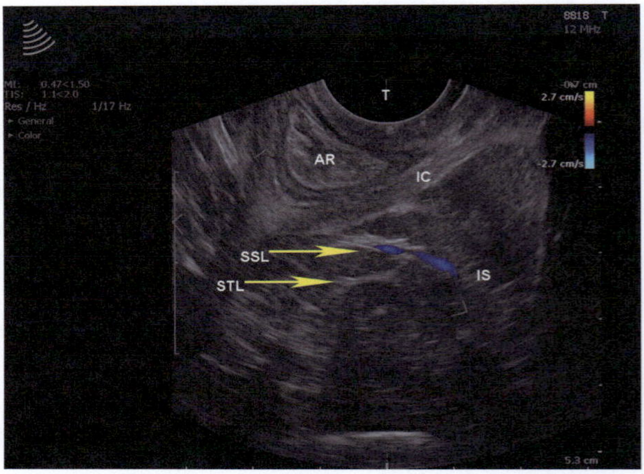

Fig. 10.16 2D endovaginal view of the sacrospinous complex obtained with a BK triplane 8818 transducer (BK Ultrasound, Analogic, Peabody, MA, USA); the pudendal nerve which goes between the sacrospinous ligament and sacrotuberous ligament travels along the neurovascular bundle *(blue)*. Transducer (T), anorectum (AR), iliococcygeus (IC), sacrospinous ligament (SSL), sacrotuberous ligament (STL), ischial spine (IS). (© Shobeiri)

intervention. In some situations, the mesh is clearly tight and tender, and the pain can be clinically reproduced by palpation of a tight band of mesh on vaginal examination. In these patients, surgical removal of the mesh may be preferred, since the removal often has rates of improvement in pelvic pain and dyspareunia exceeding 70% [58]. Dyspareunia related to mesh exposure should typically be treated with surgical revision.

Although clinical examination and urodynamic study are the basic methods in the diagnostics of incontinent women, the significance of perineal pelvic floor ultrasound (pPFUS) is often mentioned in many more recent publications as the method enabling the assessment of the position of the urethra, its anatomical relations, mobility, and hyper-rotation. pPFUS is a widely available diagnostic method that may be performed by every clinician involved in pelvic floor diagnostics; it does not require special transducers and sophisticated scanners. The equipment used for pPFUS is widely accessible in obstetrics, radiology, gynecology, urology, surgery, and other specialties; thus the access is easy and no extra investment is needed. Ultrasound has been used in the office or the operating room for drainage of hematomas and seromas. This anatomical access, however, does not allow for getting complete information about the complex anatomy of the urethra and its relations to the bladder, elements of the levator ani, and the vaginal walls, including pubocervical fascia. With this knowledge comes the ability to detect the cause of problems that have eluded us and to invent different ways of correcting the root cause of these problems. 2D or 3D EVUS has become widely available. In a patient with vaginal tenderness and implanted vaginal mesh, one can use an endovaginal or an endoanal probe and map the vagina in a blinded fashion with a long Q-tip. With an endovaginal probe, a long Q-tip is introduced alongside the probe into the vagina. With an endoanal probe, the Q-tip is visualized vaginally (Fig. 10.17).

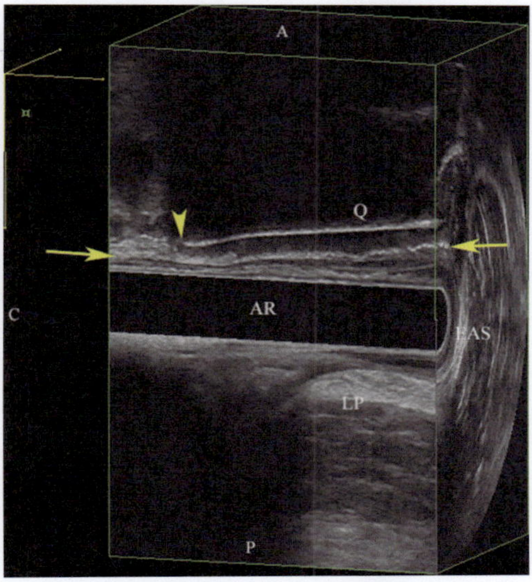

Fig. 10.17 2D endoanal view of Q-tip mapping of vagina to locate painful area. Anterior (A), cephalad (C), posterior (P), Q-tips (Q), anorectum, external anal sphincter (EAS), levator plate (LP). *Yellow arrows* outline the beginning and end of the mesh. *The yellow arrow tip* points to the tip of the Q-tips. (© Shobeiri)

One of the frequently encountered complications of vaginal mesh kits is pelvic floor spasm and pain. Recent applications of botulinum toxin A (BoNt-A) have included treatment of refractory pelvic pain and pelvic floor spasm [59, 60]. Electrophysiological or ultrasound guidance can facilitate BoNt-A injection accuracy, but clinical landmarks and palpation are often used for superficial muscles. In a study evaluating the accuracy of manual needle placement in the gastrocnemius muscles (GC) guided only by anatomical landmarks and palpation, bilateral limbs from 30 cadavers were used to evaluate ink injection into the GC. One anatomist and one orthopedic surgeon verified the accuracy of manual needle placement postinjection by calf muscle dissection. Injection was considered a failure if the ink was not located in the head of the target GC. One hundred twenty-one practitioners were evaluated. Fifty-two injections were successful (43%), and 69 failed (57%). This result was unrelated to injector experience ($P = 0.097$). The findings showed a poor success rate, regardless of injector experience. Therefore, muscle palpation and anatomical landmarks were insufficient to ensure the accuracy of BoNt-A injections, even for large, superficial muscles [61]. There has been reported variability in patient response with this levator ani muscle (LAM) BoNt-A injection, and response rates may vary due to anatomic variations of the pelvic musculature (Fig. 10.18). 3D EVUS-guided injection to the LAM is a novel application of injecting BoNt-A in patients with levator ani spasm (Fig. 10.19). Using the endovaginal probe, the needle is readily visualized in real time and injections can be performed in a directed fashion. The potential advantages of this method are many and include direct visualization of adjacent anatomical structures; direct visualization of the targeted muscle, with the possibility of repositioning the needle in cases of misdistribution or distortion of anatomy; and avoidance of potential intravascular injections. The long-term efficacy of this approach is currently the subject of an ongoing study.

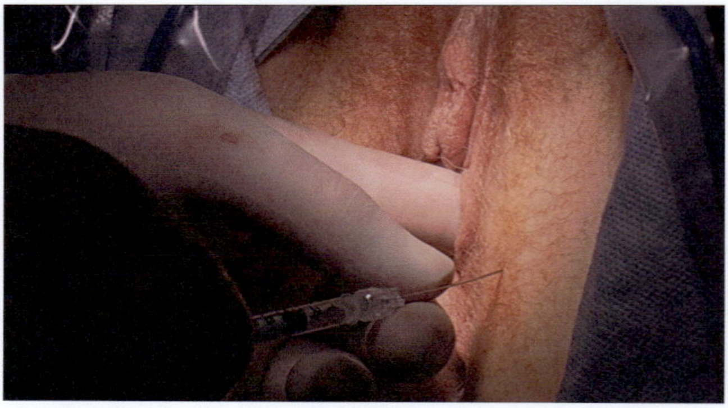

Fig. 10.18 Blind finger guided injection of the levator ani muscle via a transperineal approach. We prefer this method as it has decreased bleeding as the needles do not traverse the vascular vaginal epithelium. The needle is placed in location via US guidance and then botulinum toxin injection is carried out. (© Shobeiri)

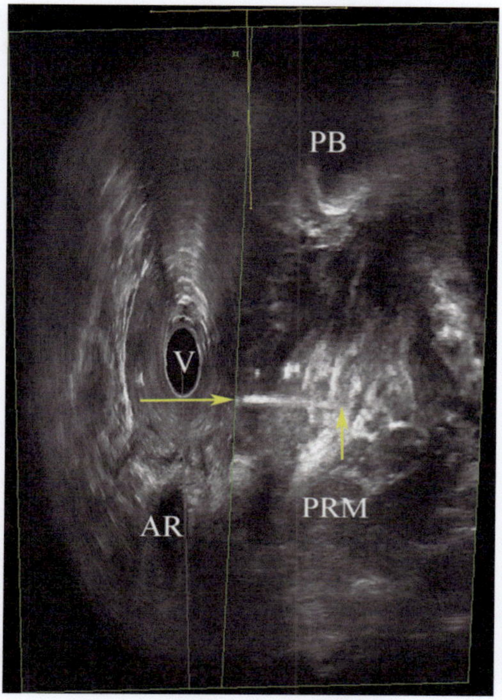

Fig. 10.19 3D volume from BK 8838 probe (BK Ultrasound, Analogic, Peabody, MA, USA) showing left (L) sagittal view of the needle in the puborectalis muscle in the same patient as Fig. 15.3. Vagina (V), pubic bone (PB), anorectum (AR), puborectalis muscle (PRM). The *arrows* show the path of the needle. (© Shobeiri)

Conclusions

Some technologies such as 3D pelvic floor ultrasound find their "calling" after invention. The 3D endoluminal/endocavitary probes were originally designed for colorectal surgeons to visualize the colorectal cancers. The editor of this book adapted this technology for endovaginal imaging in order to visualize pelvic floor muscles through a series of elaborate studies [28, 29, 62, 63]. During the course of its use, it was discovered that vaginal cysts and masses, which ordinarily would have been diagnosed using MRI, were better visualized with 3D EVUS [64]. Also the technology was able to visualize the urethral bulking agents and predict their failure [65, 66]. Ultrasound imaging became the method of choice for visualization of polypropylene mesh used for POP repair when patients presented with mesh complications; unless there was significant surrounding tissue inflammation, the area could not be visualized by MRI or CT scans. Ultrasound on the other hand produced unmistakable vivid images of shrunken, malformed, or migrated vaginal mesh and slings [5, 55]. Furthermore, it was shown that ultrasound was much more reliable than the digital exam to detect mesh remnants in the vaginal area [3]. In trained hands, ultrasound can be considerably helpful in identifying the location and integrity of vaginal mesh in patients with postoperative symptoms or mesh complications related to adjacent tissue or organs. It revolutionized understanding of the pathophysiology of vaginal mesh kit complications and helped properly to manage individual complications and to plan any needed intervention. The use of pelvic floor ultrasound is on the rise among urogynecologists and is rapidly becoming a required competency for trainees.

References

1. Schuettoff S, Beyersdorff D, Gauruder-Burmester A, Tunn R. Visibility of the polypropylene tape after tension-free vaginal tape (TVT) procedure in women with stress urinary incontinence: comparison of introital ultrasound and magnetic resonance imaging in vitro and in vivo. Ultrasound Obstet Gynecol. 2006;27(6):687–92.
2. Fischer T, Ladurner R, Gangkofer A, Mussack T, Reiser M, Lienemann A. Functional cine MRI of the abdomen for the assessment of implanted synthetic mesh in patients after incisional hernia repair: initial results. Eur Radiol. 2007;17(12):3123–9.
3. Manonai J, Rostaminia G, Denson L, Shobeiri SA. Clinical and ultrasonographic study of patients presenting with transvaginal mesh complications. Neurourol Urodyn. 2016;35(3):407.
4. Tunn R, Picot A, Marschke J, Gauruder-Burmester A. Sonomorphological evaluation of polypropylene mesh implants after vaginal mesh repair in women with cystocele or rectocele. Ultrasound Obstet Gynecol. 2007;29(4):449–52.
5. Denson L, Shobeiri SA. Three-dimensional endovaginal sonography of synthetic implanted materials in the female pelvic floor. J Ultrasound Med. 2014;33(3):521.
6. Velemir L, Amblard J, Fatton B, Savary D, Jacquetin B. Transvaginal mesh repair of anterior and posterior vaginal wall prolapse: a clinical and ultrasonographic study. Ultrasound Obstet Gynecol. 2010;35(4):474–80.
7. Santoro GA, Wieczorek AP, Dietz HP, Mellgren A, Sultan AH, Shobeiri SA, et al. State of the art: an integrated approach to pelvic floor ultrasonography. Ultrasound Obstet Gynecol. 2011;37(4):381–96.
8. Dietz HP. Mesh in prolapse surgery: an imaging perspective. Ultrasound Obstet Gynecol. 2012;40(5):495–503.
9. Svabík K, Martan A, Masata J, El-Haddad R, Hubka P, Pavlikova M. Ultrasound appearances after mesh implantation–evidence of mesh contraction or folding? Int Urogynecol J. 2011;22(5):529–33.
10. Wong V, Shek K, Goh J, Krause H, Martin A, Dietz H. Cystocele recurrence after anterior colporrhaphy with and without mesh use. Eur J Obstet Gynecol Reprod Biol. 2014;172:131–5.
11. Lo T, Ashok K. Combined anterior trans-obturator mesh and sacrospinous ligament fixation in women with severe prolapse-a case series of 30 months follow-up. Int Urogynecol J. 2011;22(3):299–306.
12. Babalola E, Bharucha A, Melton LJ, Schleck C, Zinsmeister A, Klingele C, et al. Utilization of surgical procedures for pelvic organ prolapse: a population-based study in Olmsted County, Minnesota, 1965–2002. Int Urogynecol J Pelvic Floor Dysfunct. 2008;19(9):1243–50.
13. Olsen AL, Smith VJ, Bergstrom JO, Colling JC, Clark AL. Epidemiology of surgically managed pelvic organ prolapse and urinary incontinence. Obstet Gynecol. 1997;89(4):501–6.
14. Whiteside JL, Weber AM, Meyn LA, Walters MD. Risk factors for prolapse recurrence after vaginal repair. Am J Obstet Gynecol. 2004;191(5):1533–8.
15. Smith FJ, Holman CD, Moorin RE, Tsokos N. Lifetime risk of undergoing surgery for pelvic organ prolapse. Obstet Gynecol. 2010;116(5):1096–100.
16. Margulies RU, Lewicky-Gaupp C, Fenner DE, McGuire EJ, Clemens JQ, Delancey JO. Complications requiring reoperation following vaginal mesh kit procedures for prolapse. Am J Obstet Gynecol. 2008;199(6):678.e1–4.

17. Brincat C, Lewicky-Gaupp C, Patel D, Sampselle C, Miller J, Delancey JOL, et al. Fecal incontinence in pregnancy and post partum. Int J Gynaecol Obstet. 2009;106(3):236–8.
18. Maher C, Feiner B, Baessler K, Schmid C. Surgical management of pelvic organ prolapse in women. Cochrane Database Syst Rev. 2013;30(4):CD004014.
19. U.S. Food and Drug Administration. Update on serious complications associated with transvaginal placement of surgical mesh for pelvic organ prolapse. FDA Safety Communication. 13 Jul 2011.
20. Murphy M, Holzberg A, van Raalte H, Kohli N, Goldman HB, Lucente V, Pelvic Surgeons Network. Time to rethink: an evidence-based response from pelvic surgeons to the FDA Safety Communication: "UPDATE on serious complications associated with Transvaginal placement of surgical mesh for pelvic organ prolapse". Int Urogynecol J. 2012;23(1):5–9.
21. Jakus S, Shapiro A, Hall C. Biologic and synthetic graft use in pelvic surgery: a review. Obstet Gynecol Surv. 2008;63(4):253–66.
22. Horak TA, Guzman-Rojas RA, Shek KL, Dietz HP. Pelvic floor trauma: does the second baby matter? Ultrasound Obstet Gynecol. 2014;44(1):90–4.
23. Fleischer AC, Harvey SM, Kurita SC, Andreotti RF, Zimmerman CW. Two−/three-dimensional transperineal sonography of complicated tape and mesh implants. Ultrasound Q. 2012;28(4):243–9.
24. Rostaminia GMJ, Leclaire E, Omoumi F, Marchiorlatti M, Quiroz LH, Shobeiri SA. Interrater reliability of assessing levator ani deficiency with 360° 3D endovaginal ultrasound. Int Urogynecol J. 2014;25(6):761–6.
25. Rostaminia G, White D, Quiroz L, Shobeiri SA. Is a new high-resolution probe better than the standard probe for 3D anal sphincter and levator ani imaging? Ultrason Imaging. 2015;37(2):168–75.
26. Rostaminia G, White DE, Quiroz LH, Shobeiri SA. Visualization of periurethral structures by 3D endovaginal ultrasonography in midsagittal plane is not associated with stress urinary incontinence status. Int Urogynecol J. 2013;24(7):1145–50.
27. Rostaminia G, Peck JD, Quiroz LH, Shobeiri SA. How well can levator ani muscle morphology on 3D pelvic floor ultrasound predict the levator ani muscle function? Int Urogynecol J. 2015;26(2):257–62.
28. Shobeiri SA, Leclaire E, Nihira MA, Quiroz LH, O'Donoghue D. Appearance of the levator ani muscle subdivisions in endovaginal three-dimensional ultrasonography. Obstet Gynecol. 2009;114(1):66–72.
29. Shobeiri SA, Rostaminia G, White DE, Quiroz LH. The determinants of minimal levator hiatus and their relationship to the puborectalis muscle and the levator plate. BJOG. 2012;120(2):205–11.
30. Rogowski A, Bienkowski P, Tosiak A, Jerzak M, Mierzejewski P, Baranowski W. Mesh retraction correlates with vaginal pain and overactive bladder symptoms after anterior vaginal mesh repair. Int Urogynecol J. 2013;24(12):2087–92.
31. Staack A. Translabial ultrasonography for evaluation of synthetic mesh in the vagina. Urology. 2014;83(1):68–74.
32. Khatri G, Carmel ME, Bailey AA, Foreman MR, Brewington CC, Zimmern PE, Pedrosa I. Postoperative imaging after surgical repair for pelvic floor dysfunction. Radiographics. 2016;36(4):1233–56.
33. Maher CM, Feiner B, Baessler K, Glazener CM. Surgical management of pelvic organ prolapse in women: the updated summary version Cochrane review. Int Urogynecol J. 2011;22(11):1445–57. Review
34. Barski D, Otto T, Gerullis H. Systematic review and classification of complications after anterior, posterior, apical, and total vaginal mesh implantation for prolapse repair. Surg Technol Int. 2014;24:217–24. Review
35. Haylen BT, Freeman RM, Swift SE, Cosson M, Davila GW, Deprest J, International Urogynecological Association; International Continence Society, Joint IUGA/ICS Working Group on Complications Terminology, et al. An International Urogynecological Association

(IUGA)/International Continence Society (ICS) joint terminology and classification of the complications related directly to the insertion of prostheses (meshes, implants, tapes) and grafts in female pelvic floor surgery. Neurourol Urodyn. 2011;30(1):2–12.
36. Miklos J, Chinthakanan O, Moore R, Mitchell G, Favors S, Karp D, et al. The IUGA/ICS classification of synthetic mesh complications in female pelvic floor reconstructive surgery: a multicenter study. Int Urogynecol J. 2016;27(6):933–8.
37. Feiner B, Maher C. Vaginal mesh contraction: definition, clinical presentation, andmanagement. Obstet Gynecol. 2010;115(2 Pt 1):325–30.
38. Letouzey V, De Tayrac R, Deffieux X, Fernandez H. Longterm anatomical and functional results after trans-vaginal cystocele repair using a tension-free polypropylene mesh. Int Urogynecol J Pelvic Floor Dysfunct. 2008;19:S82–S3.
39. Hammett J, Peters A, Trowbridge E, Hullfish K. Short-term surgical outcomes and characteristics of patients with mesh complications from pelvic organ prolapse and stress urinary incontinence surgery. Int Urogynecol J. 2014;25(4):465–70.
40. Jeffery ST, Brouard K. High risk of complications with a single incision pelvic floor repair kit: results of a retrospective case series. Int Urogynecol J. 2014;25(1):109–16.
41. Lee D, Bacsu C, Zimmern PE. Meshology: a fast-growing field involving mesh and/or tape removal procedures and their outcomes. Expert Rev Med Devices. 2015;12(2):201–16.
42. Lee D, Zimmern PE. Management of complications of mesh surgery. Curr Opin Urol. 2015;25(4):284–91.
43. Pickett SD, Barenberg B, Quiroz LH, Shobeiri SA, O'Leary DE. The significant morbidity of removing pelvic mesh from multiple vaginal compartments. Obstet Gynecol. 2015;125(6):1418–22.
44. Araco F, Gravante G, Sorge R, De Vita D, Piccione E. Risk evaluation of smoking and age on the occurrence of postoperative erosions after transvaginal mesh repair for pelvic organ prolapses. Int Urogynecol J. 2008;19(4):473–9.
45. de Tayrac R, Sentilhes L. Complications of pelvic organ prolapse surgery and methods of prevention. Int Urogynecol J. 2013;24(11):1859–72.
46. Huffaker RK, Shull BL, Thomas JS. A serious complication following placement of posterior Prolift. Int Urogynecol J Pelvic Floor Dysfunc. 2009;20(11):1383–5.
47. Firoozi F, Goldman H. Transvaginal excision of mesh erosion involving the bladder after mesh placement using a prolapse kit: a novel technique. Urology. 2010;75(1):203–6.
48. Alvarez Garzon HJ, Jacquemet B, Mottet N, Kleinclauss F, Riethmuller D, Ramanah R. Endoscopic lithotripsy and vaginal excision of a calcified bladder-mesh extrusion. Int Urogynecol J. 2016;27(7):1113.
49. Firoozi F, Goldman HB. Pure transvaginal excision of mesh erosion involving the bladder. Int Urogynecol J. 2013;24(6):925.
50. Ostergard D, Azadi A. To mesh or not to mesh with polypropylene: does carcinogenesis in animals matter? Int Urogynecol J. 2014;25(5):569–71.
51. Goldman H, Dwyer P. Polypropylene mesh slings and cancer: an incidental finding or association? Int Urogynecol J. 2016;27(3):345–6.
52. King AB, Zampini A, Vasavada S, Moore C, Rackley R, Goldman H. Is there an association between polypropylene midurethral slings and malignancy? Urology. 2014;84(4):789–92.
53. Linder B, Trabuco E, Carranza D, Gebhart J, Klingele C, Occhino J. Evaluation of the local carcinogenic potential of mesh used in the treatment of female stress urinary incontinence. Int Urogynecol J. 2016;27(9):1333–6.
54. Lone FW, Sultan AH, Stankiewicz A, Thakar R, Wieczorek AP. Vascularity of the urethra in continent women using colour doppler high-frequency endovaginal ultrasonography. 2015. Springerplus 2014;3:619.
55. Javadian P, Quiroz LH, Shobeiri SA. In vivo ultrasound characteristics of vaginal mesh kit complications. Female Pelvic Med Reconstr Surg. 2017;23(2):162–7.
56. Javadian P, Shobeiri SA. The disability impact and associated cost per disability in women who underwent surgical revision of transvaginal mesh kits for prolapse repair. Female Pelvic Med Reconstr Surg. 2017 Sept 13; https://doi.org/10.1097/SPV.0000000000000489. [Epub ahead of print], 1.

57. Neville CE, Fitzgerald CM, Mallinson T, Badillo S, Hynes C, Tu F. A preliminary report of musculoskeletal dysfunction in female chronic pelvic pain: a blinded study of examination findings. J Bodyw Mov Ther. 2012;16(1):50–6.
58. Abed H, Rahn DD, Lowenstein L, Balk EM, Clemons JL, Rogers RG, et al. Incidence and management of graft erosion, wound granulation, and dyspareunia following vaginal prolapse repair with graft materials: a systematic review. Int Urogynecol J. 2011;22(7):789–98.
59. Thomson AJ, Jarvis SK, Lenart M, Abbott JA, Vancaillie TG. The use of botulinum toxin type A (BOTOX) as treatment for intractable chronic pelvic pain associated with spasm of the levator ani muscles. BJOG. 2005;112(2):247–9.
60. Rao A, Abbot J. Using botulinum toxin for pelvic indications in women. Aust N Z J Obstet Gynaecol. 2009;49(4):352–7.
61. Schnitzler A, Roche N, Denormandie P, Lautridou C, Parratte B, Genet F. Manual needle placement: accuracy of botulinum toxin a injections. Muscle Nerve. 2012;46(4):531–4.
62. Shobeiri SA, White D, Quiroz LH, Nihira MA. Anterior and posterior compartment 3D endovaginal ultrasound anatomy based on direct histologic comparison. Int Urogynecol J. 2012;23(8):1047–53.
63. Rostaminia G, White D, Hegde A, Quiroz LH, Davila GW, Shobeiri SA. Levator ani deficiency and pelvic organ prolapse severity. Obstet Gynecol. 2013;121:1017–24.
64. Shobeiri SA, Rostaminia G, White D, Quiroz LH, Nihira MA. Evaluation of vaginal cysts and masses by 3-dimensional endovaginal and endoanal sonography. J Ultrasound Med. 2013;32(8):1499–507.
65. Denson L, Shobeiri SA. Imaging of urethral bulking agents: a sonographer's perspective. J Diagn Med Sonogr. 2013;29(6):255–9.
66. Yune JJ, Quiroz L, Nihira MA, Siddighi S, O'Leary DE, Santiago A, et al. The location and distribution of transurethral bulking agent: 3-dimensional ultrasound study. Female Pelvic Med Reconstr Surg. 2016;22(2):98–102.

Chapter 11
Surgical Considerations for Vaginal Mesh Complications

Farzeen Firoozi and Howard B. Goldman

Introduction

Surgical innovation has been a hallmark of female pelvic medicine and reconstructive surgery for pelvic organ prolapse. The introduction of newer techniques and materials to augment weak tissues has been borne of necessity dictated by high rates of recurrence associated with native tissue repairs [1]. The use of transvaginal augmented repairs of pelvic organ prolapse was developed with the intent to improve both subjective and objective outcomes.

The very first augmented repairs began with biologic grafts or absorbable synthetic mesh. A recent Cochrane review of these studies demonstrated that these types of augmented repairs showed neither subjective nor objective improvement [2]. The next step in the evolution of augmented repairs involved synthetic mesh. The use of synthetic mesh for pelvic organ prolapse was merely thought of as an extension of the already-established successful use of synthetic mesh in slings used to treat incontinence [3]. This logical application was deemed necessary due to the failure of augmented repairs with the use of biologic grafts and absorbable mesh. These materials simply lacked the efficacy and durability that synthetic mesh had shown in slings used for urinary incontinence. These newly designed synthetic mesh kit procedures were first approved by the US Food and Drug Administration (FDA) in 2003. A virtual tidal wave of mesh kit procedures from multiple device

F. Firoozi (✉)
Center for Female Pelvic Medicine & Reconstructive Surgery, The Arthur Smith Institute for Urology, Northwell Health, Lake Success, NY, USA

Zucker/Northwell School of Medicine of Hofstra University, Hempstead, NY, USA
e-mail: ffiroozi@northwell.edu

H. B. Goldman
Glickman Urological and Kidney Institute, Cleveland Clinic, Cleveland, OH, USA

S. A. Shobeiri (ed.), *The Innovation and Evolution of Medical Devices*,
https://doi.org/10.1007/978-3-319-97073-8_11

companies followed. The common goal of these "me too" mesh kits was to improve efficacy and durability when compared to native tissue repairs.

There have been many studies that have shown benefit, to varying degrees, in the use of synthetic mesh to augment transvaginal prolapse repairs. A well-designed randomized controlled trial in 2008 by Nguyen et al. demonstrated that the traditional repair arm had a recurrence rate of 45%, versus 13% in the synthetic mesh augmentation group [4]. A few years later, another randomized controlled trial of transvaginal mesh kit repair versus traditional colporrhaphy for anterior vaginal wall prolapse was published in the *New England Journal of Medicine* by Altman et al. The overall rate of objective success, based on pelvic organ prolapse quantification (POP-Q) stages, was significantly higher in the mesh group (60%) compared to the traditional colporrhaphy group (35%) [5]. The purported benefit in most of these studies was the objective superiority of repairs involving synthetic mesh augmentation. In addition, many of these studies showed trends toward improvements in subjective outcomes in those with mesh, but these findings were not always statistically significant.

On the heels of these studies came the controversy surrounding these newly designed commercial mesh kits. As the use of these kits rose over the years, so did the complications unique to transvaginal mesh repairs. The core complications that gave rise to the most concerned opponents were mesh extrusion, mesh visceral erosion/perforation, pain, and dyspareunia. These specific complications frequently warranted redo surgery, further casting a shadow on these new repairs. Finally, some credence was awarded to these concerns when the FDA published its first public health notification and additional patient information on the use of transvaginal mesh for incontinence and prolapse surgery in 2008 [6]. The FDA had noted that synthetic mesh for the use in transvaginal prolapse repair carried significant risks and potentially required further study. Several subsequent updates to the initial warning separated synthetic mesh for incontinence from that used for prolapse repair.

When considering the higher rate of complications related to the use of synthetic mesh for vaginal prolapse, there have been two main schools of thought. The first school of thought subscribes to the general belief that synthetic mesh placed inside the vagina is prone to causing pain and extrusion/erosion. The other camp believes that the lion's share of issues related to synthetic mesh lies squarely on the shoulders of poor surgical technique at the hands of improperly trained or inexperienced surgeons [7]. Irrespective of which group one may identify with at this point, synthetic mesh used in the surgical treatment of pelvic organ prolapse does require special consideration. In this chapter, we will review techniques for avoiding complications, recognizing technical issues intraoperatively, and managing complications postoperatively.

Avoiding Complications of Transvaginal Mesh Repairs

Preoperative Considerations

Many recommend the initiation of vaginal estrogen supplementation 4–6 weeks preoperatively to improve perioperative tissue quality. Options include Premarin® vaginal cream (Pfizer, New York, NY, USA), Estrace® cream (Allergan, Madison,

NJ, USA), Vagifem® vaginal inserts (Novo Nordisk Health Care AG, Plainsboro, NJ, USA), and Estring® vaginal ring (Pfizer, New York, NY, USA). The continued use of local hormone replacement postoperatively is often recommended to maintain tissue quality and to facilitate tissue healing.

Certain patient populations with impaired wound healing or damaged vaginal skin may be at greater risk for mesh extrusion. Some examples include patients who have had pelvic radiotherapy, those on steroids, and, possibly, smokers. Very careful consideration of risk profiles and an acknowledgment of increased rates of extrusion should be undertaken before surgery is performed in this population.

Intraoperative Considerations

Developing the proper plane of dissection is the cornerstone of transvaginal mesh repair. An excellent way to accomplish this is with copious hydrodissection of the vaginal wall to aid in the actual sharp and blunt dissection that follows. The vaginal wall incision is made through the viscerofascial layer into the potential space between the fascial layer, either pubocervical or prerectal, and the underlying viscera. This plane is much deeper than the typical superficial plane external to the viscerofascial layer used for a traditional repair. If the superficial plane is inadvertently utilized for mesh placement, vaginal wall necrosis and ulceration or extrusion may be more likely to ensue. In addition to vaginal wall extrusion, the risk for vaginal/pelvic pain and dyspareunia may be increased by dissection and mesh placement in too superficial a plane.

Hemostasis is of utmost importance. Initial postoperative pain following transvaginal mesh repairs can be secondary to perioperative bleeding. This is typically in the form of a hematoma, which can exert pressure on the vaginal tissues eliciting pain. In addition to pain, hematomas can also delay healing and promote wound separation. Wound separation in the setting of mesh use may result in extrusion of the synthetic material. For these reasons, it is paramount that adequate hemostasis is achieved at the completion of the case. We typically place a tight vaginal pack overnight as well to reduce bleeding.

Dissection should be adequate to allow the mesh to lay flat over the defect both side to side and proximal to distal. When a trocar-based system is used, one must take care to make the lateral dissection wide enough to allow the arms to be spread as they pass through that area to avoid bunching of the mesh. Pain and extrusion may occur with buckling or bunching of the mesh material.

Similar to placement of synthetic mesh slings, the mesh placed during transvaginal repair is meant to be placed without tension. The main reason for this surgical tenet is the avoidance of postoperative vaginal/pelvic pain. This can be done by loosening the arms if they are present and making a releasing incision in the body of the mesh if necessary. Again, the goal is placement of a tension-free system.

Prior to closure, the practice of vaginal wall trimming, commonly used in traditional repairs, should be avoided in transvaginal mesh repairs. Only excoriated areas should be removed and only in a very judicious fashion. The reasoning behind minimization of vaginal wall trimming relates to the competency of the wound. A wound under tension has the increased risk of developing a possible separation or compromised coverage of the underlying mesh predisposing to extrusion of the synthetic graft.

Postoperative Considerations

A Foley catheter and vaginal packing are typically left indwelling at the completion of the case. The vaginal packing serves to tamponade the vagina and reduce the risk of postoperative bleeding and can be removed within 24 h after surgery.

Intraoperative Complications

With correct dissection, bleeding involving the vaginal wall or the tissue remaining deep to this dissection plane should be minimal during transvaginal mesh repairs. If bleeding does occur on either the vaginal wall or plane of mesh placement, hemostasis can typically be achieved with electrocautery. If bleeding persists, absorbable suture placed in figure-of-eight interrupted fashion can be used as a further means of hemostasis. Bleeding can also occur with passage of external trocars or internal trocars with both anterior and posterior approaches. The first maneuver should be direct compression at the site of bleeding. If bleeding persists, optimal exposure of the site of bleeding is paramount. Typically, the source of bleeding is an aberrant vessel that cannot be managed with compression alone. Once further dissection is performed and exposure of the bleeding vessel is achieved, judicious placement of small clips may be performed to halt further bleeding. Some surgeons use hemostatic agents such as Floseal (Baxter Healthcare, Deerfield IL, USA), if there is venous oozing in a deep area where it is difficult to see. If significant bleeding cannot be controlled, packing followed by embolization must be considered.

Another potential intraoperative complication of transvaginal mesh repair is injury to other pelvic organs including the bladder or rectum. If bladder injury occurs, multilayer closure of the cystotomy should be performed with absorbable suture. A Foley catheter should be left indwelling for approximately 10 days prior to cystogram for confirmation of bladder healing. If a rectal injury is encountered, consultation with surgery is recommended. The ultimate decision of primary repair of rectal injury versus repair with diversion is at the discretion of the consultant surgeon. With either bladder or rectal injury, placement of mesh at the same setting is typically discouraged. The main concern for mesh placement would be a risk for mesh perforation of the organ given compromised tissue healing and infection after an injury.

Evaluation of Mesh Complications

History

There is a litany of complaints that patients can present with after transvaginal mesh repair. We will concentrate on patients who present with mesh extrusions and perforations. In 2010 the International Continence Society (ICS) and the International Urogynecological Association (IUGA) created a classification system to help promote a universal language that could be used by all pelvic floor surgeons in order to aid in the reporting of mesh complications [8, 9]. The new classification system uses three components to describe complications related to the use of prosthesis/grafts, which include the category (C), time (T), and site (S). The C includes the anatomical site that the graft/prosthesis complication involves and identifies the degree of exposure. More severe complications would involve increasing migration/protrusion into surrounding anatomical structures, opening into surrounding organs, and systemic compromise. The T for the complication is when it is clinically diagnosed. There are three time periods used: intraoperative to 48 h, 48 h to 6 months, and over 6 months. The S selection of this division incorporates the current sites where the graft/prosthesis complications have been noted.

The first step in taking a history from a patient involves documenting the presenting complaint, which can include dyspareunia, prolonged vaginal discharge, severe incontinence, rectal discharge, recurrent prolapse, urinary tract infection, bowel dysfunction, and thigh drainage or infection.

A complete review of systems should be performed, specifically those symptoms that have occurred since the time of surgery. If the original case was performed by another surgeon, the preoperative records, operative reports, and any other hospital reports should be reviewed. Any intraoperative issues such as bleeding or injury to pelvic organs or problems that occurred postoperatively such as prolonged bladder catheterization, blood transfusion, or need for reoperation should be closely reviewed. These issues tend to signify a complicated postoperative course, which may relate to the complication at hand. Finally, a detailed history of any events that followed surgery is useful in any future medical or surgical management of mesh complications. Good documentation of one's findings is critical as these cases may end up under medicolegal review.

Physical Exam

The focused physical exam involves a complete genitourinary exam. This includes a thorough pelvic exam with a speculum. Before the speculum exam, careful initial palpation can be performed to elicit any areas of pain. These areas can be associated with folded-over mesh, contracted mesh, or taut arms of the mesh if present. Care should be taken to evaluate each vaginal compartment in mapping out all areas of pain. Often it is easier to palpate extruded mesh than to see it, and thus a very careful palpation of the entire vaginal surface should be performed.

In terms of the speculum exam, systematic evaluation of the entire vagina should be carried out. Any areas of mesh extrusion should be documented. If a patient complains of pain over the mesh, the specific sites of pain should be mapped out. Other important findings such as fistulae should be evaluated closely. Other urologic testing, such as cystoscopy to rule out mesh perforation, cystogram or methylene blue test to confirm the presence of fistula, and urodynamics for bladder dysfunction, may also be performed based on presenting symptoms. Patients who present with rectal bleeding or discharge should be evaluated with proctoscopy.

Management of Mesh Complications

Mesh Extrusion

Complications from transvaginal mesh repairs may present days to years after initial surgery. Vaginal mesh extrusion typically occurs as a result of wound separation, infection, or vaginal atrophy. Typically, mesh extrusion noted in the immediate postoperative period, usually within 6 weeks, is a result of wound separation. If the wound does not appear infected, additional attempt at wound closure may be offered under local anesthesia with or without sedation. If the wound appears infected, a short course of antibiotics may rectify the issue, with close observation to ensure closure of the wound. Vaginal estrogens should be applied during this time. If the infection persists, then excision of the exposed area is recommended.

Vaginal mesh extrusion noted more than 6 weeks after surgery may be due to technical error, local infection, vaginal atrophy, or wound separation secondary to hematoma. Initial conservative therapy with local estrogen may be offered in order to avoid reoperation. If conservative therapy fails, partial or complete mesh excision should be pursued. Typically, only the areas of mesh that are involved in an extrusion need to be excised; much of the uninvolved mesh can usually be safely left behind. Some very small extrusions can be excised under local anesthesia in the office by just cutting the exposed portion and allowing the vaginal skin to heal over the area. Many patients with point tenderness can be treated in a similar fashion with just those areas causing tenderness excised. In such cases one must carefully map out the areas of pain preoperatively, as there will be no extruded mesh to guide you at the time of operation.

Surgical Technique for Excision of Mesh Extrusion Under either intravenous sedation or general anesthesia, the patient is placed in the dorsal lithotomy position, and the vagina and lower abdomen are prepped and draped in standard fashion. One percent lidocaine with 1:200,000 epinephrine is used to infiltrate under the vaginal skin around the site of the extrusion. Bilateral vaginal flaps are created extending at least 2 cm lateral to the visible mesh. One centimeter of skin immediately around the mesh is often discarded if of poor quality. The mesh is then incised in the midline and dissected off of the bladder or rectum in either direction at least 1–2 cm lateral to where the skin will be closed. Once the lateral extent of the mesh is dissected, the mesh is excised. The vaginal wall is then closed in a single layer with absorbable suture. A vaginal packing is placed and removed later in the recovery room.

Mesh Perforation

Once mesh perforation of the bladder or rectum has been diagnosed, mapping of the areas of perforation must be documented. Mesh perforation of the bladder is typically seen at the bladder base or lateral bladder walls where mesh arms can sometimes be found (Fig. 11.1). If the mesh has been in the bladder for an extended period of time, calcification of the synthetic material may occur. We have described the purely transvaginal excision of bladder and rectal mesh perforation as safe and efficacious [10] and feel that often the easiest way to remove the mesh is via the same route it was placed.

Surgical Technique for Excision of Mesh Perforation of the Bladder Under general anesthesia, the patient is placed in the dorsal lithotomy position, and the vagina and abdomen are prepped and draped in standard fashion. Retrograde pyelograms are performed to rule out ureteral involvement. If there is ureteral involvement, a JJ stent is placed retrograde, or a percutaneous nephroureteral stent is left indwelling to maintain continuity of the urinary tract during reconstruction. If no ureteral involvement is noted, temporary bilateral open-ended ureteral stents are inserted. One percent lidocaine with 1:200,000 epinephrine mixture is infiltrated under the vaginal skin, and an inverted U-shaped incision is made. The vaginal wall is dissected to create an inverted U-flap, which serves as the final layer of closure for the repair (in cases where there is a vesicovaginal fistula [VVF] closer to the vaginal apex, a true [noninverted] U-flap is created with the bottom of the U at the VVF site) (see Fig 11.1a). Dissection of the vaginal skin is performed laterally from the U-flap toward the pelvic sidewall (see Fig. 11.1b). When only a small area of mesh has eroded into the bladder, the remainder may be found relatively superficially under the vaginal wall. If a substantial volume of mesh has eroded into the bladder, the mesh may not be as easy to find, and the detrusor muscle may need to be incised vertically in the area of the mesh (which can be determined with cystoscopic guidance) until one comes across it. A right-angle clamp can be used to mobilize the mesh off the bladder in the midline (see Fig. 11.1c). An incision is made in the midline of the mesh after which the lumen of the bladder is visible (see Fig. 11.1d). Any remaining overlying tissues (superficial to the mesh) are bluntly and sharply dissected. By grasping on the midline (incised edge) of the mesh and pulling laterally, the bladder wall underneath the mesh is carefully peeled off using both sharp and blunt dissection. If there is a fistula present, it can be seen in its entirety at this point (see Fig. 11.1e). The mesh is incised as far laterally as feasible and removed (see Fig. 11.1f). The ureteral catheters can be both palpated and visualized.

The mucosal layer is re-approximated using 3-0 absorbable suture, taking care to stay medial to the ureteral catheters. The detrusor layer is then closed in two layers using 2-0 Vicryl suture (see Fig. 11.1g). The anterior vaginal wall is closed with 2-0 Vicryl suture (see Fig. 11.1h). Although not mandatory, the open-ended ureteral stents can be replaced with JJ ureteral stents to prevent any potential ureteral obstruction from inflammation and edema involving the bladder. A vaginal packing is placed and an 18 French Foley catheter is left per urethra.

Another option for removal of mesh perforation of the bladder would be a transabdominal approach. A Pfannenstiel incision is made in the lower abdomen. The incision is carried down to the level of the rectus fascia using electrocautery. The rectus fascia is incised transversely and the space of Retzius is entered. The bladder is filled via the indwelling Foley catheter to aid in identification. The bladder

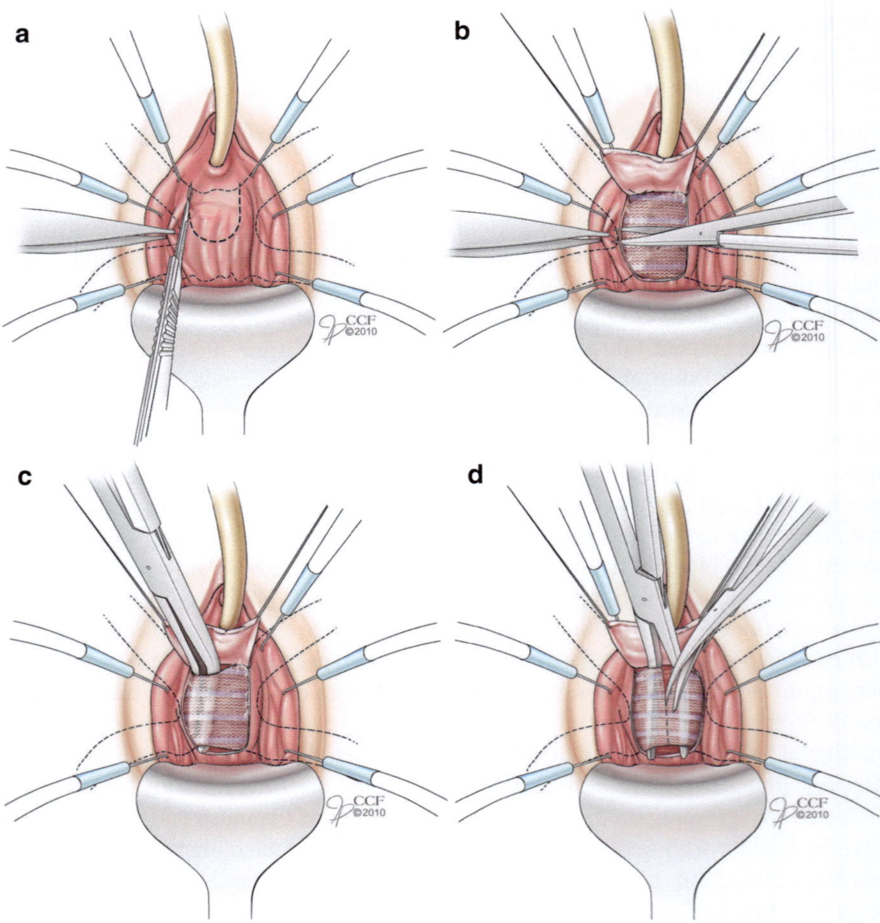

Fig. 11.1 Excision of transvaginal mesh (see text). (© Cleveland Clinic Foundation, with permission)

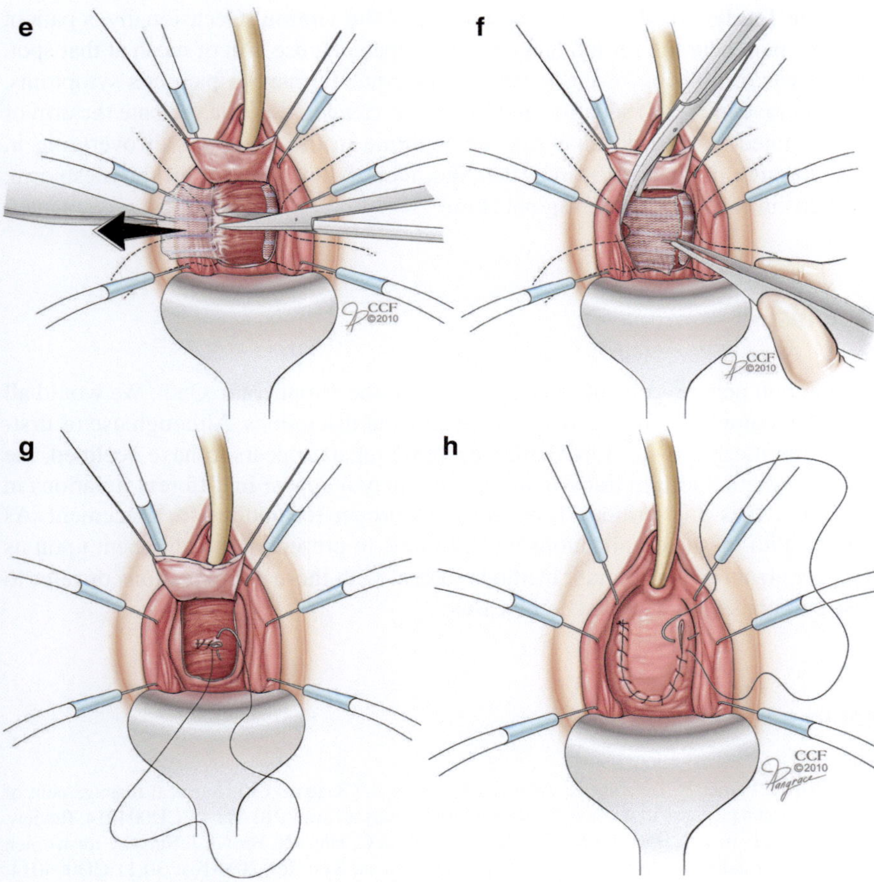

Fig. 11.1 (continued)

is then bivalved with a vertical incision using electrocautery. The mesh can now be visualized. The incision is carried down to the mesh. Bladder flaps are now created lateral to the body of the mesh. The mesh is then excised. The vaginal wall is closed using 2-0 absorbable suture. A portion of omentum may be mobilized and placed as an interposition graft between the vagina and bladder. The bladder is then closed in two layers with 2-0 absorbable suture. A vaginal packing is placed and an 18 French Foley catheter is left per urethra.

Surgical Technique for Excision of Mesh Perforation of the Rectum Under general endotracheal anesthesia, the patient is placed in the jackknife position, the perineum and buttocks are prepped, and the rectum is cleaned with betadine irrigation. A Hill Ferguson retractor is placed to aid in visualization. Mucosal flaps are developed around the exposed mesh. The mesh is then dissected off of the underlying rectal wall and excised. The mucosal flaps are closed with Vicryl suture.

Palpable Tender Mesh Arm in the Fornix of the Vagina Occasionally, a patient will note pain near the fornix, and one can palpate a tense arm of mesh at that spot. In such cases, division of the mesh arm may ameliorate the patient's symptoms. Under intravenous (IV) sedation and local or general anesthesia, palpate the arm of interest, inject some lidocaine with epinephrine in the vaginal wall overlying it, incise through the vaginal skin at that site, identify and dissect out the mesh arm, and then cut it and close the vaginal skin.

Conclusion

Primum non nocere – one of the basic tenets of the Hippocratic Oath. We would all agree that complications can occur in all surgical disciplines. Although use of first-generation mesh kits for transvaginal prolapse repair appears to have declined, the use of synthetic mesh in transvaginal repairs may reappear in different iterations in the future. It is thus critical to be aware of proper techniques for placement. As patients with mesh complications will continue to present, it is incumbent upon us to be cognizant of appropriate methods to deal with these complications or refer to those surgeons with expertise in this area.

References

1. Maher C, Feiner B, Baessler K, Adams EJ, Hagen S, Glazener CM. Surgical management of pelvic organ prolapse in women. Cochrane Database Syst Rev. 2010 Apr 14;CD004014. Review.
2. Maher C, Feiner B, Baessler K, Christmann-Schmid C, Haya N, Brown J. Surgery for women with anterior compartment prolapse. Cochrane Database Syst Rev. 2016 Nov 30;11:CD004014. Review.
3. Ulmsten U, Petros P. Intravaginal slingplasty (IVS): an ambulatory surgical procedure for treatment of female urinary incontinence. Scand J Urol Nephrol. 1995;29:75–82.
4. Nguyen JN, Burchette RJ. Outcome after anterior vaginal prolapse repair: a randomized controlled trial. Obstet Gynecol. 2008;111:891–8.
5. Altman D, Vayrynen T, Engh ME. Anterior colporrhaphy versus transvaginal mesh for pelvic-organ prolapse. N Engl J Med. 2011;364:1826–36.
6. U.S Food and Drug Administration. FDA public health notification: serious complications associated with transvaginal placement of surgical mesh in repair of pelvic organ prolapse and stress urinary incontinence. 20 Oct 2008. https://wayback.archive-it.org/7993/20170111190506/http://www.fda.gov/MedicalDevices/Safety/AlertsandNotices/PublicHealthNotifications/ucm061976.htm. Accessed 15 Sep 2017.
7. Goldman HB, Fitzgerald MP. Transvaginal mesh for cystocele repair. J Urol. 2010;183:430–2.
8. Haylen BT, Freeman RM, Swift SE, Cosson M, Davila GW, Deprest J, et al. An International Urogynecological Association (IUGA) / International Continence Society (ICS) joint terminology and classification of the complications related directly to the insertion of prostheses (meshes, implants, tapes) & grafts in female pelvic floor surgery. Int Urogynecol J. 2011;22(1):3–15.
9. The International Continence Society. ICS-IUGA complication calculator. https://www.ics.org/complication. Accessed 15 Sept 2017.
10. Firoozi F, Ingber MS, Moore CK, Vasavada SP, Rackley RR, Goldman HB. Purely transvaginal/perineal management of complications from commercial prolapse kits using a new prostheses/grafts complication classification system. J Urol. 2012;187(5):1674–9.

Chapter 12
Complications of Transobturator Synthetic Slings

Melissa R. Kaufman, Laura Chang-Kit, Elizabeth T. Brown, and Roger R. Dmochowski

Introduction

Female stress urinary incontinence (SUI) is estimated to affect up to half of adult women, although exact prevalence is unknown [1, 2]. Patient underreporting due to social embarrassment and differences in the characterization of SUI between studies contribute to the probable substantial underestimation of SUI in the population [3]. Confounding our capacity to create meaningful estimates are the varied measurement tools and definitions for both prevalence as well as complications. Additionally, the current climate of mesh litigation may drive both initial patient presentation and clinician management of complications [4]. Estimated costs for SUI, from both a social and societal perspective, are complex to quantify and unlikely to account completely for the nuances of management of mesh complications [2].

Due to the relatively short operative time, generally limited morbidity, rapid convalescence, and long-term efficacy, the synthetic midurethral sling (MUS) remains the most widely employed procedure for surgical correction of female SUI [5]. Since 1995, when Ulmsten and Petros pioneered the first retropubic (RP) synthetic MUS, a vast array of approach techniques, including transobturator (TOT) and single-incision, have emerged to accommodate MUS placement.

M. R. Kaufman (✉) · R. R. Dmochowski
Department of Urology, Vanderbilt Medical Center, Nashville, TN, USA
e-mail: melissa.kaufman@vanderbilt.edu

L. Chang-Kit
Department of Urology, Albany Medical Center, Albany, NY, USA

E. T. Brown
Department of Urology, MedStar Georgetown University Hospital, Washington, DC, USA

S. A. Shobeiri (ed.), *The Innovation and Evolution of Medical Devices*,
https://doi.org/10.1007/978-3-319-97073-8_12

In 2001, Delrome described the initial TOT approach for MUS placement [6]. As this novel approach did not violate the retropubic space in close proximity to the bladder, the risks of injury to vicus organs were therefore presumed to be diminished. Indeed, many initial proponents advocated that cystoscopy following sling placement was not mandated as the risk of bladder or urethral perforation was theoretically low. However, as outlined in the following sections, the risks of TOT placement may be both unique and significant with several anatomic compartments at immediate and long-term risk.

This chapter will focus on the diagnosis, evaluation, and management of complications specific to TOT sling placement. Although many of the principles of MUS management and complications are ubiquitous across surgical approach, the notable exceptions with TOT placement will be highlighted. Detailed elsewhere in this volume is an in-depth discussion of incidence and medicolegal aspects of mesh complications, although special mention of the role of MUS technology is warranted. In 2013, the US Food and Drug Administration (FDA) updated their previously issued Public Health Notification regarding transvaginal mesh to indicate the current iterations of MUS, including TOT technologies but with the exception of single-incision slings, were deemed safe and effective with an appropriate risk-to-benefit profile [7, 8]. Joint position statements from the Society of Urodynamics, Female Pelvic Medicine and Urogenital Reconstruction (SUFU) and the American Urogynecologic Society (AUGS) also strongly support standard of care use of polypropylene mesh MUS for the treatment of female SUI [9].

General Attributes of TOT Slings

In general, TOT slings are composed of type I synthetic polypropylene monofilamentous mesh, with a pore size between 75 and 150 μm. This pore size is critical to allow fibrous tissue ingrowth as well as leukocyte and macrophage entry in order to reduce bacterial colonization. Understanding of how midurethral support with synthetic slings corrects SUI continues to evolve. In general, the aim of any SUI surgery is to augment the urethral closure pressures to prevent involuntary urinary leakage when there are increases in abdominal pressures [10]. Mechanisms of sling efficacy may contribute to the complication profiles outlined in following sections. TOT slings, akin to other MUS, are placed in a "tension-free" fashion and hypothesized to stabilize the midurethral complex, where urethral closure pressure is maximal. If the posterior wall of the urethra lacks such support, "shear forces" during periods of intraabdominal pressure can cause the anterior wall of the urethra (attached to the pubic bone by pubourethral ligaments and endopelvic fascia) to move independently of the posterior wall, promoting urinary incontinence [11]. Another mechanism proposes that the MUS obstructs the downward movement of the urethra, in effect, kinking the urethra during stress maneuvers [12]. A combination of mechanisms likely contributes to efficacy and may manifest in an individualized fashion dependent on the patient's unique pathologies provoking SUI.

Indications and Contraindications

Fundamental to avoidance of the perioperative complications of TOT slings is appropriate patient selection and evaluation. A 2006 prospective study examined reasons for 328 complications requiring surgical intervention after MUS in four European urogynecology centers [13]. Incorrect indication for the initial procedure was determined to be the second most common cause of complications (38%), following poor surgical technique (45%). This data highlights the critical necessity for the surgeon treating SUI to be facile with indications and contraindications for sling placement.

The American Urological Association (AUA) guidelines for the surgical management of female SUI indicate the goal of evaluation is to characterize the type of incontinence, assess contributing comorbid medical conditions, elucidate the differential diagnosis, and uncover prognostic information to aid in the selection of treatment [14]. Mandated aspects of the exam include a thorough history critically elucidating the urgency component, focused neurological and pelvic examinations, urinalysis, and measurement of post-void residual. Although there remains debate regarding the use of further functional or anatomic evaluations, in any patient whom a definitive diagnosis of SUI is unclear, or if there exists a substantial urgency component, urodynamics and possibly cystoscopy may illuminate pathology and drive appropriate treatment strategies.

In general, patients with an untreated poorly compliant bladder or urge urinary incontinence without demonstrated stress incontinence are unsuitable candidates for any sling procedure. Likewise, according to the AUA guidelines, synthetic slings are contraindicated in the setting of concurrent urethrovaginal fistula, urethral erosion, intraoperative urethral injury, and/or urethral diverticulum. Such patients are considered higher risk for subsequent urethral erosion, vaginal extrusion, urethrovaginal fistula, and foreign body granuloma formation. Autologous fascia and alternative biologic slings are preferred in these complex patients for treatment of concomitant SUI.

Patient comorbidities must also be considered when choosing the type of sling to employ. It may prove prudent to avoid synthetic TOT slings in patients with estrogen deficiency, previous surgery, or history of pelvic radiation, as well as in very young patients (<30 years old), because of the suspected increased risk of late complications such as erosion into the lower urinary tract. For young women who desire future vaginal deliveries, sling placement in general is a controversial topic, and it is generally recommended to avoid placement of synthetic slings in this population. In patients appropriate for synthetic MUS, one distinct advantage of the TOT approach includes avoidance of the retropubic space. Vectors for placement outside the retropubic space may be particularly beneficial for patients with suspected significant fibrosis in the area secondary to multiple prior surgeries or radiation.

Complication Rates

Multiple retrospective and case control studies have estimated the complication rate of MUS, although in general this data is plagued by lack of standardization of definitions and inadequate long-term follow-up. In the randomized controlled Trial of

Midurethral Slings (TOMUS), efficacy and complication rates between RP and TOT MUS were compared in 597 women [15]. Results suggested subjective and objective equivalence between the two surgical approaches. However, at 2-year follow-up, a higher rate of voiding dysfunction was witnessed in the RP arm. Alternately, the TOT approach resulted in increased neuromuscular complaints such as leg weakness, pain, and groin numbness when compared to RP MUS (9.7 versus 5.4%). These special considerations for the TOT complication profile will be expanded upon in the following sections.

Classification of Complications

The first standardized classification and terminology system for complications arising from the insertion of synthetic and biological materials in female pelvic floor surgery was recently reported by the International Continence Society (ICS)/ International Urogynecological Association (IUGA) [16]. Each complication is classified according to three aspects: category, time, and site. The aim of the classification is to improve communication among providers and allow standardization of research registries. Suggested changes to current terminology include avoidance of the terms "erosion," in favor of the terms "extrusion" or "perforation" when referring to mesh involvement in the vagina or lower urinary tract. Inter-observer and intra-observer reliability of the classification is yet to be tested, and widespread adoption is not yet accomplished. As all currently published references use the older nomenclature, this chapter will generally reflect traditional descriptions as well as ICS/IUGA nomenclature to avoid any potential discord in data.

Anatomy of TOT Sling

Critical to understanding of the potential unique complications of TOT is a basic understanding of the anatomy of this surgical approach (Fig. 12.1) [17]. Whether placed in an in-to-out or out-to-in vector, TOT MUS surgery begins with dissection in the vesicovaginal space. This dissection is carried out lateral to the urethra until the inferior border of the ischiopubic rami and pubic symphysis can be easily palpated. A trocar must traverse the obturator internus muscle, obturator membrane, and obturator externus muscle through the obturator foramen. Lateral to the obturator foramen are the adductor muscles (gracilis and adductor brevis muscles) of the thigh [18]. Presumably protected from normal trocar passage, the obturator nerve and vessels are located in the obturator canal at the superior aspect of the obturator foramen. It is certainly feasible that slight differences in patient positioning, including rotation and hyperflexion of the hip, as well as body habitus, may alter the vector of the helical needle and potentially impact location of sling placement and risk to structures within the urinary tract and obturator canal.

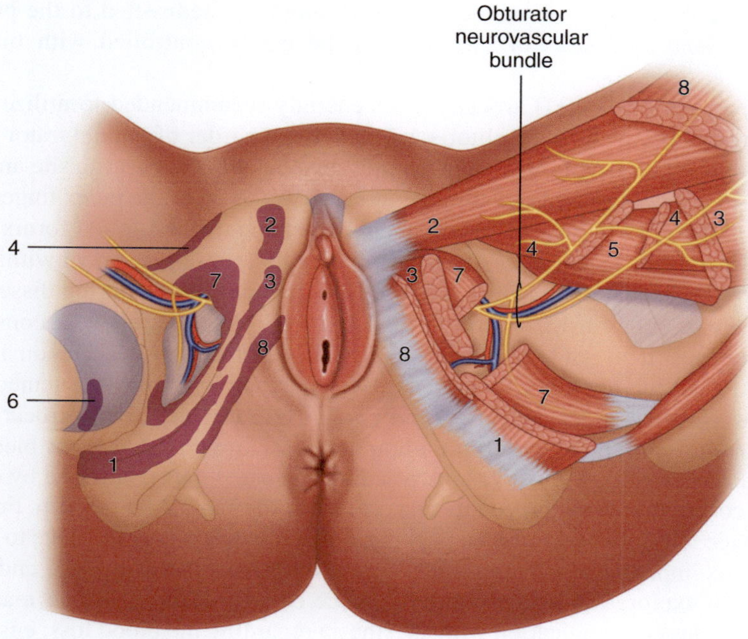

Fig. 12.1 Illustration of inner thigh anatomy in region of obturator foramen: medial thigh muscles and attachments. Muscle identification: (1) adductor magnus; (2) adductor longus; (3) adductor brevis; (4) pectineus; (5) iliopsoas; (6) quadratus femoris; (7) obturator internus; (8) gracilis (From Karram and Pancholy [17], with permission. © Elsevier)

Intraoperative Complications

Hemorrhage

Significant bleeding during procedures for SUI is infrequent and transfusion rates range from 1% to 4% [14]. Major vascular injuries to iliac, femoral, obturator, and epigastric vessels during sling surgery have been reported in the literature [19]. Even for the TOT approach, pelvic vessels coursing along the pelvic sidewall and within the vascular pedicle of the bladder can also be injured during dissection or passage of trocars. Solid knowledge of the relative pelvic anatomy and adherence to good surgical technique are paramount in avoiding perioperative hemorrhage.

During vaginal dissection, the source of bleeding can be difficult to identify and control due to lack of direct visualization. During dissection of the vaginal flap from the underlying pubocervical fascia, it is uncommon to encounter significant bleeding if the dissection planes are correct. Initial hydrodissection of the vaginal epithelium with either injectable saline or lidocaine with epinephrine generally helps to better elucidate this plane. Bleeding at this stage likely signifies an excessively deep incision through the pubocervical fascia into the detrusor or urethra. If this occurs, the dissection should be redirected to the proper surgical plane and areas of bleeding can be gently controlled with bipolar cautery.

For passage of the TOT trocars, it is generally recommended to utilize anatomic landmarks such as the clitoris and define the border of the obturator foramen with a seeker needle. A stab incision is created over the passage site and the outside-in trocar is passed with direct guidance on the tip of the index finger or a helical passer for the inside-out approach. Inspection of the vaginal fornix with the trocar in place is a critical step to avoid potential mesh placement within the lumen of the vagina. Blind entry into the transobturator space during dissection or passage of either inside-out or outside-in trocars can manifest with considerable bleeding. It is not unusual for some venous bleeding to occur on initial perforation of the obturator membranes, which generally settles spontaneously. However, substantial maneuvering and manipulation of the helical trocars can result in substantial damage to the obturator muscle with subsequent bleeding and should be avoided. Most venous bleeding can usually be controlled by expeditious conclusion of the procedure and closure of the vaginal epithelium. Further tamponade is gained with vaginal packing. Bleeding that is unresponsive to these maneuvers implies major vessel injury due to inaccurate trocar passage and warrants open exploration of the obturator space or embolization. Initial management includes communication with anesthesia regarding the blood loss, ensuring adequate availability of blood products and excellent exposure and lighting. Possible intraoperative consultation with an orthopedic or vascular surgeon should be considered. Pelvic bleeding is especially problematic to control because of the confined working space, depth of field, potential for rapid, massive bleeding, and close proximity and high anatomic variation. Vascular control can be accomplished by repairing larger vessels with 4–0 or 5–0 permanent sutures such as Prolene, whereas en bloc ligation is performed with absorbable 3–0 Vicryl sutures. Hemostatic agents can be applied over slowly oozing areas if no definite bleeding vessels are identified. If bleeding still cannot be controlled, the obturator foramen can be packed and the patient brought back after resuscitation. In addition, angiography and arterial embolization by Interventional Radiology colleagues may be considered. Successful outcomes using embolization have been reported for cases of profuse hemorrhage with the TOT approach where direct visualization of vessels is limited [20].

Urinary Tract Perforation

During any procedure for SUI, the urinary tract is at high risk for direct injury. Although urinary tract perforation with TOT MUS is reported to be <0.5%, the surgeon must maintain vigilance and suspicion for potential injury must remain high [19, 21]. Immediate intraoperative detection and management of these injuries can mitigate a myriad of possible debilitating complications such as vesicovaginal fistula or bladder/urethral erosion. Paramount to prevention of injury is utilization of a urethral catheter or sound and emptying of the bladder prior to trocar passage. With the trocars in place, performance of intraoperative cystourethroscopy to detect intraoperative urinary tract injuries is considered standard of practice [14]. A rigid or flexible cystoscope should be used to inspect the bladder and urethra prior to the conclusion of the procedure. Optimal visualization of the female urethra is accomplished by using a short beak rigid cystoscope or flexible fiberoptic cystoscope. If a rigid cystoscope is used, both 30° and 70° lenses provide optimal surveillance of the bladder, bladder neck, and ureteral orifices. The bladder must be examined while full, with special attention being paid to the bladder neck at the 3 and 9 o'clock positions, where TOT trocar injuries may be postulated to occur. Redirection of the trocars and repeat cystoscopy is mandated for any bladder perforation. Placement of synthetic MUS at the time of an intraoperative urethral injury is contraindicated due to the higher risk of urethral erosion.

Ureteral Injury

Ureteral injury during transvaginal SUI procedures are rare and usually reported in conjunction with concomitant prolapse repairs. During transvaginal operations, the distal third of the ureter is at highest risk. If ureteral injury is suspected after cystoscopy, intraoperative retrograde pyelogram should be conducted to better assess ureteral integrity. Delayed ureteral injuries can present with flank pain, fever, and wound leakage. Appropriate imaging includes CT urography or retrograde pyelogram. The advantage to retrograde pyelography is that ureteral stenting, if necessary, can be conducted in the same setting.

Postoperative Complications

Voiding Dysfunction

The true incidence of voiding dysfunction and iatrogenic bladder outlet obstruction (BOO) after sling surgery is unknown owing to under diagnosis, misdiagnosis, lack of standard definitions, and underreporting. A Cochrane review involving 14 trials of MUS indicated postoperative voiding dysfunction occurred significantly less frequently with the TOT route compared to the RP route (4% versus 7%) [19]. In most patients, postoperative voiding dysfunction is transient and resolves with conservative treatments such as catheter drainage or short-term pharmacological therapy. Surgery may be required for patients with severe or prolonged voiding dysfunction refractory to these conservative treatments.

Evaluation of Voiding Dysfunction

Patients with persistent voiding dysfunction after sling surgery must be evaluated with a focused history, physical examination, urinalysis, urine culture, and cystoscopy. A post-void residual volume should be documented. Important factors in the history include preoperative and postoperative storage and voiding symptoms, the temporal relationship of the surgery to the symptoms, and type of sling surgery. Preoperative urodynamic data or flow studies become particularly useful when evaluating postoperative voiding complaints. Physical examination should evaluate for signs of a hyper-elevated, fixed bladder neck or urethra, urethral hypermobility, stress incontinence, new or worsened pelvic organ prolapse, and vaginal exposure of mesh. Urine studies are critical to rule out urinary tract infection. Cystoscopy is essential to evaluate for stones, sling erosion, and other urinary tract injury or pathology including a hyper-suspended bladder neck or midurethra, fibrosis, diverticula, or fistula (Fig. 12.2).

In select cases, urodynamic evaluation provides useful information about sensation, bladder capacity, compliance, stress incontinence, detrusor overactivity, and coordination of sphincter activity. However, the role of urodynamic studies to evaluate for female BOO is controversial. The diagnosis of female BOO is complex and requires consideration of several limiting factors. First, there is no accepted gold standard nomogram for female BOO, although several nomograms exist. Secondly, some female patients void primarily by pelvic floor relaxation, with barely any rise in their intravesical pressures and with possible Valsalva maneuvers. These patients can be obstructed by a very slight increase in urethral closure pressures. These women may not generate a significant contraction on urodynamic studies but are still obstructed. Thus, although the classic urodynamic "high pressure-low flow" pattern indicative of BOO in men confirms the diagnosis of BOO in women, if present, its absence does not rule out obstruction. To date, there are no consistent preoperative parameters or urodynamic findings which predict success or failure of urethrolysis for BOO [22]. Indeed, patients who have failed to generate a detrusor contraction and those with non-diagnostic urodynamic studies have had the same

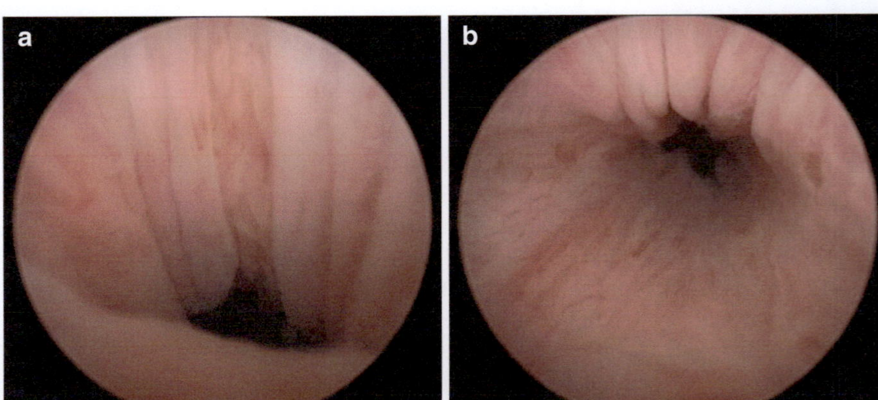

Fig. 12.2 Cystoscopic images of urethral hypersuspension of transobturator sling before (**a**) and after (**b**) mesh excision

outcome after urethrolysis as those patients who demonstrated the classic "high pressure-low flow" pattern [23].

How then should the diagnosis of female BOO after TOT sling surgery be made? The diagnosis is obvious in patients with absolute prolonged urinary retention or who produce the classic urodynamic pattern of obstruction. However, without these, in patients who had normal preoperative voiding function, a culmination of the history, physical exam, temporal relationship of the surgery to the symptoms, and supporting cystoscopic findings should raise the suspicion of BOO.

Urinary Retention and Obstruction

Iatrogenic obstruction secondary to sling surgery is the most common cause of female BOO. Outlet obstruction classically presents with storage symptoms of frequency, urgency, and urge incontinence along with obstructive voiding symptoms and elevated PVR [24]. Interestingly, in a study of 51 women undergoing urethrolysis, 75% presented with storage (irritative) symptoms, 61% with voiding (obstructive) symptoms, 55% with de novo urge incontinence, and 24% with persistent retention [25]. Therefore, patients complaining of de novo postoperative storage symptoms, even in the absence of voiding symptoms, should be evaluated for possible obstruction.

Temporary urethral obstruction may result from postoperative edema of the bladder neck or urethra. Retention after nonradical pelvic surgery may also be attributed to a lack of urethral relaxation due to increased sympathetic response to pain, local irritation, anxiety, and trauma [26]. Other possible causes for postoperative retention include use of narcotic or anticholinergic medications, constipation, immobility, and hematoma. A successful strategy which settles most cases of postoperative retention is to address all the reversible risk factors, while instituting short-term (typically a few days) urethral catheter drainage or clean intermittent catheterization (CIC). Patients should always be counseled preoperatively about the potential need for catheterization postoperatively.

The incidence of postoperative retention lasting more than a month or requiring intervention has been reported in 3% of women after synthetic MUS placement [14]. No robust data exists to identify definite risk factors for postoperative obstruction. Once the diagnosis of obstruction is established or suspected and the patient has failed nonsurgical therapies, surgical options for management of prolonged obstruction include sling incision, transvaginal urethrolysis, retropubic urethrolysis, suprameatal transvaginal urethrolysis, and interposition grafts. Although urethral dilation and attempts to loosen with traction an obstructing biologic pubovaginal sling in the very early postoperative period can be successful, we do not advocate the use of dilation techniques for synthetic mesh MUS due to the risk of urethral erosion.

The timing of surgical intervention is debated in the literature and is dependent on the type of procedure, symptom severity, patient bother, and expectation of outcome. Historically, expectant management with catheter drainage or intermittent catheterization for up to 3 months has been employed. However, to avoid long-term voiding dysfunction, in our experience significant incomplete emptying and urinary retention after 4–6 weeks usually mandates operative intervention.

MUS Incision

Following MUS, 66–100% of temporary voiding dysfunction resolves by 6 weeks, and most patients will empty fairly normally after 72 h [27]. If the transvaginal incision of the MUS is conducted within the early postoperative period, there is little tissue ingrowth into the sling, and the procedure can be done with minimal manipulation. Although this can be done in the office setting under local anesthetic, we prefer the more controlled setting of the operating room where vaginal exposure can be maximized (Fig. 12.3) [28]. The vaginal wall is infiltrated with local anesthetic, and the suture used to close the vaginal wall is opened. The sling can usually be easily visualized. A right-angle clamp is then placed behind the sling, and the sling is loosened by either downward traction or spreading of the right-angle clamp. Caution must be taken to avoid urethral injury when passing the clamp between the urethra and an over-tensioned sling. If the sling is already incorporated into the tissue or has been in place for more than 2 weeks, it may be cut in the midline. In select instances, it may be prudent to excise the cut ends of the sling or actually remove the suburethral portion to prevent any potential exposure through the vaginal wall.

Indeed, if the clinical presentation is delayed and significant tissue ingrowth has occurred, it is our practice to perform a complete mesh excision of the vaginal portion of the TOT with removal of the maximum amount of mesh outside of

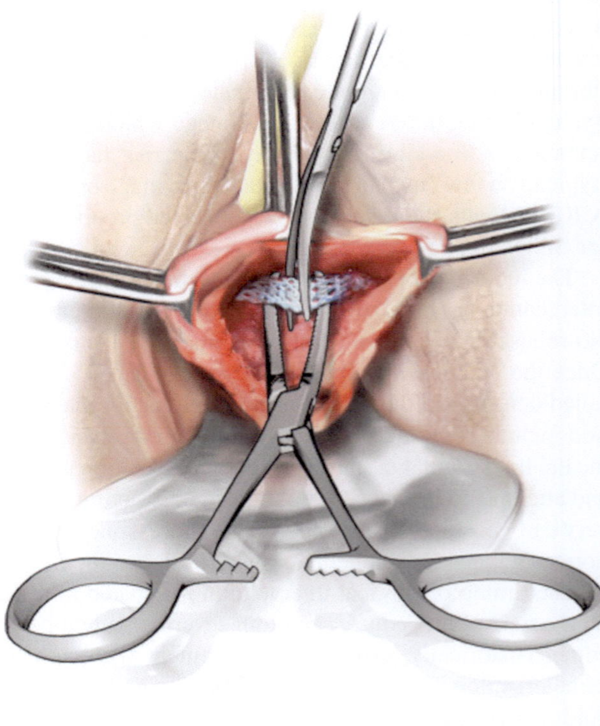

Fig. 12.3 Technique for incision of synthetic transobturator sling. The sling is identified, a right-angle clamp is placed between the sling and urethra, and the sling is transected at the midline. (From Dmochowski et al. [28], with permission. © Elsevier)

the obturator foramen (Fig. 12.4) [28]. It has been the author's experience that the location of the TOT slings in patients requiring removal for refractory symptoms or obstruction is rarely seated at the midurethra and is more likely placed at the proximal urethra or bladder neck. Translabial ultrasound may be useful to

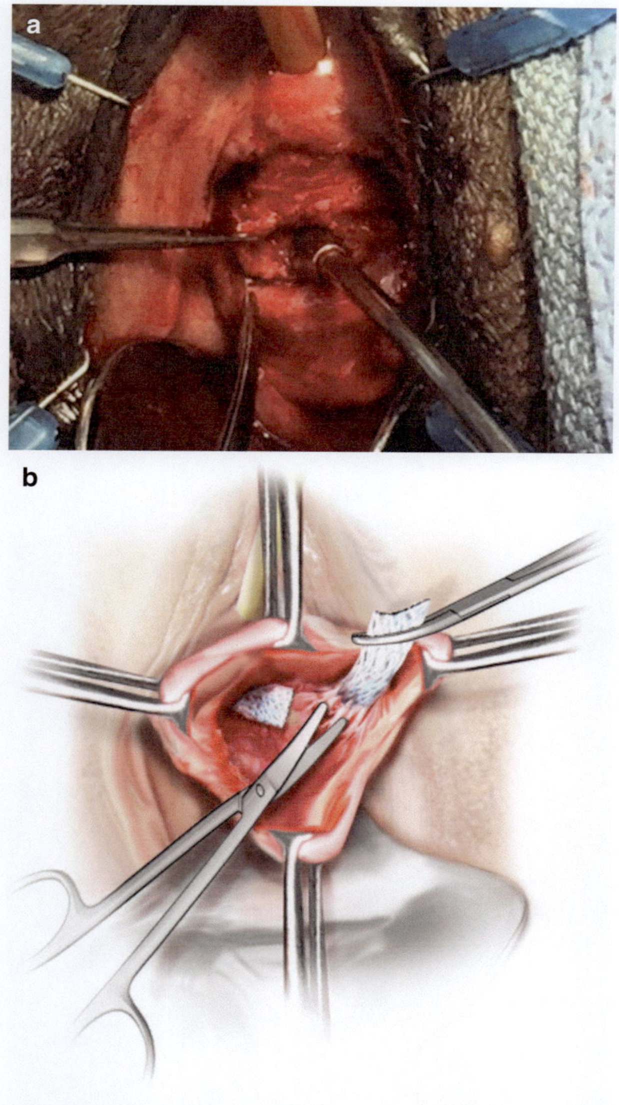

Fig. 12.4 Technique for sharp dissection off the ventral urethra. When the sling is adherent to the urethra, the sling is transected at midline over a sound, and sharp dissection is used for mobilization off the urethra (**a**, **b**). (The latter image from Dmochowski et al. [28], with permission. © Elsevier)

accurately locate the position of the TOT sling in these settings [29]. Although exceedingly rare following TOT removal, in patients who fail transvaginal sling excision, urethrolysis can be performed with success rates ranging from 65% to 84% [15, 30].

Mesh Excision and Transvaginal Urethrolysis

To perform a complete mesh excision or transvaginal urethrolysis, an inverted U-shaped anterior vaginal wall flap is created with the apex at the midurethra and base at the bladder neck (Fig. 12.5). The dissection is taken along the plane of pubocervical fascia up to the pubic bone laterally. The endopelvic fascia is perforated sharply with Metzenbaum scissors to enter the retropubic space (Fig. 12.6). Blunt and sharp dissection is used to free the urethra from its attachments to the pubic bone. Any scar or sling encountered in the retropubic space is divided. The urethra

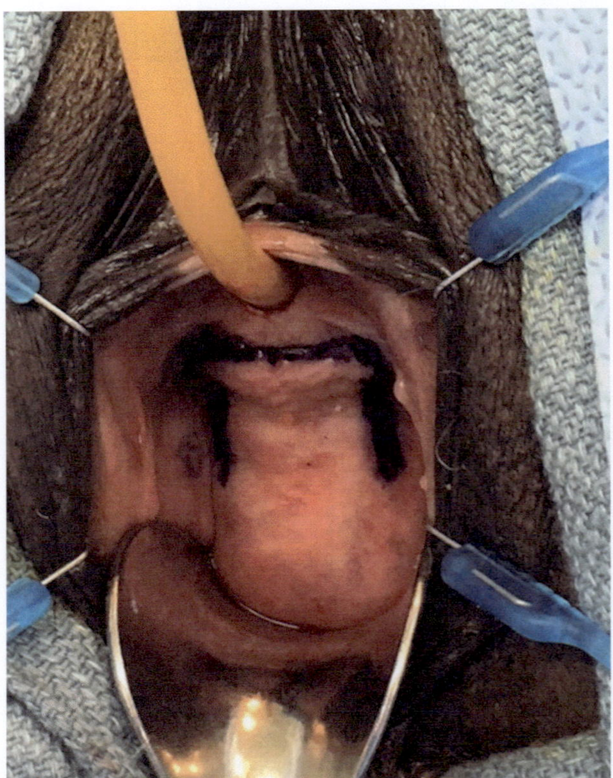

Fig. 12.5 Inverted U vaginal incision for mesh excision or transvaginal urethrolysis

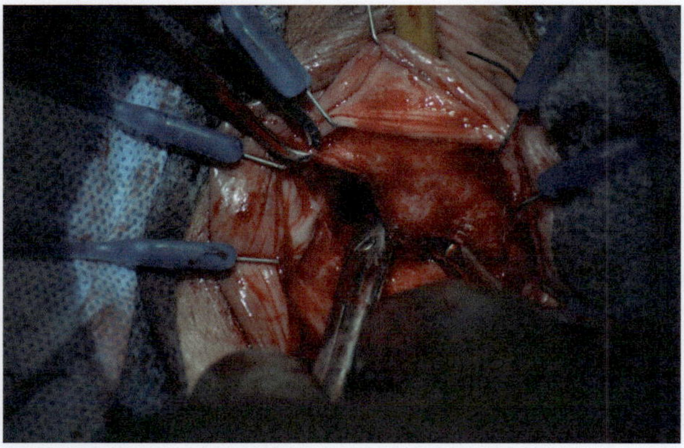

Fig. 12.6 Passage of scissors through fascia during transvaginal urethrolysis

is freed proximally to the bladder neck. The inverted U incision is advocated as it can accommodate flap coverage in the event the necessity for urethral or bladder reconstruction is encountered.

De Novo Urgency

Anti-incontinence surgery may either resolve or aggravate urge symptoms and lead to de novo urgency and detrusor overactivity. Urgency symptoms following incontinence surgery is unpredictable and a major cause of patient dissatisfaction. Meta-analysis of studies of patients undergoing sling surgery without concomitant prolapse repair estimated median rates of de novo urge incontinence to be 9% in pubovaginal groups and 6% in MUS groups; however the MUS groups were not separated according to route of sling placement [14]. In a Cochrane review, there was no statistical difference in de novo urgency and urge incontinence between TOT and RP MUS groups in the 14 trials compared (7% versus 6%, respectively, RR 1.08, 95% CI 0.75 to 1.56); however, the confidence interval was wide [19].

As alluded to previously, it is critical to be aware that storage symptoms such as de novo urgency, even with complete emptying may be a manifestation of urethral obstruction [25]. If diagnosed, relief of obstruction is the primary goal of treatment, while urge symptoms may be alleviated in a similar treatment algorithm as uncomplicated overactive bladder [31]. In the absence of obstruction (or any other reversible anatomic cause of the urgency such as sling erosion), initial treatment of urgency and urge incontinence consists of fluid management, timed voiding and antimuscarinic or beta-3 agonist medications. The majority of sling patients will have cure or control of their symptoms with these conservative measures. Refractory cases can be treated with botulinum toxin, peripheral nerve stimulation, sacral neuromodulation and peripheral nerve stimulation, and, in more extreme cases, augmentation cystoplasty or urinary diversion.

Delayed Postoperative Complications

Often patients present after a significant time delay from placement of the TOT, either due to evolution of symptoms or difficulty in identifying a provider with sophisticated knowledge of treating TOT complications. Clinical evaluation should, as always, begin with a detailed clinical history and a high index of suspicion for mesh-related complications. In addition to the aforementioned voiding dysfunction, patients should be assessed for dyspareunia, partner pain with intercourse, vaginal discharge or bleeding, pelvic/groin pain, urinary incontinence, hematuria, and recurrent urinary tract infections. Acquiring previous operative records is paramount to understanding of the potential pathology. Focused physical exam is performed, particularly with regard to understanding the focal areas of pain in the vagina and groin. As mentioned previously, cystourethroscopy is mandated if there is any possibility of mesh perforation of hypersuspension. Urodynamics may be utilized to elucidate obstruction and refractory irritative symptoms or to document recurrent/persistent SUI. In select cases, particularly with vaginal discharge, bleeding, or groin pain following TOT, imaging with CT or MRI of the pelvis may be warranted. Additionally, as discussed in several complementary chapters, ultrasound imaging may elucidate mesh location and suggest pathologic mechanisms. Pelvic imaging is of particular utility when there exists concern for a pelvic abscess or infection.

Meta-analysis has estimated the urethral erosion rate for synthetic slings between 2% and 4% [14]. Underreporting and variability in terminology likely cause underestimation of this complication in the literature. Urinary tract erosion can be a devastating complication for patients and frequently requires primary surgical management. It remains unclear whether erosions represent missed intraoperative perforations into the urinary tract or result from passive migration of the material into the urinary tract postoperatively. As discussed above, intraoperative cystoscopy during sling surgery is considered standard of care in order to identify iatrogenic urinary tract injuries. Potential contributing factors to urethral erosion include compromised urethral blood supply (from radiation or estrogen deficiency), excessive sling tension, extensive dissection too close to the urethra with subsequent devascularization, missed intraoperative urethral injury, and traumatic catheterization or dilation postoperatively.

Patients can present with irritative and obstructive voiding complaints, urinary incontinence, hematuria, recurrent urinary tract infections, and pain. Diagnosis is often delayed with one analysis reporting a mean of 9 months from sling placement to diagnosis of urethral erosion [32]. Definitive diagnosis is made endoscopically. Synthetic mesh erosions typically mandate complex open exploration, removal of all the exposed material, closure of the urinary tract, placement of an interposition graft material, and adequate postoperative drainage. Occasionally, small intravesical erosions in select patients may be treated with endoscopic scissor or laser excision and/or ablation [33, 34]. Due to complex nature of these repairs, preoperative counseling should emphasize realistic goals of anatomical and functional outcomes.

Exposure/Extrusion

The incidence of exposure or extrusion of synthetic slings into the vagina is 2–9% [14]. Extrusions may result from subclinical or overt infection, wound dehiscence, unrecognized vaginal wall perforation, devascularized vaginal flaps, wound compromise secondary to early local trauma (such as early intercourse), or the physical properties of the graft itself. Several earlier types of mesh were taken off the market due to high rates of encapsulation and subsequent extrusion yet may still be encountered in clinical practice [35].

Patients are typically symptomatic and may present with malodorous vaginal discharge, vaginal pain, dyspareunia, vaginal spotting, and partner discomfort during intercourse. Patients also frequently report that they can palpate mesh in the vagina. The exposed mesh is often palpable and visible on physical exam and can be associated with granulomatous tissue.

Unlike perforations or erosions into the urinary tract, management of mesh extrusion is usually straightforward and is associated with a high success rate and resolution of symptoms. Small extrusions can be initially treated conservatively with the application of topical estrogen creams to promote healing of the vaginal epithelium over the extruded material. Except in select instances of asymptomatic patients who are not surgical candidates, these exposures only be observed for a brief period of time before considering surgical intervention. Larger extrusions and those failing conservative treatment can be treated by raising vaginal flaps and covering the exposed mesh. We prefer to excise the exposed sling before covering the defect with the vaginal flaps to prevent future extrusions.

Recurrent Urinary Tract Infections

Up to 15% of patients undergoing sling procedures report urinary tract infections (UTI), and 8% of women undergoing urethrolysis after sling surgery presented with recurrent UTI [14, 25]. However, there exist inconsistencies in the detection and reporting of UTI after SUI procedures. Patients presenting after a routine sling procedure with symptoms suggestive of UTI such as frequency, urgency, and hematuria should be evaluated with a history, physical exam, urinalysis, and urine culture. Routine dipstick may be difficult to interpret immediately postoperatively, especially if the patient is being catheterized. Post-void residual urine volume may additionally suggest mechanism for infection or storage symptoms. A short course of antibiotics can be instituted empirically while awaiting culture results.

Patients with severe, ascending, or systemic symptoms such as abdominal or flank pain and fever and persistent or recurrent UTI warrant more thorough investigation. This includes a full history, physical exam, and appropriate urine and blood studies including cultures. Cross-sectional imaging and cystoscopy are essential in diagnosing sources of infection such as abscess, upper urinary tract obstruction, stones, foreign bodies, erosion of slings, or other occult bladder diseases. Post-void residual measurement and urodynamic studies can be used to rule out obstruction as a cause of the recurrent UTI.

Wound-Related Infections

Due to the unique anatomy of TOT placement, wound infections may become particularly problematic and present as leg pain, difficulty with ambulation, cellulitis, or overt infection. The literature is replete with case reports of thigh infection and abscesses, even progression to necrotizing fasciitis following TOT placement [36–40]. As is mandated in the majority of such severe infections, most mandate exploration and drainage which often includes mesh removal from multiple compartments.

Pain

Vaginal, pelvic, and groin pain, associated with or without dyspareunia, is one of the most problematic clinical scenarios to evaluation and manage following TOT sling. Pain in the context of the MUS may occur from a myriad of etiologies, including mesh contraction, excessive tensioning, fibrosis with nerve entrapment, and subclinical or overt infection, or may be completely unrelated to the sling itself. The intricacies of groin pain associated specifically with TOT slings can be debilitating and complex with regard to surgical management. In the majority of cases, the postoperative groin or leg pain is transient and may be managed with conservative treatment such as rest, physical therapy, or nonsteroidal anti-inflammatory medications. Progression to use of local anesthetic may necessitate collaboration with pain management specialists and consideration for progression to surgical excision.

Unfortunately, MUS excision may not be curative with regard to pain resolution. However, studies estimate that between 67% and 73% of women report improvement in pain symptoms following mesh excision [41, 42]. However, up to 18% of patients reported worsening pain symptoms with 19% indicating their pain was unchanged.

Groin Pain

Groin pain is a recognized complication of all MUS techniques, but particularly prevalent with the TOT approach. Such devastating groin pain has been reported in between 4% and 24% of patients following TOT MUS [43, 44]. Additional

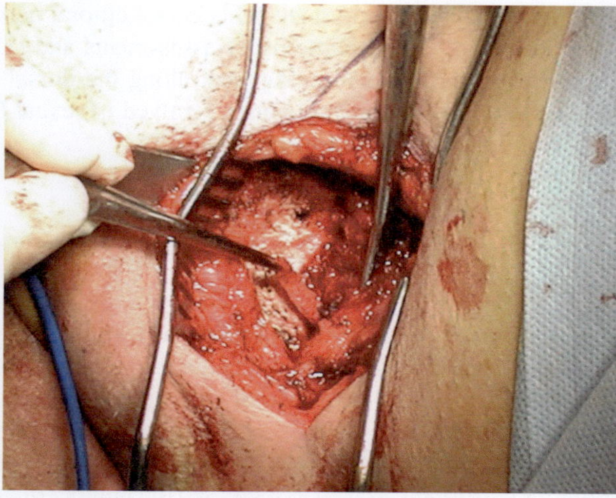

Fig. 12.7 Transobturator removal of transobturator sling arm for refractory thigh pain

analyses of women undergoing sling removal for mesh-related complications indicated 21% of their TOT population experienced groin pain, which was five times higher risk than RP slings [45]. Fifteen percent of these TOT patients required unilateral or bilateral groin mesh removal. Such intractable groin and leg pain typically requires a dual approach with both thigh and vaginal dissection to optimize complete mesh excision and pain symptoms [46, 47]. Obturator dissection and mesh excision are typically performed through a lateral groin incision over the inferior pubic ramus at the level of the obturator foramen (Fig. 12.7). The incision is located approximately 2 cm lateral to the pubic ramus and 3 cm inferior to the adductor longus tendon insertion. The adductor brevis and gracilis are divided for maximal exposure of the obturator membrane. A vaginal incision with dissection medial in the obturator foramen may be useful even when the vaginal component of the mesh was previously excised. Often it is prudent to involve consultant orthopedic surgeons outside of exceptionally high-volume centers where routine mesh excision is performed.

Dyspareunia

Dyspareunia is a frequently reported complication of all types of MUS but appears in some studies to have a higher incidence with TOT placement. In an evaluation of late sling complications, compared to the 3% rate of dyspareunia with RP slings, 18% of women reported persistent dyspareunia following TOT placement [48]. Alternately, a follow-up analysis from the TOMUS trial reported significant improvement in dyspareunia, incontinence during sex, and fear of incontinence during sex for both TOT and RP approaches [49].

One particularly striking case report documents dorsal clitoral nerve injury following TOT sling placement [50]. Neurosensory assessments and selective nerve blocks were utilized to trace the nerve entrapment along the dorsal nerve of the clitoris. This case highlights that many structures involved in sexual function may be vulnerable to injury during TOT placement.

Conclusion

TOT sling surgeries for female SUI are widely performed with generally high rates of success and low rates of morbidity. Complications from these procedures are likely underreported in the literature because of variability of definitions, lack of mandatory reporting vehicles and the need for studies with longer follow-up. Enthusiasm for minimally invasive MUSs has substantially increased the number of incontinence surgeries performed, as well as increased the number of and variability in the practitioners implanting these devices. Many complications can be prevented by first ensuring that the indication for the particular type of sling is appropriate and, second, by adhering to good surgical technique. Patients must be well-counseled preoperatively about all the potential risks of the procedure, as well as the realistic expected outcomes. Practitioners should remain attentive to patient symptoms postoperatively, in order to promptly identify potential complications. Unique aspects to TOT complications may require specialized evaluation and therapy, particularly with regard to management of refractory pain symptoms.

References

1. Reynolds WS, Dmochowski RR, Penson DF. Epidemiology of stress urinary incontinence in women. Curr Urol Rep. 2011;12(5):370–6.
2. Lemack G, Anger J. Urinary incontinence and pelvic prolapse: epidemiology and pathophysiology. In: Wein AJ, Kavoussi LR, Partin AW, Peters CA, editors. Campbell-Walsh urology, vol. 3. 11th ed. Philadelphia: Elsevier; 2016. p. 1743–60.
3. van Geelen J, Hunskaar S. The epidemiology of female urinary incontinence. Eur Clin Obstet Gynecol. 2005;1:3.
4. Koski ME, Chamberlain J, Rosoff J, Vaughan T, Kaufman MR, Winters JC, et al. Patient perception of transvaginal mesh and the media. Urology. 2014;84(3):575–82.
5. Wood LN, Anger JT. Urinary incontinence in women. BMJ. 2014;349:g4531.
6. Delorme E. Transobturator urethral suspension: mini-invasive procedure in the treatment of stress urinary incontinence in women. Prog Urol. 2001;11:1306–13.
7. U.S. Food & Drug Administration. Medical devices. Urogynecologic surgical mesh implants. FDA's role and activities. Updated 4 Jan 2016. http://www.fda.gov/MedicalDevices/ProductsandMedicalProcedures/ImplantsandProsthetics/UroGynSurgicalMesh/ucm262301.htm. Accessed 15 Sept 2017.
8. U.S. Food & Drug Administration. Medical devices. Considerations about surgical mesh for SUI. Updated 27 Mar 2013. http://www.fda.gov/MedicalDevices/ProductsandMedicalProcedures/ImplantsandProsthetics/UroGynSurgicalMesh/ucm345219.htm. Accessed 15 Sept 2017.

9. American Urogynecologic Society (AUGS) and the Society for Urodynamics, Female Pelvic Medicine and Urogenital Reconstruction (SUFU). Position Statement. Mesh midurethral slings for stress urinary incontinence. Jan 2014; updated Jun 2016. http://sufuorg.com/docs/news/augs-sufu-mus-position-statement.aspx. Accessed 15 Sept 2017.
10. Dmochowski RR, Osborn DJ, Reynolds WS. Slings: autologous, biologic, synthetic, and midurethral. In: Wein AJ, Kavoussi LR, Partin AW, Peters CA, editors. Campbell-Walsh urology. 11th, vol. 3. Philadelphia: Elsevier; 2016. p. 1987–2038.
11. Tash J, Staskin DR. Artificial graft slings at the midurethra: physiology of continence. Curr Urol Rep. 2003;4(5):367–70.
12. Fritel X, Zabak K, Pigne A, Demaria F, Benifla JL. Predictive value of urethral mobility before suburethral tape procedure for urinary stress incontinence in women. J Urol. 2002;168(6):2472–5.
13. Petri E, Niemeyer R, Martan A, Tunn R, Naumann G, Koelbl H. Reasons for and treatment of surgical complications with alloplastic slings. Int Urogynecol J Pelvic Floor Dysfunct. 2006;17(1):3–13.
14. Dmochowski RR, Blaivas JM, Gormley EA, Juma S, Karram MM, Lightner DJ, et al. Female Stress Urinary Incontinence Update Panel of the American Urological Association Education and Research, Inc, Whetter LE. Update of AUA guideline on the surgical management of female stress urinary incontinence J Urol. 2010;183(5):1906–14.
15. Richter HE, Albo ME, Zyczynski HM, Kenton K, Norton PA, Sirls LT, et al. Retropubic versus transobturator midurethral slings for stress incontinence. N Engl J Med. 2010;362(22):2066–76.
16. Haylen BT, Freeman RM, Swift SE, Cosson M, Davila GW, Deprest J, et al. An International Urogynecological Association (IUGA) / International Continence Society (ICS) joint terminology and classification of the complications related directly to the insertion of prostheses (meshes, implants, tapes) & grafts in female pelvic floor surgery. Int Urogynecol J. 2011;22(1):3–15.
17. Karram M, Pancholy A. Synthetic midurethral slings for the correction of stress urinary incontinence. In: Baggish MS, Karram MM, editors. Atlas of pelvic anatomy and gynecologic surgery. 3rd ed. St. Louis: Elsevier Saunders; 2011. p. 747–80.
18. Corton MM. Critical anatomic concepts for safe surgical mesh. Clin Obstet Gynecol. 2013;56(2):247–56.
19. Ogah J, Cody JD, Rogerson L. Minimally invasive synthetic suburethral sling operations for stress urinary incontinence in women. Cochrane Database Syst Rev. 2009 Oct 07(4):CD006375.
20. Ko JK, Ku CH. Embolization for pelvic arterial bleeding following a transobturator tape procedure. J Obstet Gynecol Res. 2013;40(3):865–8.
21. Daneshgari F, Kong W, Swartz M. Complications of mid urethral slings: important outcomes for future clinical trials. J Urol. 2008;180(5):1890–7.
22. Shah SR, Nitti VW. Diagnosis and treatment of obstruction following incontinence surgery—urethrolysis and other techniques. In: Cardoza L, Staskin D, editors. Textbook of female urology and urogynecology. 3rd ed. London: Informa UK Ltd; 2010. p. 749–62.
23. Nitti VW, Raz S. Obstruction following anti-incontinence procedures: diagnosis and treatment with transvaginal urethrolysis. J Urol. 1994;152(1):93–8.
24. Gomelsky A, Nitti VW, Dmochowski RR. Management of obstructive voiding dysfunction after incontinence surgery: lessons learned. Urology. 2003;62(3):391–9. Review
25. Carr LK, Webster GD. Voiding dysfunction following incontinence surgery: diagnosis and treatment with retropubic or vaginal urethrolysis. J Urol. 1997;157(3):821–3.
26. FitzGerald MP, Brubaker L. The etiology of urinary retention after surgery for genuine stress incontinence. Neurourol Urodyn. 2001;20(1):13–21.
27. Mishra VC, Mishra N, Karim OM, Motiwala HG. Voiding dysfunction after tension-free vaginal tape: a conservative approach is often successful. Int Urogynecol J Pelvic Floor Dysfunct. 2005;16(3):210–4; discussion: 4.
28. Dmochowski RR, Karram MM, Reynolds WS. Surgery for urinary incontinence: female pelvic surgery video atlas series. Expert consult: online and print, Female pelvic video surgery atlas series. Philadelphia: Elsevier Saunders; 2013.

29. Staack A, Vitale J, Ragavendra N, Rodriguez LV. Translabial ultrasonography for evaluation of synthetic mesh in the vagina. Urology. 2014;83(1):68–74.
30. Chang-Kit L, Kaufman MR, Dmochowski RR. Complications of biologic and synthetic slings and their management. In: Goldman HB, editor. Complications of female incontinence and pelvic reconstructive surgery, Current clinical urology. New York: Springer Science+Business Media; 2013. p. 115–32.
31. Gormley EA, Lightner DJ, Burgio KL, Chai TC, Clemens JQ, Culkin DJ, et al. Diagnosis and treatment of overactive bladder (non-neurogenic) in adults: AUA/SUFU guideline. J Urol. 2012;188(6 Suppl):2455–63.
32. Amundsen CL, Flynn BJ, Webster GD. Urethral erosion after synthetic and nonsynthetic pubovaginal slings: differences in management and continence outcome. J Urol. 2003;170(1):134–7. discussion 7
33. Oh TH, Ryu DS. Transurethral resection of intravesical mesh after midurethral sling procedures. J Endourol. 2009;23(8):1333–7.
34. Doumouchtsis SK, Lee FY, Bramwell D, Fynes MM. Evaluation of holmium laser for managing mesh/suture complications of continence surgery. BJU Int. 2011;108(9):1472–8.
35. Yamada BS, Govier FE, Stefanovic KB, Kobashi KC. High rate of vaginal erosions associated with the mentor ObTape. J Urol 2006;176(2):651–4; discussion: 4.
36. Roth TM. Serratia marcescens thigh infection after transobturator sling without associated mesh exposure. Female Pelvic Med Reconstr Surg. 2015;21(2):e19–20.
37. Kim TH, Lee HH, Kim JM. Chronic vaginal discharge and left leg edema after a transobturator tape procedure. Int Urogynecol J. 2014;25(5):695–7.
38. Choi H, Bae JH, Lee JG. Severe thigh abscess two years after transobturator sling operation. Low Urin Tract Symptoms. 2011;3(1):51–4.
39. Rardin CR, Moore R, Ward RM, Myers DL. Recurrent thigh abscess with necrotizing fasciitis from a retained transobturator sling segment. J Minim Invasive Gynecol. 2009;16(1):84–7.
40. Goldman HB. Large thigh abscess after placement of synthetic transobturator sling. Int Urogynecol J Pelvic Floor Dysfunct. 2006;17(3):295–6.
41. Danford JM, Osborn DJ, Reynolds WS, Biller DH, Dmochowski RR. Postoperative pain outcomes after transvaginal mesh revision. Int Urogynecol J. 2015;26(1):65–9.
42. Hou JC, Alhalabi F, Lemack GE, Zimmern PE. Outcome of transvaginal mesh and tape removed for pain only. J Urol. 2014;192(3):856–60.
43. Laurikainen E, Valpas A, Kivela A, Kalliola T, Rinne K, Takala T, et al. Retropubic compared with transobturator tape placement in treatment of urinary incontinence: a randomized controlled trial. Obstet Gynecol. 2007;109(1):4–11.
44. Brubaker L, Norton PA, Albo ME, Chai TC, Dandreo KJ, Lloyd KL, et al. Adverse events over two years after retropubic or transobturator midurethral sling surgery: findings from the Trial of Midurethral Slings (TOMUS) study. Am J Obstet Gynecol. 2011;205(5):498.e1–6.
45. Chinthakanan O, Miklos JR, Moore RD, Karp DR, Nogueiras GM, Davila GW. The indication and surgical treatment of 286 midurethral synthetic sling complications: a multicenter study. Surg Technol Int. 2016;29:167–71.
46. Reynolds WS, Kit LC, Kaufman MR, Karram M, Bales GT, Dmochowski RR. Obturator foramen dissection for excision of symptomatic transobturator mesh. J Urol. 2012;187(5):1680–4.
47. King AB, Tenggardjaja C, Goldman HB. Prospective evaluation of the effect of thigh dissection for removal of transobturator mid urethral slings on refractory thigh pain. J Urol. 2016;196(4):1207–12.
48. Petri E, Ashok K. Comparison of late complications of retropubic and transobturator slings in stress urinary incontinence. Int Urogynecol J. 2012;23(3):321–5.
49. Zyczynski HM, Rickey L, Dyer KY, Wilson T, Stoddard AM, Gormley EA, et al. Sexual activity and function in women more than 2 years after midurethral sling placement. Am J Obstet Gynecol. 2012;207(5):421.e1–6.
50. Moss CF, Damitz LA, Gracely RH, Mintz AC, Zolnoun DA, Dellon AL. Dorsal clitoral nerve injury following transobturator midurethral sling. J Pain Res. 2016;9:727–30.

Chapter 13
Vaginal Mesh and Pain Complications

Ghazaleh Rostaminia, Tanaz Ferzandi, and S. Abbas Shobeiri

Introduction

In pelvic reconstructive surgery, the school of thought that fascial defects are a primary etiology for development of genital prolapse has led to increased graft utilization to augment fascial strength in an attempt to promote repair longevity and permanence [1]. Grafts serve to strengthen attenuated tissue and enhance healing in areas with compromised tissue integrity. However, the use of synthetic mesh or biologic grafts in pelvic organ prolapse surgery is associated with unique complications not seen in repairs with native tissue including pain that can be debilitating for patient. Pain can be a result of direct nerve injury during mesh placement or delayed neuropathy due to fibrosis, or mesh shrinkage. There is also a human factor involved in reactivity to mesh in vivo. Some individuals are "high responders," and others are "low responders" in the formation of fibrous tissue as stimulated in the presence of the mesh [2]. Treating pain complication after mesh placement requires complete work up and can be challenging in presence of neuropathy. Another issue to consider is the surgeon factor. Some surgeons are "high performers" who can identify and resolve device related complications quickly, while the "low performer"

G. Rostaminia
Female Pelvic Medicine and Reconstructive Surgery NorthShore University Health System/University of Chicago, Skokie, IL, USA

T. Ferzandi
Division of Urogynecology and Pelvic Reconstructive Surgery, Department of Obstetrics and Gynecology, Tufts Medical Center, Boston, MA, USA

S. A. Shobeiri (✉)
INOVA Health System, Falls Church, VA, USA
e-mail: Abbas.shobeiri@inova.org

S. A. Shobeiri (ed.), *The Innovation and Evolution of Medical Devices*,
https://doi.org/10.1007/978-3-319-97073-8_13

surgeons fail to recognize when the device has malfunctioned. In this chapter, we will discuss acute and chronic mesh, vaginal mesh kit and trocar complications.

The lifetime risk for requiring pelvic surgery for pelvic floor dysfunction symptoms for a woman in the United States is 11%, with a reoperation risk of 29% [3]. The management of advanced and symptomatic prolapse or incontinence is primarily surgical; however, the route and method of operation are a matter of debate. Despite many attempts at standardization of surgical techniques, pelvic reconstructive surgery is still somewhat of an art that requires intimate understanding of pelvic floor anatomy.

Given the high reoperation rate, grafts have been widely promoted for use in reconstructive surgeries, and the use of artificial implanted materials to enhance tissue repair has long been a hallmark of general surgery. Based on pervious data collected from hernia procedures, the use of grafts in pelvic reconstructive surgery has increased in the past decades. In pelvic reconstructive surgery, the school of thought that fascial defects are a primary etiology for development of genital prolapse has led to increased graft utilization to augment fascial strength in an attempt to promote repair longevity and permanence [1]. Grafts are supposed to serve to strengthen attenuated tissue and enhance healing in areas with compromised tissue integrity. This mindset overlooks the fact that the pelvic floor is not made entirely of fascia but also of muscles, tendons, and nerves.

Grafts are available in biologic and synthetic forms. Regardless of their origin, the properties of ideal grafts should be similar to that of an ideal suture. They should be non-carcinogenic, durable, chemically inert, and overall resistant to infection, although cost can be a factor. Unlike sutures, the grafts create a large foreign body burden that may overcome body defenses. Perhaps like sugar, a little is sweet and too much becomes poison. Randomized controlled trials have revealed improved anatomic outcomes after vaginal reconstructive surgery utilizing polypropylene mesh when compared with traditional vaginal prolapse repairs for the anterior compartment [4, 5]. However, the use of synthetic mesh or biologic grafts in pelvic organ prolapse surgery is associated with unique and at times irreversible complications not seen in repair with native tissue. A systematic review of seven randomized controlled trials comparing native tissue repair with synthetic mesh vaginal prolapse repairs found that more women in the mesh group required repeat surgery for the combined outcome of prolapse, stress incontinence, or mesh exposure (RR, 2.40; 95% CI, 1.51–3.81) [6]. Abbott et al., in a large multicenter review, described the management of mesh-related complications at four tertiary referral centers. Of 347 patients presenting with mesh-related complications, the majority (79.3%) underwent a surgical intervention, and approximately one-quarter (26.2%) underwent more than one procedure. TVM-related complications were typically described as severe, managed surgically with the majority (60%) undergoing two or more interventions [7]. In a long-term follow-up of 79 patients undergoing mesh removal at least 2 years after initial implant (mean 4 years), 27% (21 patients) required one or more additional treatments for pain symptoms after mesh removal, and 20% (16 patients) underwent additional surgery [8]. During a 75-month period, a total of 398 procedures were performed for the removal of vaginally placed mesh. A total of 326 (82%) patients underwent single-compartment surgery, 48 (12%) underwent multicompartment surgery, and in 26 (6%), the type of surgery was unclear. The indications for mesh removal included pain (63%), dyspareunia (57%), mesh exposure (54%), and voiding dysfunction (39%). The mean length of mesh removed was 4 cm (standard deviation±2.8). Those with multicompartment surgery had approximately three times higher estimated blood loss compared with single-compartment surgery ($P < 0.001$). The odds of blood transfusion after multicompartment surgery were more than nine times higher than the odds of transfusion after a single-compartment surgery (odds ratio 9.7, 95% confidence interval 2.1–44.6; $P < 0.01$) [8].

The International Urogynecology Association and International Continence Society developed a classification of complications related to the insertion of grafts (Fig. 13.1 and Table 13.1) [9]. Our general approach to patients with vaginal mesh complications at the INOVA Women's Hospital is detailed in Fig. 13.2. All patients with mesh complications benefit from a 3D pelvic floor ultrasonography. If the presenting complication is recurrent prolapse, then they would be evaluated for a restrictive repair such as colpocleisis or a reconstructive repair using their own tissue, depending on their age and desire for sexual activity. The phenomenon of recurrent prolapse after a giant piece of mesh is inserted can be explained by mesh reorganization and contraction. We have seen prolapses that slide posterior or anterior to the prolapse. If the patient has extrusion/erosion, we remove as much mesh as possible to arrive at fresh tissue and edges for tissue approximation. If the tissue reapproximation results in undesired vaginal stenosis, we harvest tissue from the fascia lata to perform an anterior or posterior hammock procedure. If pain is primary or part of the presenting symptom, one of the major reasons may be mesh contraction that is easily seen on ultrasound as roping, folding, bunching, or a mesh that is flat and stretched to the maximum. Removal of mesh can be more complicated if pudendal neuralgia is part of the etiology. Full removal of mesh causing pudendal neuralgia requires transgluteal (Fig. 13.3) or the ischiorectal approach. In some cases obturator exploration may be required to remove the mesh arms (Fig. 13.4) [10]. If pain is persistent despite mesh removal, the patient may be facing a lifelong treatment with nerve injections and medical management.

Pain is a less commonly acknowledged and yet most distressing complication of vaginal mesh kit surgeries, and its clinical manifestation varies greatly. It is not that pain occurs much more frequently in vaginal mesh kit surgeries than in uterosacral suspension, but it is the fact that it is varied and frequently irreversible (Table 13.2) [11]. In this chapter, we aim to review the pathophysiology of pain after pelvic reconstructive surgeries utilizing vaginal mesh kits. Understanding the contributing factors to pain complications after vaginal mesh kit surgery is essential for treatment algorithms.

Host Response to Synthetic Graft (Mesh)

Use of mesh for pelvic reconstructive surgery is not new, as multiple materials have been used for vaginal prolapse and stress incontinence management in the past. Synthetic mesh is classified into four types based primarily on its pore size (Table 13.3) [12]. Recognition of the frequent occurrence of healing abnormalities

CATEGORY

	General Description	A (Asymptomatic)	B (Symptomatic)	C (Infection)	D (Abscess)
1	**Vaginal:** no epithelial separation Include prominence (e.g. due to wrinkling or folding), mesh fibre palpation or contraction (shrinkage)	**1A:** Abnormal prosthesis or graft finding on clinical examination	**1B:** Symptomatic e.g. unusal discomfort/pain; dyspareunia (either partner); bleeding	**1C:** Infection (suspected or actual)	**1D** = Abscess
2	**Vaginal:** smaller ≤ 1cm exposure	**2A:** Asymptomatic	**2B:** Symptomatic	**2C:** Infection	**2D** = Abscess
3	**Vaginal:** larger >1cm exposure, or any extrusion	**3A:** Asymptomatic 1-3Aa if no prosthesis or graft related pain	**3B:** Symptomatic 1-3B (*b-e*) if prosthesis or graft related pain	**3C:** Infection 1-3C/1-3D (*b-e*)if prosthesis or graft related pain	**3D** = Abscess
4	**Urinary Tract:** compromise or perforation including prosthesis (graft) perforation, fistula and calculus	**4A:** Small intraoperative defect e.g. bladder perforation	**4B:** Other lower urinary tract complication or urinary retention	**4C:** Ureteric or upper urinary tract complication	
5	**Rectal or Bowel:** compromise or perforation including prosthesis (graft) perforation and fistula	**5A:** Small intraoperative defect (rectal or bowel)	**5B:** Rectal injury or compromise	**5C:** Small or Large bowel injury or compromise	**5D** = Abscess
6	**Skin and/or musculoskeletal:** complications including discharge pain lump or sinus tract formation	**6A:** Asymptomatic, abnormal finding on clinical examination	**6B:** Symptomatic e.g. discharge, pain or lump	**6C:** Infection e.g. sinus tract formation	**6D** = Abscess
7	**Patient:** compromise including hematoma or systemic compromise	**7A:** Bleeding complication including haematoma	**7B:** Major degree of resuscitation or intensive care*	**7C:** Mortality* ^(additional complication - no site applicable - **S 0**)	

TIME (clinically diagnosed)

T1: Intraoperative to 48 hours	**T2:** 48 hours to 2 months	**T3:** 2 months to 12 months	**T4:** over 12 months

SITE

S1: Vaginal: area of suture lines	**S2:** Vaginal: away from from area of suture line	**S3:** Trocar passage Exception: Intra-abdominal **(S5)**	**S4:** other skin or musculoskeletal site	**S5:** Intra-abdominal

N.B

1. Multiple complications may occur in the same patient. There may be early and late complications in the same patient. i.e. All complications to be listed. Tables of complications may often be procedures specific.
2. The highest final category for any single complication should be used if there is a change over time. (patient 888)
3. Urinary tract infections and functional issues (apart from 4B) have not been included.

CODE ☐☐☐ - T ☐ - S ☐

Fig. 13.1 International Urogynecological Association (IUGA) vaginal mesh complication classification. (From Haylen et al. [9], with permission)

Table 13.1 Terminology of vaginal mesh. The International Urogynecology Association and International Continence Society classification of complications related to the insertion of grafts

Terms Used	Definition
Prosthesis	A fabricated substitute to assist a damaged body part or to augment or stabilize a hypoplastic structure
A. Mesh	A (prosthetic) network fabric or structure
B. Implant	A surgically inserted or embedded prosthesis
C. Tape (sling)	A flat strip of synthetic material
Graft	Any tissue or organ for transplantation. This term will refer to biological materials inserted
A. Autologous grafts	From the woman's own tissues, e.g., dura mater, rectus sheath, or fascia lata
B. Allografts	From postmortem tissue banks
C. Xenografts	From other species, e.g., modified porcine dermis, porcine small intestine, bovine pericardium
Complication	A morbid process or event that occurs during the course of a surgery that is not an essential part of that surgery
Contraction	Shrinkage or reduction in size
Prominence	Parts that protrude beyond the surface (e.g., due to wrinkling or folding with no epithelial separation)
Separation	Physically disconnected (e.g., vaginal epithelium)
Exposure	A condition of displaying, revealing, exhibiting, or making accessible, e.g., vaginal mesh visualized through separated vaginal epithelium
Extrusion	Passage gradually out of a body structure or tissue
Compromise	Bring into danger
Perforation	Abnormal opening into a hollow organ or viscus
Dehiscence	A bursting open or gaping along natural or sutured line

From Haylen et al. [9], with permission

associated with microporous, multifilament materials (i.e., Gore-Tex, WL GORE, Newark DE, USA; Protogen, Boston Scientific, Natick MA, USA) as compared to macroporous, monofilament polypropylene has led to exclusive use of the latter (Type 1 mesh) for vaginal surgery. Polypropylene in mesh form is commonly considered inert and without adverse reactions after implantation in humans. The literature suggests otherwise as it pertains to the vaginal mesh kits for pelvic organ prolapse, with reports of various degrees of degradation including depolymerization, cross-linking, and oxidative degradation by free radicals, additive leaching, hydrolysis, stress cracking, and mesh shrinkage along with infection, chronic inflammation, and the stimulation of sclerosis. Gristina [13] stated in 1987 that minutes after insertion there is a "race for the surface" of the mesh between host cells and bacteria. If the host cells win, then the surface is protected from bacterial colonization, whereas if the bacteria win and manage to secrete their "slime" that envelops them so that host defenses cannot get to them, then the graft is irreversibly contaminated. These bacteria can remain quiescent for long periods of time with the possibility of establishing an actual tissue infection at any time. In 1998, Klinge reported shrinkage of mesh by 30–50% after 4 weeks [14]. Because the

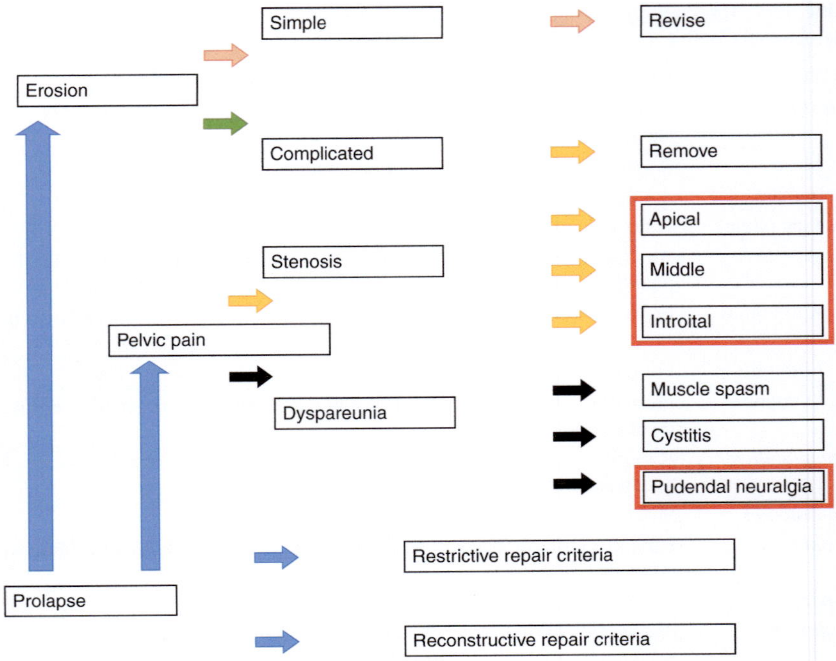

Fig. 13.2 The mesh treatment pathway as utilized by the senior author

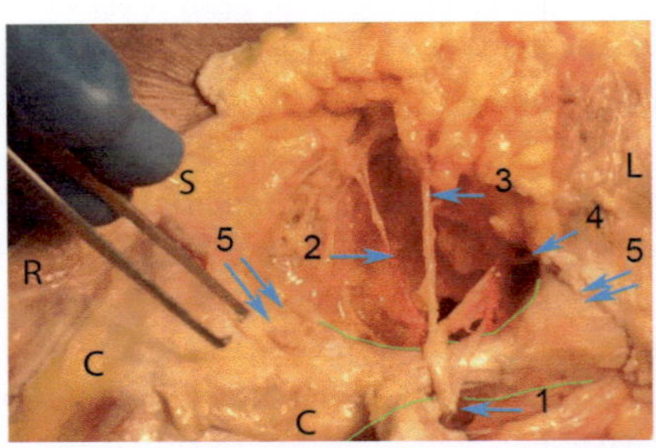

Fig. 13.3 Transgluteal view of a pudendal nerve dissection in a fresh cadaver in prone position with head toward the bottom of the picture and feet toward the top. Gluteus maximus and minimus muscles have been removed. (1) The *green line* outlines the sacrospinous ligament. (2) The inferior rectal nerve. (3) The perineal branch. (4) The vulvar/clitoral branch entering the Alcock's canal. (5) The sacrotuberous ligament has been cut to unroof the sacrospinous ligament underneath. (C) Cephalad. (R) Right. (L) Left. (S) Sacrum. (© Shobeiri)

vagina is a tubular structure, a decreased caliber and shortening can result, and as such, dyspareunia can be explained by such mesh shrinkage, as well as by tension on mesh arms (often implanted with trocars) with neuroma formation (Fig. 13.5) [15]. There is also a human factor involved in reactivity to mesh in vivo. Some individuals may be "high responders," and others are "low responders" in the

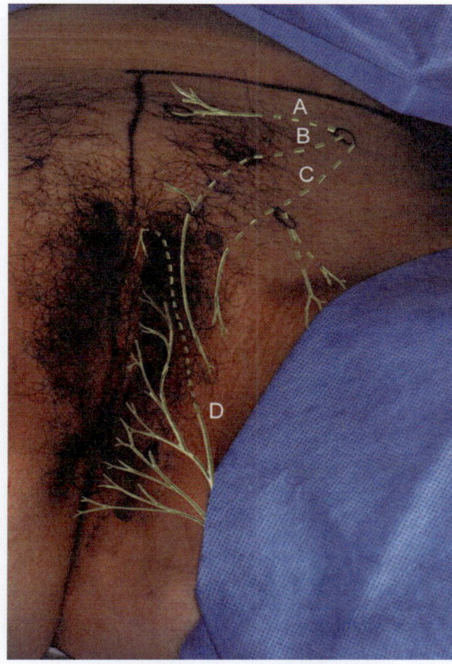

Fig. 13.4 (A) Anterior cutaneous branches of the iliohypogastric nerve. (B) Anterior labial branches of the ilioinguinal nerve. (C) Genitofemoral nerve (both the genital and femoral branches). (D) Dorsal nerve of the clitoris (continuation of pudendal nerve shown as dashed lines deeper in the muscles of the urogenital diaphragm). The course of the specified nerves is delineated based on quantitative sensory testing and selective nerve block in this patient. (From Parnell et al. [10], with permission)

Table 13.2 Intraoperative and postoperative complications

Variables	VMP ($n = 206$)	USLS ($n = 231$)	*P* Value	ASC ($n = 305$)	*P* value
Bladder injury, no. (%)	2 (1.0)	6 (2.6)	NS	14 (4.6)	<0.02[a]
Small bowel injury, no. (%)	0 (0.0)	1 (0.4)	NS	1 (1.03)	NS
Rectum injury, no. (%)	1 (0.5)	2 (0.9)	NS	1 (1.03)	NS
Hemorrhage, > 500 mLno. (%)	0 (0.0)	11 (4.8)	<0.01[a]	12 (3.9)	<0.01[a]
Transfusion, no. (%)	1 (0.5)	8 (3.5)	0.04[a]	7 (2.3)	NS
Fever, no. (%)	0 (0.0)	4 (1.7)	NS	14 (4.6)	<0.01[a]
Return to OR, no. (%)	6 (2.9)	10 (4.3)	NS	4 (1.3)	NS
Urinary tract infection, no. (%)	11 (5.3)	22 (9.6)	NS	17 (5.6)	NS
Urinary retention, no. (%)	12 (5.9)	9 (3.9)	NS	6 (2.0)	<0.03[a]
Vaginal hematoma, no. (%)	1 (0.5)	1 (0.4)	NS	0 (0)	NS
Thromboembolism, no. (%)	0 (0.0)	1 (0.4	NS	1 (0.3)	NS
Groin pain, no. (%) ←	22 (10.7)	3 (1.3)	<0.01[a]	6 (2.0)	<0.01[a]
Buttock pain, no. (%) ←	14 (6.8)	9 (3.9)	NS	0 (0)	<0.01[a]
Defecatory pain, no. (%) ←	5 (2.4)	4 (2.1)	NS	2 (0.7)	NS
Erosion, no. (%)	1 (0.5)	0 (0.0)	NS	1 (0.3)	NS
Vaginal extrusion, no. (%)	9 (4.4)	19 (8.3)	NS	16 (5.3)	NS
Dyspareunia, no. (%) ←	10 (4.9)	14 (6.4)	NS	13 (4.3)	NS

From Sanses et al. [11], with permission

ASC abdominal sacrocolpopexy, *NS* not statistically significant, *OR* operating room, *USLS* uterosacral ligament suspension, *VMP* vaginal mesh procedure

NS = $P > 0.05$

[a]Fisher exact test

Table 13.3 Classification of synthetic mesh

Type	Fiber	Porosity	Pore size	Polymer example
I	Monofilament	Macroporous	>75 μm	Polypropylene
II	Multifilament	Microporous	<10 μm	Expanded polytetrafluoroethylene
III	Multifilament	Microporous/Macroporous	Varies	Polyethylene
IV	Monofilament	Submicronic	<1 μm	Polypropylene sheet with silicone

Data from Amid [12]

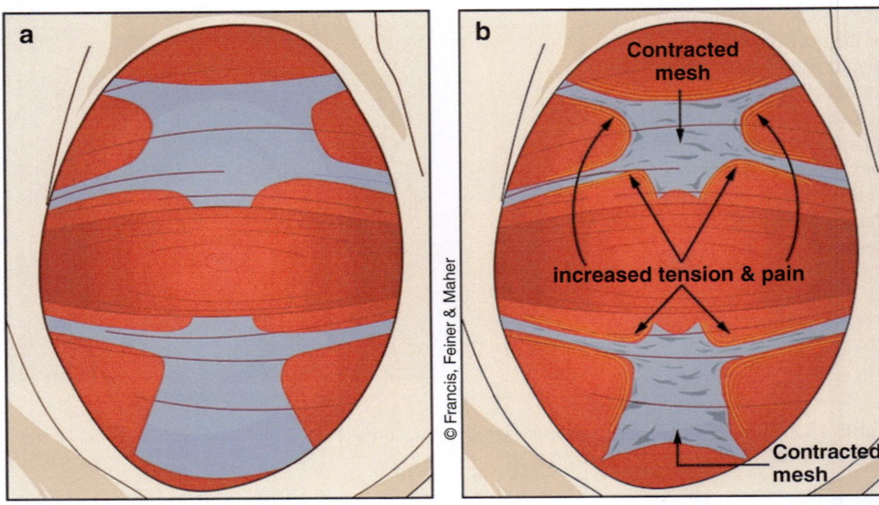

Fig. 13.5 Vaginal mesh after anterior and posterior placement and after reorganization leading to increased tension on the arms. Illustration: Stephen Francis. (From Feiner and Maher [15], with the kind permission of Christopher Maher)

formation of fibrous tissue as stimulated by the presence of the mesh [2]. "High responders" reaction is summarized in (Fig. 13.6) [2]. Overcoming host response to mesh and applying other clinical factors combined with a mechanism to detect "high responders" for fibrous tissue formation are needed to properly select individual patients who will benefit from the insertion of permanent mesh prostheses while minimizing adverse events. Another issue to be discussed is the mesh load, defined as the amount of mesh required in the body for the host to mount a response that is deleterious. Why is that much fewer patients with vaginally placed mesh slings have inflammatory response compared to vaginally placed mesh kits? Obviously the answer is different for each patient as the immune response is individualized based on genetics and the patient's protoplasm. The concept of genomics as a companion diagnostics to mesh insertion to see which patient it may be inappropriate for is in its infancy. Understanding the host response mechanism and the personalized unfavorable response to a polypropylene mesh device that is generally viewed as inert may be critical for individuals who develop chronic debilitating immunologic diseases subsequent to mesh implantation.

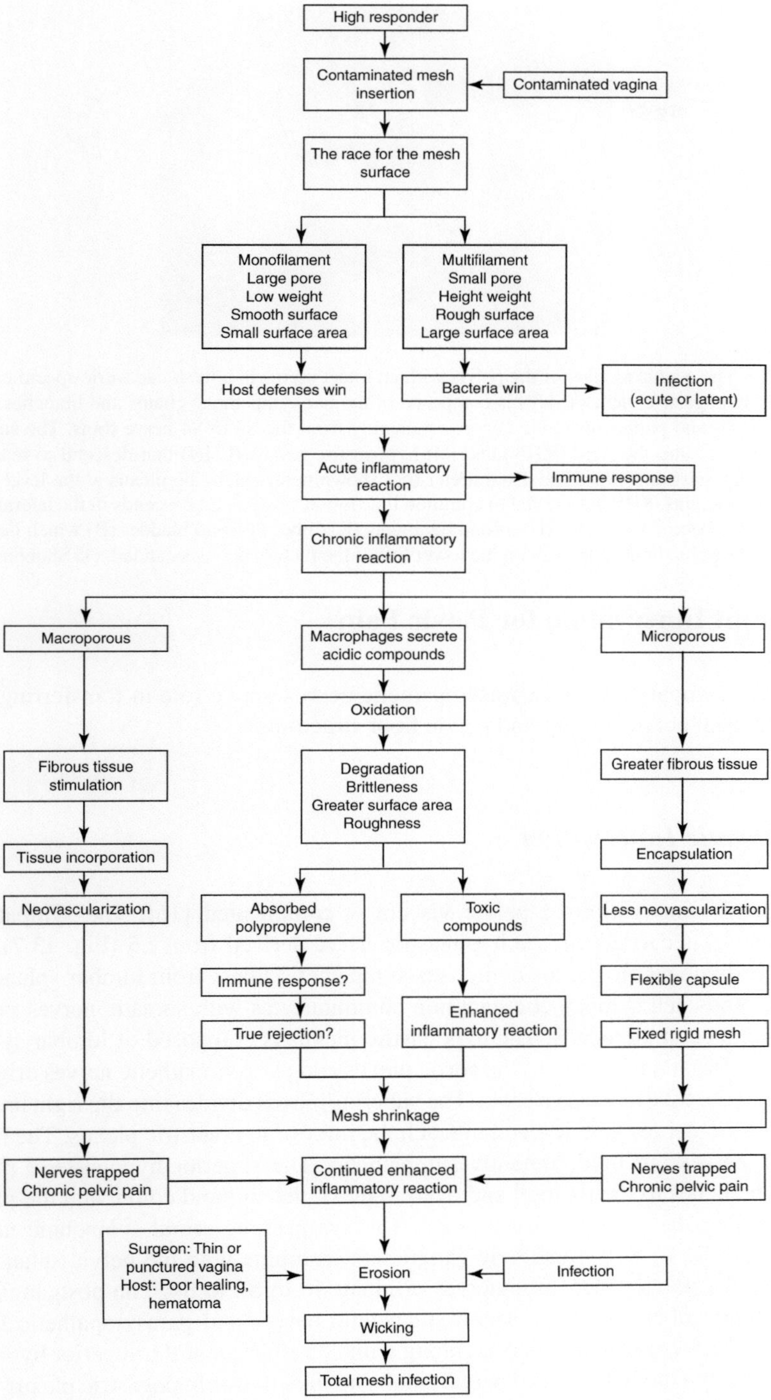

Fig. 13.6 The progression of fibrous tissue formation in individuals who are "high responders" to vaginal mesh graft. (From Ostergard [2], with permission)

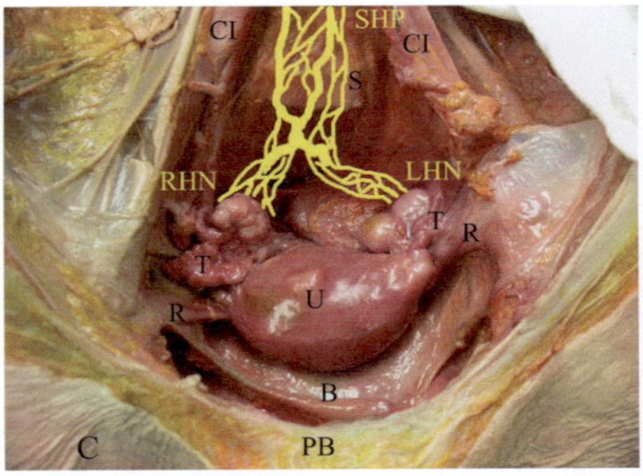

Fig. 13.7 The cephalad view of the pelvis with an intact uterus in a fresh cadaveric specimen. The superior hypogastric plexus (SHP) is composed of lumbar sympathetic chains and branches of the aortic plexus and parasympathetic nerves originating from the S2 to S4 nerve roots. The superior plexus divides into the right (RHN) and left hypogastric nerves (LHN) that descend to reach the inferior hypogastric plexus. The distal ureter (not shown here) enters the plexus at the level of the cardinal ligaments. SHP lies medial to common iliac blood vessels and descends in the lateral walls of the pelvis behind the uterus (U), round ligaments (R), tubes (T), and bladder (B) which lies posterior to the pubic bone (PB). (C) on the lower left of the picture denotes caudad. (© Shobeiri)

Afferent Innervation for Pelvic Pain

Somatic, sympathetic, and parasympathetic nerves play a role in transferring pain signals from pelvic viscera and pelvic floor structures.

Autonomic Innervation

Autonomic innervation of pelvic viscera is complicated [16]. The sympathetic innervation is carried via the hypogastric nerve derived from L5 (Fig. 13.7). The superior hypogastric plexus comprises sympathetic fibers from lumbar splanchnic nerves, and each sympathetic ganglion communicates with somatic nerves via the gray ramus communicans. The hypogastric plexus is composed of lumbar sympathetic chains and branches of the aortic plexus and parasympathetic nerves originating from the S2 to S4 nerve roots. The superior plexus divides into the right and left hypogastric nerves that descend to reach the inferior hypogastric plexus. The hypogastric nerves are predominantly sympathetic. The superior hypogasteric plexus sends branches to the ureteral and ovarian plexi, the sigmoid colon, and the plexus surrounding the internal iliac arteries. The sympathetic sacral splanchnic nerves arise from S1 to S4 sympathetic ganglia and combine with the pelvic splanchnic nerves. The pelvic splanchnic nerves originate from S2 to S4. The postganglionic sympathetic fibers from the sacral splanchnic nerves and parasympathetic fibers from the pelvic splanchnic nerves, along with contribution of the superior hypogastric plexus via the hypogastric nerves, make up the inferior hypogastric plexus [17].

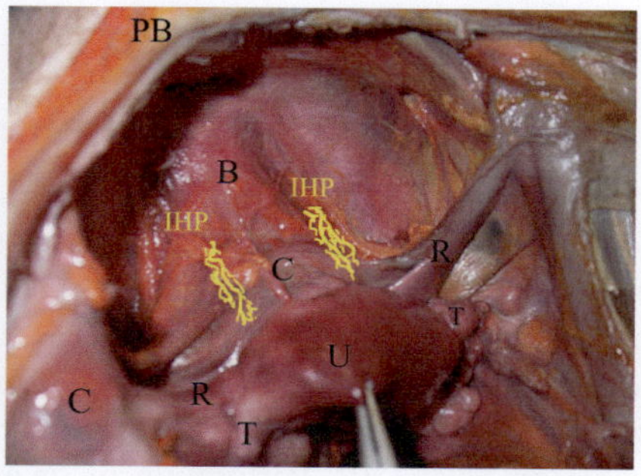

Fig. 13.8 The caudad view of the pelvis with an intact uterus in a fresh cadaveric specimen. The inferior hypogastric plexus (IHP) lies in the cardinal ligament inferior to the point where the uterine branch of iliac artery crosses the distal ureter. In this retropubic view the cervix (C), bladder (B), pubic bone (PB), round ligaments (R), and tubes (T) are visualized. (C) on the lower left of the picture denotes cauded while C in the center of the picture is the location of cervix covered by the bladder. (© Shobeiri)

The inferior hypogastric plexus lies in the cardinal ligament inferior to the point where the uterine branch of iliac artery crosses the distal ureter (Fig. 13.8).

Somatic Innervation

The somatic innervation of the pelvic area is the iliophypogastric, ilioinguinal, lateral femoral cutaneous, and genitofemoral nerves originating from T12 to L3, as well as the nerve to the levator ani and pudendal nerves originating from S2 to S5. These nerves share the same spinal cord levels as the pelvic organs innervated by the superior and inferior hypogastric plexi. Thus, it infers that nerve entrapments can refer pain to the pelvic region [17].

Understanding of the innervation of the pelvic floor, particularly the close relationship of somatic and visceral nerves within the pelvis and pelvic floor, is very important. The levator ani nerve (S3 to S5) consistently innervates the levator ani muscle, whereas the pudendal nerve does not. The pudendal nerve innervates the external urethral and anal sphincters, perineal muscles (bulbospongiosus, ischiocavernosus, deep and superficial transverse perineal muscles), clitoris, and skin [18, 19]. The coccygeal plexus is formed from the anterior division, primarily of S5 with a small contribution from S4 that joins with the coccygeal nerve. The plexus lies anterior to the sacrum and coccyx and posterior to the pelvic organs, and this area is rich in somatic and autonomic nerve endings. The autonomic structures are the ganglion impar and the superior and inferior hypogastric plexi. The S4, S5, and coccygeal nerves are sensory nerves, where stimulation of S4 might evoke vaginal pain and stimulation of S4, S5, and coccygeal roots may evoke anal and coccygeal pain. In some patients, the coccyx pain is experienced in the S3 distribution because of the S3 innervation of vascular structures in this area.

Mesh-Related Pain

Type 1, Direct Injury of Muscle, Nerve, or Viscera

Mesh-related pain refers to the pain exceeding the routine postoperative pain when its pattern and duration do not correlate with the nature of surgery performed.

Fluid collection around mesh (hematoma or abscess) is an example of pathologies that can result in pain complications that can be identified on initial exam with palpation or radiography. Up to 25% of patients undergoing retropubic slings have postoperative hematomas visible on MRI [20]. Perforation of or extrusion into adjacent viscera also can cause early postoperative pain that can often be resolved with removing mesh in a timely fashion.

Mesh may penetrate the bladder or urethra, bowel, levator ani or anal sphincter, primarily due to incorrect initial design and subsequent placement at the time of surgery, hence causing direct injury. A tight sling may cut through the urethra or roll under the urethra to a more cephalad position under the bladder. Anterior rectus muscle trauma can be a result of retropubic mesh placement if the trocar deviates from anticipated placement, while a transobturator tape can injure the internal obturator muscle and nerves.

Coccygeus muscle that overlies the sacrospinous ligament can be traumatized during sacrospinous ligament fixation procedures and placement of mesh or sutures into that ligament. Additionally, Patients who undergo posterior compartment mesh repair with trocar-guided lateral mesh arms may experience pain in the levator muscles or gluteus maximus.

Bone-related mesh pain may be another etiology of pain. Bone pain after retropubic sling is caused by trocar passage along the posterior aspect of the superior pubic rami posterior to the obturator grove, while trocar passage during placement of a transobturator mesh is in close proximity to the inferior pubic rami. Anterior vaginal wall mesh placed with trocar guidance travels along the lateral inferior aspect of the ischial rami until emerging medially into the vaginal canal just posterior to the descending rami. It is recommended that during placement, surgeons avoid the superior pubic rami, which is in close proximity to the obturator artery and nerve. This is perhaps easier said than done. Almost none of the mesh kits removed by the senior author has followed a prescribed path, which proves that reliable placement of vaginal mesh kits may not be possible, leading to injury and pain. Other areas of concern include pain following placement of sutures (to secure mesh); ischial spines and ischial tuberosities may be injured during vaginal approaches to posterior compartment repair. Placement of posterior mesh arms in close proximity to these prominences may cause pain by direct trauma or mesh fixation.

Somatic nerves including iliohypogastric, ilioinguinal, lateral femoral cutaneous, genitofemoral, and pudendal nerves can be injured directly during mesh placement by trocar or later being entrapped with suture of fibrosis around mesh. Table 13.4 summarizes procedures that can potentially harm somatic nerves and cause acute or chronic pain.

Table 13.4 Somatic nerve injury during pelvic mesh augmented surgeries

Nerve	Root	Procedures
Iliohypogastric	T12-L1	Retropubic sling
Ilioinguinal	L1	Retropubic sling
Lateral femoral cutaneous	L2–L3	Transobturator sling
Pudendal	S2–S5	Sacrospinous suspension Transobturator sling

Type 2: Fibrosis and Mesh Shrinkage-Related Injury

Surgeons have used implantable mesh for decades (albeit only more recently in vaginal reconstructive surgery). However, there is much debate about the implication of mesh and chronic pain with increasing emerging data.

The process by which pelvic pain develops after mesh implant surgery is likely multifactorial, and host response may have significant role, specifically in cases of chronic pain. Polypropylene mesh, in particular low-density large pore monofilament variety, is the most commonly used material in the pelvic floor reconstructive surgery at present. It is generally considered an inert material [21], but studies have shown that mesh undergoes degradation following insertion [22] which can potentially contribute to pain after procedures. During the immediate postoperative period, inflammation is followed by the formation of granular tissue. This granular tissue foundation is critical to strength and stability as it is converted into dense fibrous tissue beginning 4–6 weeks following insertion, peaking at approximately 6–12 weeks. Tissue incorporation occurs concurrently with mesh shrinkage. Ultrasound data demonstrates 30–60% decrease in mesh size at 4–12 weeks compared to size at insertion [23]. Using pelvic floor ultrasound, the dimensions of grafts can be accurately assessed postoperatively and compared with the original mesh. Feiner et al. studied symptoms in women with vaginal mesh contraction [15]. All the women included in this series had palpable painful mesh contraction. In the majority of cases, the most severe tenderness on examination was present at the junction between the central mesh graft and the fixation arms, presumably as a result of excessive tension after shrinkage of the main body of the mesh against the serrated arms that remain fixated and unmovable in the tissue. Palpation of the contracted mesh reproduced the pain these women experienced with movement and sexual intercourse.

Vaginal mesh contraction is a serious complication after pelvic organ prolapse repair using armed polypropylene mesh, and surgical intervention is often required to alleviate symptoms. It involves mobilization of the mesh, division of the fixation arms, and excision of contracted mesh or removal of the mesh en bloc. Concerted research and development efforts are needed for newer graft materials with diminished shrinkage properties.

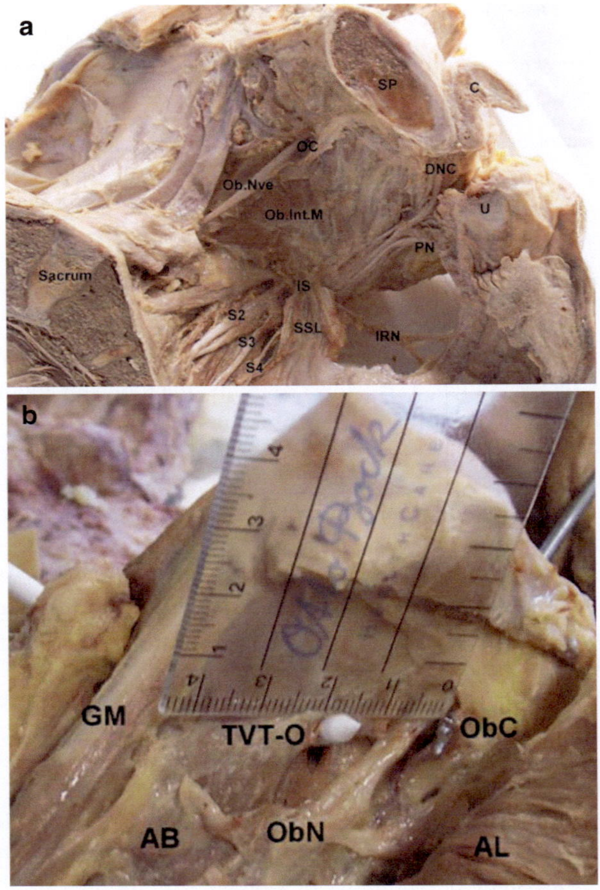

Fig. 13.9 (**a**) Left hemipelvis; (**b**) distance between the transobturator device and obturator canal. (From Achtari et al. [24], with permission)

Obturator Neuropathy

With the use of obturator kits, the primary issue has been of medial groin and leg pain, but there are patient reports of the injury to the obturator nerve with a retropubic approach as well [17, 18]. While obturator nerve injury can occur during delivery or in lithotomy position, iatrogenic injury can occur with passage of trocars (Fig. 13.9) [24]. Obturator neuralgia generally presents as a sharp, electric, or burning pain in the groin and in the anterior and internal surface of the thigh aggravated by certain movements such as walking. The pain can be clinically reproduced on exam by internal rotation and extension that is localized anteroinferior to the inguinal region and thigh. Diagnosis is usually based on clinical findings, and denervation findings in electromyography (EMG) are not more specific. Other imaging such as CT or MRI is helpful only if one suspects a tumor or hematoma causing a mass effect. Pelvic floor ultrasound is the diagnostic modality of choice for documenting the course and pattern of mesh slings. Improvement of symptoms by infiltration of local anesthetic to the area is an effective manner in which to ascertain the diagnosis. Additionally, case reports have illustrated resolution of said pain after surgical removal and the findings of improper position of the mesh arms [19].

Pudendal Neuropathy

The pudendal nerve is a small nerve with few branches, crossing the sacrospinous ligaments very close to the ischial spine as earlier described. Its location is close to where the posterior trocars pass and where posterior meshes might be placed in posterior compartment surgery. Pudendal nerve capture has been described following sacrospinous ligament fixation where the sutures pass very close to the ligament, near where the pudendal nerve cross. Hence, the correct anatomic placement of said sutures is critical. The Nantes criteria for the diagnosis of pudendal neuralgia include:

(a) Pain in the anatomic region of the pudendal nerve
(b) Pain exacerbated by sitting
(c) No waking up at night due to pain
(d) No objective sensory loss on clinical examination
(e) Positive anesthetic pudendal nerve block [20]

Unfortunately, Nantes criteria were not developed for vaginal mesh complications, and as such many patients cannot sleep at night because of constant mesh pain or may not respond to anesthetic block due to dense scarring which may prevent the anesthetic from dispersing around the nerve. Pain at the level of Alcock's canal or a tight mesh bridge between sacrospinous ligaments during rectal exam can also help identify a pudendal nerve injury or entrapment [21]. The best time to note pudendal neuralgia will be in the immediate postoperative period. The pudendal nerve branches may be affected variably, and the vaginal mesh kit implanters may not be familiar with subtle mesh kit-related pudendal neuralgia presentation such as urethritis, inability to void, rectal pain, and such which may be unilateral or different on each side. By the time the patient has persistent pain after 2 weeks, the nerve capture and scarring have set in, and the longer the condition continues, it is more likely that the condition becomes irreversible. The patient's pudendal pain metastasizes to the adjacent organs, and the patient will have a more difficult to treat chronic pain syndrome. Since healthcare professionals are not used to evaluating or treating this pain etiology, such patients go from physician to physician helplessly. The patient's prognosis may be better the sooner the mesh arms are removed from the pudendal or the obturator nerve territory.

Conclusion

In reconstructive pelvic surgery for pelvic organ prolapse, the use of biological and synthetic grafts for the transabdominal of pelvic organ prolapse has improved long-term support and function. The same is not true of vaginal mesh. The potential benefits of using grafts needs to be carefully balanced against the risks of using implant materials. The newer kits that do not pass the trocar through the sacrospinous ligament likely have less problems with pudendal neuralgia. Ultimately, clear informed consent should include all the risks including the chronic pain syndromes.

Innovation of a medical device must undergo many reiterations before a device is ready to be safely released to the market. In the absence of due diligence in testing of the device or thoroughly assuring its safety before release, innovations occur in response to the device malfunction. Such has been the case with the vaginal mesh kits and the field of pain management in response to vaginal mesh kit pain.

References

1. Patel H, Ostergard DR, Sternschuss G. Polypropylene mesh and the host response. Int Urogynecol J. 2012;23(6):669–79.
2. Ostergard DR. Polypropylene vaginal mesh grafts in gynecology. Obstet Gynecol. 2010;116(4):962–6.
3. Olsen AL, Smith VJ, Bergstrom JO, Colling JC, Clark AL. Epidemiology of surgically managed pelvic organ prolapse and urinary incontinence. Obstet Gynecol. 1997;89(4):501–6.
4. Nguyen JN, Burchette RJ. Outcome after anterior vaginal prolapse repair: a randomized controlled trial. Obstet Gynecol. 2008;111(4):891–8.
5. Withagen MI, Milani AL, den Boon J, Vervest HA, Vierhout ME. Trocar-guided mesh compared with conventional vaginal repair in recurrent prolapse: a randomized controlled trial. Obstet Gynecol. 2011;117(2, Part 1):242–50.
6. Maher C, Feiner B, Baessler K, Christmann-Schmid C, Haya N, Marjoribanks J. Transvaginal mesh or grafts compared with native tissue repair for vaginal prolapse. Cochrane Database Syst Rev. 2016;2:CD012079.
7. Abbott S, Unger CA, Evans JM, Jallad K, Mishra K, Karram MM, et al. Evaluation and management of complications from synthetic mesh after pelvic reconstructive surgery: a multicenter study. Am J Obstet Gynecol. 2014;210(2):163.e1–8.
8. Pickett SD, Barenberg B, Quiroz LH, Shobeiri SA, O'Leary DE. The significant morbidity of removing pelvic mesh from multiple vaginal compartments. Obstet Gynecol. 2015;125(6):1418–22.
9. Haylen BT, Freeman RM, Swift SE, Cosson M, Davila GW, Deprest J, et al. An International Urogynecological Association (IUGA)/International Continence Society (ICS) joint terminology and classification of the complications related directly to the insertion of prostheses (meshes, implants, tapes) and grafts in female pelvic floor surgery. Neurourol Urodynam. 2011;30(1):2–12.
10. Parnell BA, Johnson EA, Zolnoun DA. Genitofemoral and perineal neuralgia after transobturator midurethral sling. Obstet Gynecol. 2012;119(2 Pt 2):428–31.
11. Sanses TV, Shahryarinejad A, Molden S, Hoskey KA, Abbasy S, Patterson D, Fellows' Pelvic Research Network, et al. Anatomic outcomes of vaginal mesh procedure (Prolift) compared with uterosacral ligament suspension and abdominal sacrocolpopexy for pelvic organ prolapse: a Fellows' Pelvic Research Network study. Am J Obstet Gynecol. 2009;201(5):519.e1–8.

12. Amid PK. Classification of biomaterials and their related complications in abdominal wall hernia surgery. Hernia. 1997;1(1):15–21.
13. Gristina AG, Naylor PT, Myrvik QN. Biomaterial-centered infections: microbial adhesion versus tissue integration. In: Torkel Wadström T, Eliasson I, Holder I, Ljungh A, editors. Pathogenesis of wound and biomaterial-associated infections. London: Springer-Verlag; 1990. p. 193–216.
14. Klinge U, Klosterhalfen B, Müller M, Öttinger A, Schumpelick V. Shrinking of polypropylene mesh in vivo: an experimental study in dogs. Eur J Surg. 1998;164(12):965–9.
15. Feiner F, Maher C. Vaginal mesh contraction, definition, clinical presentation, and management. Obstet Gynecol. 2010;115(2):325–30.
16. Bent AE, Cundiff GW, Swift SE, editors. Ostergard's urogynecology and pelvic floor dysfunction. 6th ed. Philadelphia: Lippincott Williams & Wilkins, Wolters Kluwer; 2008.
17. Prather H, Spitznagle TM, Dugan SA. Recognizing and treating pelvic pain and pelvic floor dysfunction. Phys Med Rehab Clin N Am. 2007;18(3):477–96.
18. Moore K, Dalley AF. Clinically oriented anatomy. 4th ed. Philadelphia: Lippincott Williams & Wilkins/Wolters Kluwer; 1999.
19. Barber MD, Bremer RE, Thor KB, Dolber PC, Kuehl TJ, Coates KW. Innervation of the female levator ani muscles. Am J Obstet Gynecol. 2002;187(1):64–71.
20. Giri SK, Wallis F, Drumm J, Saunders JA, Flood HD. A magnetic resonance imaging-based study of retropubic haematoma after sling procedures: preliminary findings. BJU Int. 2005;96(7):1067–71.
21. Debodinance P, Delporte P, Engrand J, Boulogne M. Development of better tolerated prosthetic materials: applications in gynecological surgery. J Gynecol Obstet Biol Reprod (Paris). 2002;31(6):527–40. [Article in French].
22. Clavé A, Yahi H, Hammou J-C, Montanari S, Gounon P, Clavé H. Polypropylene as a reinforcement in pelvic surgery is not inert: comparative analysis of 100 explants. Int Urogynecol J. 2010;21(3):261–70.
23. García-Ureña MÁ, Ruiz VV, Godoy AD, Perea JMB, Gómez LM, Hernández FJ, et al. Differences in polypropylene shrinkage depending on mesh position in an experimental study. Am J Surg. 2007;193(4):538–42.
24. Achtari C, McKenzie BJ, Hiscock R, Rosamilia A, Schierlitz L, Briggs CA, et al. Anatomical study of the obturator foramen and dorsal nerve of the clitoris and their relationship to minimally invasive slings. Int Urogynecol J Pelvic Floor Dysfunct. 2006;17(4):330–4.

Chapter 14
Outcomes of Vaginal Mesh Surgeries

Miles Murphy, Michael Ting, and Vincent R. Lucente

Introduction

The transvaginal placement of synthetic mesh has been used for over 20 years in an attempt to increase the durability of pelvic reconstruction, particularly in cases where the risk of failure/recurrence is high [1]. The idea of using synthetic materials to augment a defect in compromised native tissues is not unique to pelvic floor reconstruction. Synthetic materials are used to reconstruct great vessel aneurysms, orthopedic joints, and most similarly in abdominal wall hernias. The pelvic floor, however, presents atypical challenges due to the fact that the vagina is so intimately connected to sexual health and cannot be completely sterilized.

As a result, synthetic meshes have traditionally been reserved for recurrent or severe defects. Furthermore, their use has historically been restricted to physicians who sub-specialize in pelvic floor reconstruction (i.e., specialists in urogynecology or female urology). That changed with the advent of the tension-free vaginal tape (TVT) procedure in the late 1990s [2]. This procedure not only revolutionized the way female stress urinary incontinence (SUI) is treated around the world, but it changed the way people learned how to do surgery in gynecology. It was very effective in treating SUI and appeared to be relatively easy to learn to perform without extensive training. While there are some surgeons who feel that any use of mesh

M. Murphy (✉)
The Institute for Female Pelvic Medicine and Reconstructive Surgery, North Wales, PA, USA
e-mail: milesmurphy@comcast.net

M. Ting
Division of Minimally Invasive Gynecologic Surgery, Department of Obstetrics and Gynecology, St Luke's University Health Network, Bethlehem, PA, USA

V. R. Lucente
Department of Obstetrics and Gynecology, St Luke's University Health Network, Bethlehem, PA, USA

S. A. Shobeiri (ed.), *The Innovation and Evolution of Medical Devices*,
https://doi.org/10.1007/978-3-319-97073-8_14

placed through a vaginal incision is inappropriate, the vast majority of those who treat SUI on a regular basis feel that a transvaginally placed midurethral is the standard of care for female SUI.

Within 5–10 years of the introduction and success of the TVT, many surgeons sought to marry the benefits of transvaginal surgery with the durability of abdominal mesh in the treatment of pelvic organ prolapse (POP). These procedures came to be known as tension-free or transvaginal mesh (TVM) surgeries [3]. The hope was that the innovative success of TVT could be translated to POP repair. These procedures were often taught in the same manner as TVT had been taught. The success of this approach has been fervently debated. There was great enthusiasm for these TVM procedures, but some felt that innovation was moving faster than the supporting data [4].

Some surgeons still harbor these concerns. They feel that we should continue to perform traditional procedures until the scientific data that support the traditional procedures are matched by the data for the more innovative approaches. Many people with this view regard the abdominal placement of mesh, such as is done in the sacral colpopexy procedure, as the standard of care for advanced POP. And indeed, the conventional wisdom is that there are more data on abdominally placed mesh than there are on vaginally placed mesh, but the argument can be made that the opposite is true. Examination of two recent systematic reviews of these two procedures reveals 33 comparative studies of TVM versus native tissue repairs, while there were only 13 such studies of abdominal mesh [5, 6]. The goal of this chapter will be to examine the outcomes of vaginal mesh surgeries in detail.

Vaginal Mesh for Urinary Incontinence

One of the most studied procedures in all of gynecology is the 3-incision, synthetic, tension-free midurethral sling (MUS). It is widely regarded as the recommended surgical procedure for the treatment of female SUI in routine cases. As such, further studies have not been ordered by the US Food and Drug Administration (FDA) for these products to remain on the market. Outcomes for this well-established procedure will not be covered in this chapter. However, the FDA determined that single-incision slings (SIS) were different enough from the standard MUS that manufacturers must conduct further clinical (FDA 522, postmarket surveillance) trials if they want to continue marketing these types of slings.

Currently the SIS procedure is completed through one vaginal incision using polypropylene tape, which fixates into the internal obturator muscle bilaterally. These slings differ in the type/robustness of the anchorage mechanism used [7]. Several recently developed slings also allow for post-anchorage adjustment of the sling's tension. There are some theoretical advantages with SIS when compared to their retropubic and transobturator MUS. By not penetrating the space of Retzius or the obturator fossa, the limited surgical approach used to delivery single-incision slings eliminates the need for external incisions and reduces the risk of potential injury to surrounding structures. This simplified dissection reduces surgical time and anesthetic requirements, potentially allowing the procedure to be performed in an outpatient office-based setting [8].

The landscape and availability of SIS are constantly shifting, given the challenging medicolegal climate, industry changes, and FDA requirements [9]. As a result the outcome data currently available are often of shorter follow-up duration and include products that have been discontinued, which make comparisons difficult. However two recent comprehensive reviews are available.

The Cochrane database review in 2014 evaluated 31 trials involving 32,290 women. This large meta-analysis revealed that women were more likely to remain incontinent after surgery with SIS than with retropubic slings or with inside-out transobturator slings. The authors of the review acknowledge that most of these conclusions were derived from trials involving TVT Secur™ (Gynecare, Ethicon, Somerville NJ, USA) and that the higher risk of incontinence was principally associated with use of this specific device, which had been withdrawn from clinical use in March 2013. The data also were insufficient to suggest a significant difference between any of the SIS in any of the comparisons made [10].

A similar comprehensive review was also performed in 2014 by Mostafa et al. [11]. This analysis excluded data from TVT Secur™ clinical trials. The authors found no evidence of significant differences between SIS and MUS in patient-reported cure rates and objective cure rates at a mean follow-up of 18.6 months. There was also no evidence of significant differences in most perioperative complications between both groups after excluding TVT Secur™. SIS also had significantly lower postoperative pain scores and earlier return to normal activities and to work. The analysis also demonstrated a nonsignificant trend toward higher rates of repeat continence surgery, less postoperative voiding dysfunction, more de novo urgency, and/or worsening of pre-existing urgency within the SIS group.

Since the release of these two meta-analyses in 2014, several small trials with short-term follow-up have published their findings. Some of the best data available for SIS are those involving a sling that is no longer being marketed, MiniArc™ (American Medical Systems, Minnetoka MN, USA). The data include a randomized control trial (RCT) of 225 women who were randomized to receive either the MiniArc™ (SIS) or Monarc™ (American Medical Systems) transobturator MUS [12]. Objective cure was defined as negative cough stress test with a comfortably full bladder. Subjective cure was defined as no report of leakage with coughing or exercise on questionnaire. There was no statistically significant difference in the subjective or objective cure rates between MiniArc™ and Monarc™ at 12 months, respectively, with a significant improvement in overactive bladder outcomes and incontinence impact from baseline in both arms.

Medium-term outcome measures have also been collected. These data include a cohort study of 381 women with primary SUI in a single tertiary referral center [13]. Median length of follow-up was 60 months. Of 381 patients, 215 were treated with Monarc™ slings and 166 with MiniArc™. The two groups were comparable in terms of preoperative characteristics. No difference was found in cure rates between Monarc™ and Miniarc™ patients at 5-year follow-up. Monarc™ showed better overactive bladder-free rates (97% vs. 92%). No significant differences have been found in terms of sexual function, mesh exposure, and objective cure rates.

Of products still remaining on the market, 2-year data for the Altis® (Coloplast, Minneapolis MN, USA) adjustable SIS system for treatment of SUI comes from an industry-sponsored, multicenter, single-arm trial of 113 patients with primary efficacy defined as ≥50% reduction in 24 h pad weight from baseline at 6 months [14]. In this study 90.0% of patients achieved ≥50% reduction in pad weight, 81.1% were dry (pad weight ≤4.0 g), and 87.9% had a negative cough stress test. The investigators also observed significant median reductions in the Urogenital Distress Inventory and Incontinence Impact Questionnaire scores.

Finally, one retrospective trial has evaluated the safety and efficacy of the Solyx™ (Boston Scientific, Marlborough MA, USA) SIS on 69 patients with a mean follow-up of 43 months [15]. In this study, the investigators stated that 93% of the patients were subjectively dry by questionnaire and were satisfied with their outcome. Also 91% of the patients stated that they would undergo the procedure again. There were no serious adverse events and no mesh erosions or extrusions during the reported period.

For later generation SIS, long-term efficacy has not yet been determined, but short-term efficacy rates seem to be comparable to traditional MUS. Long-term follow-up is warranted, and comparative studies will help to determine their relative efficacy.

Vaginal Mesh for Pelvic Organ Prolapse

Postoperative recurrence of POP has plagued pelvic reconstructive surgeons for decades [16]. There are multiple risk factors that have been shown to be associated with prolapse recurrence. These include advanced stage (III or IV) prolapse and younger age at the time of surgery (<60 years) [17]. Furthermore, anterior compartment defects tend to be the most prone to recurrence. We now know that anterior compartment defects are often closely associated with apical defects, and failure to address the apical component of these defects may be partially responsible for the high recurrence rate seen with traditional anterior repairs [18]. The rationale for using vaginally placed synthetic mesh for the treatment of prolapse is to minimize the risk of recurrence while at the same time minimizing the greater morbidity and length of hospital stay often associated with laparotomy/laparoscopy [19, 20].

Types of Transvaginal Mesh Procedures and Associated Outcomes

One can divide TVM procedures into two basic categories: trocar-assisted placement and nontrocar-assisted repairs. For the most part, trocar-assisted procedures come packaged and are marketed by surgical device companies. Nontrocar-assisted procedures can also come as packaged "kits" but are often performed by suturing in hand-cut mesh.

Techniques for suturing mesh in place vary. Likewise there have been many varied packaged mesh delivery systems marketed for the treatment of POP. This chapter will only report on nonabsorbable synthetic mesh and will focus on the most studied systems, with special focus on those currently being marketed as of the drafting of this chapter. It will also be limited to comparative studies or series with large numbers and at least 1 year of follow-up. Later in the chapter, outcomes for all TVMs when grouped together in systematic reviews and meta-analyses will be reviewed; first, the most studied procedures and their specific outcomes will be reviewed.

Sutured-In Hand-Cut Vaginal Mesh

There is great variation in the procedures that encompass this heading. Because the meshes and their associated delivery systems are not standardized in a manufacturing process, it is hard to lump the results together. Nonetheless, this group includes the original vaginal mesh procedures and other procedures that have served as the prototypes for those performed to this day.

The first comparative study on vaginal mesh for prolapse was published by Julian in 1996 [1]. Twenty-four women with two or more postsurgical recurrences of "severe" anterior vaginal prolapse were divided into two groups (no randomization was performed). The control group underwent suture-based anterior colporrhaphy and vaginal paravaginal repair. The treatment group underwent the same repair, but the repair was augmented by sewing synthetic nonabsorbable polypropylene mesh (PPM) from the urethrovesical junction to the vaginal apex and from the junction of the obturator and lavatory fascia from one side to the other. The author followed these patients for 2 years and noted a significantly higher recurrence rate in the control group (33% vs. 0%, $P < 0.05$). However, there was a 25% mesh complication rate (2 erosions and 1 prolonged granulation tissue). Of note, while it is still considered a Type I PPM, the graft used in this series (Marlex) has a more tightly knitted pattern and heavier weight than most of the "low-weight" PPMs used in the treatment of POP today.

The first large randomized trial to compare the transvaginal use of hand-cut, low-weight PPM to native tissue repair in the treatment of anterior vaginal wall prolapse was published in 2007 [21]. In this trial the mesh had a body with four extending arms sutured into place over plicated fascia. This technique is often referred to now as a split-thickness dissection, with the mesh being placed between the vaginal epithelium and the endopelvic fascia, as opposed to a full-thickness dissection in which the mesh is placed in the vesicovaginal space as it would be in abdominally placed mesh. Over 200 patients were randomized, and the authors found that the recurrence rate was significantly higher in the no-mesh group (38.5% vs. 6.7%, $P < 0.001$) at 12 months. The erosion rate was 17.3%. The authors subsequently published 2- and 3-year follow-up studies. At 2 years, not only did the approximately 30% higher recurrence rate in the no-mesh group persist ($P < 0.001$), but they also found a greater sensation of bulge as well (17% vs. 5%, $P = 0.003$). There was one de novo mesh exposure [22]. At 3 years of follow-up, the proportion of symptomatic patients was similar between groups. However, the percentage of patients with an optimal outcome (defined as absence of anatomic recurrence and sensation of vaginal bulge) was greater in the mesh group (82% vs. 55%, $P < 0.001$). By the end of 3 years, 19% of patients had been diagnosed with mesh exposure at any visit; none experienced erosion of mesh into the bladder or other serious complications. The overall reoperation rate for POP or UI was 18% in the no-mesh and 11% in the mesh group (no *P* value given). No patients in the mesh group required reoperation for repeat anterior prolapse [23].

The most recent RCT of hand-cut vaginal mesh is the largest population studied to date [24]. In this study 1352 women were randomized to one of three arms: (a) standard repair of anterior or posterior compartment prolapse surgery (i.e., native tissue), (b) standard repair augmented with synthetic mesh, or (c) standard repair augmented with biological graft. The weights of mesh ranged from 19 g/m^2 to 44 g/m^2, and hybrid (coated) mesh was allowed. The biological graft materials were porcine acellular collagen matrix, porcine small intestinal submucosa, or bovine dermal grafts. The grafts were inserted below the fascial layer "if possible" and secured with peripheral sutures. Thirty-five centers recruited patients into the trial, and patients were reassessed at 6, 12, and 24 months. Augmentation with mesh or biological graft did not improve outcomes in terms of effectiveness, quality of life, adverse effects, or any other outcome in the short term, but the cumulative number of women with a mesh complication over 2 years was 12% (51 of 434). The authors note that only one woman had total mesh removal because of infection (0.2%). In most women the exposure of mesh into the vagina was small or asymptomatic, requiring only partial removal as a day case.

Trocar-Based Kits

The first generation of marketed kits manufactured by surgical device companies was influenced by the success of full-length, 3-incision midurethral slings in which trocars were used to deliver the implants. There were a number of different systems marketed, but this chapter will focus on the two most popularly used systems in the United States: Apogee™/Perigee™ (American Medical Systems) and Prolift® (Ethicon). These procedures involved placement of a body of mesh through a vaginal incision. These bodies of mesh were secured in place by extending arms of mesh that were placed in a tension-free manner. For anterior compartment defects, these mesh arms were placed through the distal and proximal arcus tendineus using a trocar and exiting through the obturator fossa via two small groin incisions per side. For posterior compartment defects, these mesh arms were placed through the sacrospinous ligament using a trocar and exiting through the ischiorectal fossa via one small buttock incision per side. These systems are not currently being marketed.

The Perigee™ system is used for anterior compartment defects. The first high-quality study of the Perigee™ system was a prospective clinical trial in which 76 women were randomized to either a standard anterior colporrhaphy or anterior repair with Perigee™ and followed for 1 year [25]. In this trial, the investigators found a higher rate of prolapse recurrence (≥ pelvic organ prolapse quantification system [POP-Q] stage II) in the native tissue arm, 45% vs. 13% ($P = 0.005$). Quality of life and sexual symptom score improvements were comparable in both groups. A 5% mesh extrusion rate was found. The authors concluded that nine native tissue patients would have to have recurrent prolapse to prevent one mesh extrusion.

The rest of the data on Perigee™ and Apogee™ (the posterior compartment system) is observational, composed mostly of cohort studies and case series. Some of the notable data in this vein include two studies by Moore and colleagues. The first study by Moore et al. is a 2-year prospective, multicenter trial of Perigee™ [26]. In this study of 114 women the authors found the 2-year anatomic cure rate to be 88.5% with significant improvement in domain-specific quality of life and sexual function questionnaires. The erosion rate was 10.5%, and the groin, pelvic, or vaginal pain rate was 4.4%. The second study, by Moore and Lubkan, is a retrospective cohort study of the Perigee™/Apogee™ mesh delivery system using mesh of two different densities (50 g/m^2 vs. 25.2 g/m^2) [27]. The traditional mesh was used in 371 cases and the lightweight mesh in 116. While the difference in mesh erosion was not statistically significant between the two groups, there was a 46% reduction in the lightweight arm (11.1% vs. 6.0%, $P = 0.12$). The most recent prospective study of the Perigee™/Apogee™ mesh delivery system is a single-center study of 158 patients in which both traditional and lightweight meshes were implanted [28]. The median follow-up times were 105 and 138 weeks for the anterior and posterior kits, respectively. Approximately half of the cases were for recurrent prolapse; the cure rates for these patients were 90.9% in the anterior compartment and 95.7% in the posterior. Overall success rates were 81.4% and 74.7%, respectively. The exposure rate was noted to be significantly lower in the lightweight mesh group ($P = 0.04$ for Perigee™ and $P < 0.001$ for Apogee™) in this study.

The Prolift® mesh delivery system is based on the "TVM technique," which was first described in 2004 [3] and is one of the most studied vaginal mesh procedures designed to correct prolapse. The Prolift® trocar-based mesh delivery system was marketed with three different kit options: anterior, posterior, and total. The first published report of outcomes of the Prolift® system was a French multicenter retrospective series of 110 patients [29]. Many of the surgeons involved in this study were involved in the original development of the TVM technique. All of the patients in this study had ≥ stage III prolapse: 54% underwent the total Prolift®, 26% the posterior Prolift®, and 20% the anterior Prolift® procedure. In this initial series, there were one bladder injury and two hematomas that required surgical intervention. At short-term follow-up, the mesh exposure and prolapse recurrence rates were both 4.7%. The results of this original investigation were promising enough to stimulate great interest in this technique, and soon other centers began reporting their outcomes.

One of the first and largest studies was conducted by the Nordic Transvaginal Mesh Group, a multinational group of surgeons from Sweden, Denmark, Finland,

and Norway. Between 2006 and 2007, they recruited 261 patients from 26 centers to enroll in a prospective study: 48% underwent the anterior Prolift®, 27% the posterior Prolift®, and 25% the total Prolift® procedure [30]. At 1-year the respective anatomic cure rates were 81%, 82%, and 79%. Visceral (bladder and rectal) perforations occurred in 9 of 252 (3.4%) of patients, and the 1-year erosion rate was 11% of which 7 (2.8%) required surgical intervention.

Other centers looked at specific clinical applications such as posthysterectomy and advanced prolapse. A retrospective series of 97 patients undergoing repair of posthysterectomy prolapse with the Prolift® (47% anterior, 29% posterior, and 24% total) reported on ≥1-year outcomes [31]. Anatomic success (≤ stage I in the treated compartment, including the apex) was noted in 87%, and there were significant improvements in domain-specific quality of life questionnaires. No mesh exposures were seen in this population. The same center carried out a retrospective cohort study of 90 (45 per arm) older patients (≥65 years) with severe prolapse (leading edge ≥4 cm beyond the hymen) undergoing either Prolift® of obliterative surgery (LeFort colpocleisis or total colpectomy) [32]. The rates of recurrence (prolapse beyond the hymen) (2.2% vs. 6.7%, respectively, $P = 0.30$) and patient satisfaction (86% vs. 92%, respectively, $P = 0.38$) were comparable between groups. Operative time, estimated blood loss, and complication rates were either equal or lower in the Prolift® group.

Six randomized clinical trials have been published comparing the Prolift® procedure to native tissue repair; the anatomic outcome results of these RCTs are compiled in Table 14.1 [33–38]. Overall, all but one showed a statistically significant difference in anatomic cure favoring the mesh-based repair. The Gutman et al. study [35] was the smallest study and did not meet its predetermined sample size, which may be why the difference in anatomic outcomes (14% lower cure rate in the native tissue arm) was not found to be statistically significant. Most of these differences were noted in the anterior compartment. However, two studies noted a difference in posterior compartment anatomic outcomes as well. A study of surgery only for recurrent POP showed a significantly higher posterior cure rate in the mesh arm (76.5% vs. 95.9%, $P = 0.003$) [33]. The other noted significantly different POP-Q values in both the posterior and apical compartments at 1-year follow-up [37].

Only three of the six trials looked at subjective cure. In one trial this outcome was comparable between arms [33], and in the smallest study, a difference of 11% was noted [35], but again this was not statistically significant. In the largest trial,

Table 14.1 Anatomic cure with Prolift® vs. native tissue repair

Study	Patients (*N*)	Length (mo)	Compartment studied	Mesh cure anatomic (%)	Native cure anatomic (%)	*P* value
Withagen et al. [33]	194	12	All	92.2	44.9	< 0.001
Altman et al. [34]	389	12	Anterior	82	48	< 0.001
Gutman et al. [35]	65	36	All	85	71	**0.45**
Halaska et al. [36]	168	12	All	83	61	0.003
Svabik et al. [37]	72	12	All	97	35	< 0.001
Dos Reis Brandão da Silveira et al. [38]	184	12	Anterior posterior	86.4 97.7	70.4 91.4	0.019 0.089

subjective cure was higher in the mesh arm (62% vs. 75%, $P = 0.008$) [34]. All trials reported on either de novo dyspareunia rates or Pelvic Organ Prolapse/Urinary Incontinence Sexual Questionnaire (PISQ) scores. There were no significant differences noted between arms on these outcomes in any of the studies. De novo dyspareunia rates ranged from 3.7% to 10.3% in the native tissue arm and from 3.4% to 8.1% in the mesh arm. Four studies looked at pelvic pain beyond the immediate postoperative period, and no differences were noted between groups. Pain rates ranged from 0.0% to 11.7% in the native tissue arm and from 0.5% to 10.1% in the mesh arm. De novo SUI rates were noted in five studies, these rates were comparable between study arms in all but one study that noted a significantly higher rate in the mesh arm ($P = 0.02$) [37]. Mesh exposure rates varied from 3.0% to 20.8%. Three of the studies reported the percentage of patients that needed to undergo mesh revision under anesthesia; these rates ranged from 3.0% to 7.6% [34, 36, 37].

Most of these RCTs followed patients for 12 months, but there are quite a few studies with longer-term follow-up that show comparable longer-term success rates (Table 14.2) [39–47].

Table 14.2 Studies of Prolift® with 40 or more patients with >1 year follow-up

Study	Patients (*N*)	Length of follow-up (mo)	Graft type (other surgical criteria)	Visceral injury and/or erosion	Vaginal mesh exposure (%)	Success rate (%)
Wang et al. [39]	80	36	Prolift® (severe POP, w/ hysterectomy)	1 Rectal injury	6.3	93.3
Khandwala [40]	157	13	Anterior, posterior, and total Prolift® + M	None	2.2	94
Alperin [41]	85	24	Anterior, posterior, and total Prolift®	2 Bladder and 1 rectal injury	13	91.5
Gad [42]	40	7–39	Anterior, posterior, and total Prolift®	N/A	N/A	97.5
Benbouzid et al. [43]	75	54	Anterior, posterior, and total Prolift®	N/A	5.3	85.3
de Landsheere et al. [44]	524	38	Anterior, posterior, and total Prolift®	33 Bladder and 1 rectal injury; 0 visceral erosion	2.5	97
Huang et al. [45]	65	25	Total Prolift®	1 Bladder and 1 rectal injury	2	94
Lo [46]	43	16	Anterior and posterior Prolift® (severe POP only)	None	2.3	95
Wetta et al. [47]	68	14	Anterior, posterior, and total Prolift®	2 Bladder injuries	4.4	97.8

POP pelvic organ prolapse

Single-Incision Kits

Single-incision kits include procedures whereby the mesh is implanted through a vaginal incision without the use of trocars. A number of different systems have been marketed, but this chapter will focus on the two most popularly used systems in the United States: Elevate (American Medical Systems) and Uphold™ (Boston Scientific); as of this writing only, the latter is still on the market.

The Elevate system was available in both an anterior/apical and a posterior/apical kit. In both kits, self-fixating tips (shaped like arrow heads) swedged onto mesh arms are placed into the sacrospinous ligament, which are then articulated to bodies of mesh placed into the anterior or posterior compartments through a single vertical vaginal incision. In the case of the anterior system, there are two additional self-fixating tips swedged onto the distal aspect of the body of the mesh that are inserted into the distal aspect of the arcus tendineus.

There are substantially less prospective and comparative data on the Elevate system than the Prolift®. However, there are two high-quality, multicenter prospective series looking at the Elevate. The first investigates outcomes with the posterior system [48] and the second with the anterior system [49]. The study of the posterior system followed 139 women for 12 months after surgery. This showed objective posterior wall and apical cure rates of 92.5% and 89.2%, respectively. The mesh exposure rate was 6.5% [48]. The study design of the anterior system was similar with a sample size of 128 women. This showed objective anterior wall and apical cure rates of 87.5% and 88.5%, respectively. The mesh exposure rate was similar to the posterior series at 6.3% [49]. Both studies noted significant improvement in domain-specific quality of life and sexual function questionnaires and other adverse rates of de novo SUI, dyspareunia, and hematoma formation at <5%.

While there are no RCTs involving Elevate, there are at least four retrospective cohort studies comparing Elevate to other transvaginal mesh systems. Three of these compare anterior Elevate to the Perigee™ system [50–52], and the other is a comparison to anterior Prolift® [53]. Most of the studies had sample sizes between 50 and 100 in each arm and follow-up of at least 1 year. All studies showed comparable anatomic success between the two systems studied. However, all but one, Wong et al. [50] showed lower mesh exposure rates in the Elevate group.

The second nontrocar/single-incision kit, Uphold™, is the only kit currently being marketed for prolapse in the United States. Unlike many of the other systems, Uphold™ has only one kit, and it is designed to treat anterior/apical defects. There is no posterior compartment equivalent. The mesh used in the original iteration of the Uphold™ had a weight of 45 g/m^2; the mesh used in the current kit (Uphold™ LITE) is 25 g/m^2. The mesh delivery system includes a body with two extending arms of mesh that are fixated in a tension-free manner to the sacrospinous ligaments using a push-and-catch suturing device (Capio®, Boston Scientific) that is included in the kit.

There have been five large published series of this procedure (only one of these was a comparative trial). A summary of the findings of these studies is displayed in Table 14.3 [54–58]. All followed the study population for at least 12 months, three were prospective, and three limited their population to *utero*vaginal prolapse

Table 14.3 Anatomic cure and mesh exposure rates with uphold system

Study	Study design	Length (mo)	Patients (*N*)	Population	Anatomic success (%)	Rate of mesh exposure (&)
Vu et al. [54]	Single-site retrospective	12	115	Uterovaginal and vaginal vault prolapse	93	2.6
Jirschele et al. [55]	Multicenter prospective	12	99	Uterovaginal prolapse	96.6	6.5
Letouzey et al. [56]	Retrospective	23	115	Uterovaginal prolapse	92	2.7
Altman et al. [57]	Multicenter prospective	12	207	Uterovaginal and vaginal vault prolapse	94	1.4[a]
Gutman et al. [58]	Multicenter prospective	12	76	Uterovaginal prolapse	80	6.6

[a]This was the percentage of patients who underwent surgery for mesh exposure. Total percentage of exposure not listed. Two additional patients had mesh removed for other complications

patients. All but one demonstrated an anatomic success rate of greater than 90%. The rate of mesh exposure ranged from 2.6% to 6.6%.

The first study comes from the center that helped develop the technique and product [54]. In it the authors demonstrate the efficacy of the device in both uterovaginal and posthysterectomy POP. In some of the cases of uterovaginal prolapse, the uterus was preserved, and in others a concomitant hysterectomy was performed. As with other mesh-based prolapse repairs [59], a higher rate of mesh erosion appeared to be associated with concomitant hysterectomy at the time of the Uphold™ procedure. Notably, all but one of the remaining studies limited their populations to patients with uterovaginal prolapse, with the vast majority of the subjects undergoing hysteropexy.

The first of these studies investigating Uphold™ for the treatment of uterovaginal prolapse is a multicenter, prospective trial in which all of the 99 subjects underwent hysteropexy [56]. The anatomic success rate at 12 months was 96.6%, with an exposure rate of 6.5%, and a reoperation rate of 7.5%. All of the domain-specific quality of life questionnaires showed significant pre- to postoperative improvement. In the second study, 17 (14.8%) of the 115 subjects underwent concomitant hysterectomy, and the remaining subjects underwent hysteropexy [57]. There were three patients (2.7%) who required surgery for vaginal mesh exposure in this study; one of the three patients had undergone concomitant hysterectomy. The anatomic success rate was 93% at a mean follow-up of 23 months, and no patients required surgery for recurrent prolapse. In addition to the three abovementioned patients, one other patient underwent partial mesh removal for subsequent pain attributed to pudendal neuralgia, for a total reoperation rate of 3.4% for mesh-related complications. The last study limited to patients with uterovaginal prolapse is a multicenter, prospective parallel cohort study comparing laparoscopic hysteropexy (n = 74) to vaginal mesh (Uphold™) hysteropexy (n = 76) [58]. In this study, the operative time for the laparoscopic approach was almost three times that of the vaginal ($P < 0.001$). There were no differences in blood loss, complications, and hospital stay. Anatomic and symptomatic cure rates were comparable between the laparoscopic and vaginal groups (83% vs. 80%, $P = 0.20$ and 90% vs. 95%, $P = 0.40$, respectively). The rate of mesh exposure was also similar between groups (2.7% vs. 6.6%, $P = 0.44$).

The remaining Uphold™ study is a prospective, multicenter single cohort study of 207 women with either uterovaginal or posthysterectomy POP [59]. Objective and subjective cure rates were similar to those of the previous studies: 94% and 91%, respectively. The overall rate of serious complications was 4.3%. Within 1 year of follow-up, seven (3.4%) patients underwent reoperation for prolapse recurrence, and three (1.4%) underwent surgical revision of mesh due to exposure.

Multiple prospective studies comparing Uphold™ to other types of surgical repair of POP are currently underway. These include the FDA-mandated 522 cohort study comparing 3-year outcomes between Uphold™ and vaginal native tissue repair and two randomized trials conducted by the Pelvic Floor Disorders Network: one comparing hysteropexy with Uphold™ to vaginal hysterectomy with uterosacral ligament vault suspension and, the other, a three-arm study comparing transvaginal native tissue repair, TVM with Uphold™, and sacral colpopexy. Thus, robust comparative outcome data regarding the Uphold™ procedure should be available within the next few years.

Overall Outcomes of Transvaginal Mesh for Prolapse

Many individual studies and systematic reviews exist to give us an overall appreciation regarding the various outcomes associated with vaginal mesh procedures for POP as a whole. The goal of augmenting a prolapse repair with synthetic mesh is to increase the longevity and durability of the repair. Obviously, however, anatomic cure is far from the only important outcome for prolapse surgery. Equally important are complications and subjective outcomes.

Erosion

Erosion of mesh into the vaginal lumen (exposure) or into visceral organs is a unique complication of mesh-based prolapse repairs. Fortunately, erosion into visceral organs is a rare complication [60]. But vaginal exposure is noted in most published studies of vaginal mesh.

The rate of mesh exposure has been examined in a number of systematic reviews. One such review that includes 91 (total $N = 10{,}440$) comparative and single-arm studies that have an $n \geq 30$ noted an average rate of 10.3% (95% CI 9.7–11.0) [61]. A systematic review limited to randomized trials shows an average rate of 8% of patients requiring reoperation for mesh exposure [62]. Another systematic review limited to comparative studies showed a mesh exposure rate ranging from 1.4% to 19% in the anterior compartment and 3–36% when mesh was placed in multiple compartments [5].

Risk factors that have been associated with the risk of exposure include smoking, mesh placed in multiple compartments, surgeon experience [63], multiple childbirth, somatic inflammatory disease (i.e., rheumatoid arthritis) [64], older age [65], concurrent hysterectomy, and inverted "T" colpotomy [66]. Surgical technique almost certainly plays a role in the risk of mesh exposure, given the wide range of the incidence of this outcome. In fact, one multicenter RCT demonstrated a range of mesh exposure rates from 0% to 100% at the different clinical centers, despite the use of the same mesh and mesh delivery system [63].

Other Complications

While complications such as chronic pain, dyspareunia, de novo SUI, and visceral injury are often attributed to the use of mesh in vaginal prolapse repair, these complications are certainly not unique to mesh-augmented repairs.

Pain and dyspareunia have been shown to occur postoperatively in up to 13% and 45% of mesh patients, respectively. As would be expected, pre-existing pain and dyspareunia are associated with higher rates of these conditions postoperatively [63]. However, systematic review suggests that the use of vaginal mesh in prolapse repair is not associated with a higher risk of de novo dyspareunia when compared to native tissue repairs (RR = 0.92, 95% CI 0.58–1.47) [62]. And there is no evidence from systematic review to suggest that the rate of de novo pain is any higher in mesh patients either [5].

In regard to intraoperative complications, the rates appear to be comparable between mesh and native tissue vaginal repair [5]. However, the rate of bladder injury may be higher in mesh-based repairs (RR = 3.92, 95% CI 1.62–9.5) [62].

Unmasking of occult SUI is a well-known phenomenon that occurs after surgical repair of POP. Just as correcting prolapse can lead to a resolution of incomplete bladder emptying, it can also lead to de novo SUI. It could be argued that de novo SUI is actually a marker of effective correction of prolapse. Nonetheless, de novo SUI is an unwelcome outcome of prolapse repair. The data on de novo SUI as it relates to mesh and native tissue repairs are mixed. The risk of de novo SUI is not statistically higher (RR = 0.67, 95% CI 0.44–1.01) in mesh-augmented repairs of the anterior compartment [67], but it does appear to be when all mesh procedures are combined (RR = 1.39, 95% CI 1.06–1.82) in the meta-analysis [62]. However, the risk of undergoing repeat surgery for de novo SUI is not higher in either population.

The need to undergo surgery for recurrent POP is perhaps one of the best indicators of prolapse repair failure. A meta-analysis involving outcomes from 12 RCTs suggests that the rate of repeat surgery for prolapse is lower in transvaginal mesh surgery as compared to native tissue repair (RR = 0.53, 95% CI 0.31–0.88) [62]. A similar analysis limited to anterior compartment repair suggests that the rate of need for repeat surgery for prolapse is approximately twice as high (RR = 2.03, 95% CI 1.15–3.58) following native tissue repair as compared to mesh [67]. Risk factors for recurrent prolapse include age <60 years, obesity, and preoperative stage III or IV prolapse [17, 68]; furthermore, the anterior compartment is the site most prone to recurrence [69]. It therefore follows that patients with these characteristics may be the most likely to benefit from a mesh-augmented repair.

There are no randomized studies comparing mesh-based repairs that are done abdominally with robotic assistance to those done transvaginally. However, there are two retrospective cohort studies that compare outcomes between these procedures. One looked specifically at the risk of reoperation after these two types of surgeries [70]. The median length of follow-up in the 181 women who underwent robotic surgery was 3 months, and it was 11.5 months in the 64 women who had vaginal mesh surgery. The authors found no difference in overall rate of reoperation for apical prolapse (10.3% vs. 7.8%, respectively, $P = 0.63$). They specifically found no differences in the rates of reoperation for prolapse (3.0% vs. 0%, $P = 0.33$) or mesh exposure (1.2% vs. 3.1%, $P = 0.58$). Similarly, the authors of the other study found equivalent rates (2.6% in both arms) of mesh exposure in the robotic and vaginal groups [71]. No difference was noted in blood loss, hospital stay, or time of return to normal voiding.

Anatomic Outcomes

Anatomic cure is the primary outcome that is used to calculate sample size (and thus power) for most RCTs comparing mesh to native tissue repair. As such, the data for this outcome are the most robust data we have regarding vaginal mesh outcomes. When anatomic cure is assessed in meta-analysis, it is consistently noted to be higher in mesh-based vaginal repair, particularly in regard to the anterior compartment. One review from Brazil noted an odds ratio of 1.28 (95% CI 1.07–1.53) significantly favoring mesh over native tissue [72]. The difference noted by the most recent Cochrane review was more distinct with a relative risk of 0.45 (95% CI 0.36–0.55). When the analysis was limited to studies of anterior compartment repair, the benefit in the mesh group was more pronounced (RR = 0.36, 95% CI 0.28–0.47) [62]. A similar analysis by the same group suggests that if recurrent anterior compartment prolapse occurs in 13% of women after mesh repair, 32–45% would have recurrence after native tissue repair [67].

Subjective Outcomes

While early systematic reviews noted some benefit of mesh augmentation in regard to anatomic outcomes following vaginal POP repair, there were not enough data to comment on differences in subjective outcomes [60]. However, in the last 10 years, a large increase in the number of higher-quality comparative studies of transvaginal mesh vs. native tissue surgeries has made such an analysis possible.

Two independent meta-analyses have addressed this topic and have drawn the same conclusion. The first looks at "awareness of prolapse" after surgery as the variable of interest in randomized trials [62]. The authors conclude that this outcome at one to 3 years was less likely after mesh repair (RR = 0.66, 95% CI 0.54–0.81). The second [5] used two variables to measure subjective outcomes in all comparative studies: "symptoms of bulge" (Fig. 14.1) [23, 34, 73–79] and the net change from pre- to postoperative scores on the Pelvic Organ Prolapse Distress Inventory (POPDI) subscale (Fig. 14.2) [25, 77, 79–81]. Both analyses favored mesh, with a

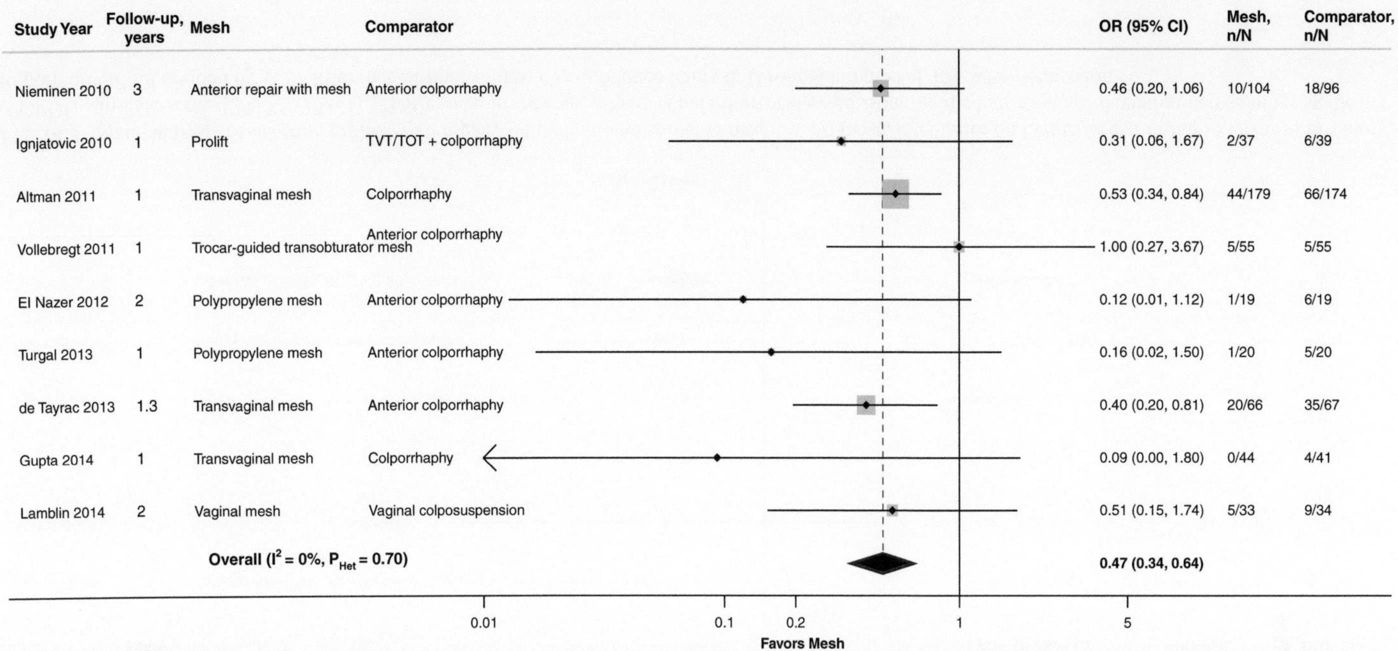

Fig. 14.1 Meta-analysis of anterior vaginal wall repair, synthetic nonabsorbable mesh vs. no mesh, subjective symptoms of a bulge postoperatively [23, 34, 73–79]. OR odds ratio, CI confidence interval, TVT/TOT tension-free vaginal tape and transobturator tape midurethral sling surgery. (From Schimpf et al. [5], with permission)

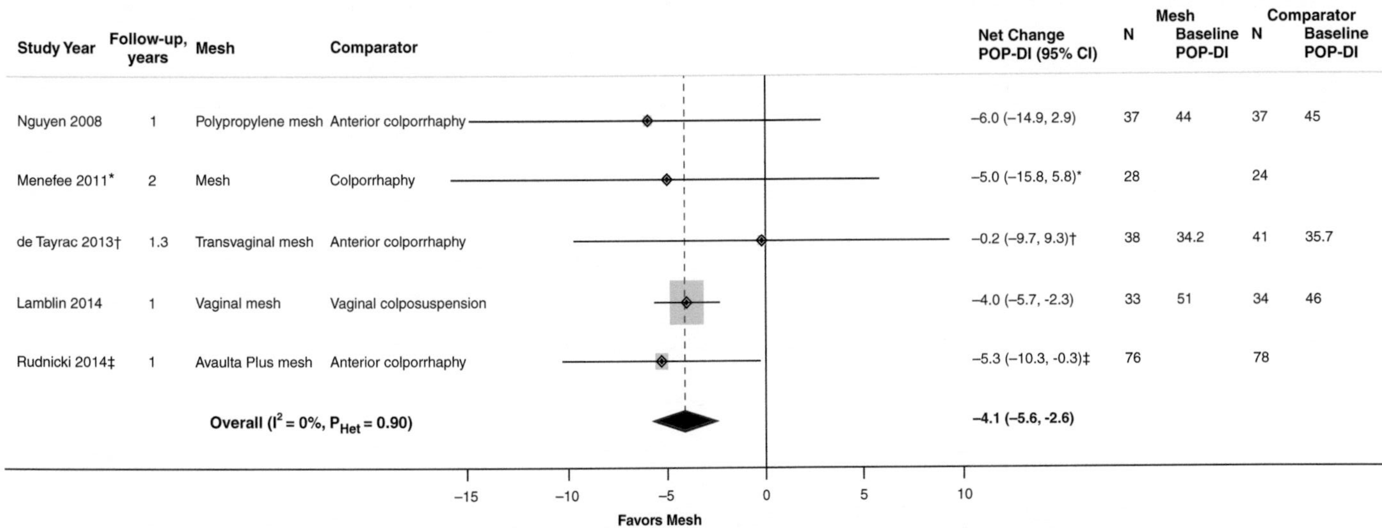

Fig. 14.2 Meta-analysis of anterior vaginal wall repair, synthetic nonabsorbable mesh vs. no mesh, total score on Pelvic Organ Prolapse Distress Inventory (POPDI) subscale score [25, 77, 79–81] (*Difference in median values; standard error derived from the median standard deviation across other studies; † Reported POP-DI divided by 3; ‡ Difference of final values; *CI* confidence interval; (From Schimpf et al. [5], with permission)

lower rate of symptoms of bulge as compared to native tissue (OR = 0.47, 95% CI 0.34–0.64) and greater improvement in POPDI score (net change = −4.1, CI −5.6 – −2.6). Sensitivity analysis of this second meta-analysis yielded similar results when limited to randomized trials. Both reviews failed to find a difference in overall quality of life and sexual function outcomes as assessed by pre- and postoperative validated questionnaires.

Conclusion

While a common criticism of vaginal mesh surgeries is a lack of data on these procedures, as this chapter demonstrates, there is actually a very large body of evidence regarding the outcomes of many of these procedures. This literature suggests that mesh use may decrease the risk of both objective and subjective prolapse recurrence, without significantly compromising the risk of sexual dysfunction or pain. However, mesh exposure is clearly a unique risk of mesh use whether it is placed vaginally or abdominally.

As such, we must continue to strive to discern in which patients this risk is outweighed by the potential benefits of vaginal mesh surgery. We know from the current data that the benefit of mesh in most patients appears to be greatest in repair of anterior compartment defects. Furthermore, the risk of recurrence is greatest in patients with more advanced (stage III and IV) defects.

When is hysterectomy indicated? And are there times when a native tissue or an abdominally placed mesh may be of greater benefit to a particular type of patient? These questions need to be addressed. Fortunately, there are number of well-designed experimental trials currently enrolling patients that should help to answer such questions. It is critical to realize, however, that while research trials give us valuable information, it is unlikely that we will ever find one single procedure that works best for every patient with POP. It is important that we continue to have a number of different surgical techniques at our disposal and that, through careful counseling with our patients, we continue to be able to tailor our surgery to best fit each individual woman suffering from pelvic floor dysfunction.

References

1. Julian T. The efficacy of Marlex mesh in the repair of severe, recurrent vaginal prolapse of the anterior midvaginal wall. Am J Obstet Gynecol. 1996;175(6):1472–5.
2. Ulmsten U, Falconer C, Johnson P, Jomaa M, Lannér L, Nilsson CG, Olsson I. A multicenter study of tension-free vaginal tape (TVT) for surgical treatment of stress urinary incontinence. Int Urogynecol J Pelvic Floor Dysfunct. 1998;9(4):210–3.
3. Debodinance P, Berrocal J, Clavé H, Cosson M, Garbin O, Jacquetin B, et al. Changing attitudes on the surgical treatment of urogenital prolapse: birth of the tension-free vaginal mesh. J Gynecol Obstet Biol Reprod (Paris). 2004;33(7):577–88. [*Article in French*].

4. Wall LL, Brown D. Commercial pressures and professional ethics: troubling revisions to the recent ACOG practice bulletins on surgery for pelvic organ prolapse. Int Urogynecol J Pelvic Floor Dysfunct. 2009;20(7):765–7.
5. Schimpf MO, Abed H, Sanses T, White AB, Lowenstein L, Ward RM, Society of Gynecologic Surgeons Systematic Review Group, et al. Graft and mesh use in transvaginal prolapse repair: a systematic review. Obstet Gynecol. 2016;128(1):81–91. https://doi.org/10.1097/AOG.0000000000001451.
6. Siddiqui NY, Grimes CL, Casiano ER, Abed HT, Jeppson PC, Olivera CK, Society of Gynecologic Surgeons Systematic Review Group, et al. Mesh sacrocolpopexy compared with native tissue vaginal repair: a systematic review and meta-analysis. Obstet Gynecol. 2015;125(1):44–55. Review
7. Gadjiev N, Tabaza R, Kirschner-Hermanns R. Mini-slings: What is known about anchorage systems? (abstract). Scientific programme, 42nd annual meeting of the international continence society, 15–19 Oct 2012, Beijing, China. Neurourol Urodyn. 2012;31(6):730–1.
8. Levi A, Nasra R, Shachar IB, Braun NM. Medium-term results of mini-arc for urinary stress incontinence in ambulatory patients under local anesthesia. Int Braz J Urol. 2016;42(6):1195–201.
9. Nager CW. Midurethral slings: evidence-based medicine vs the medicolegal system. Am J Obstet Gynecol. 2016;214(6):708.e1–5.
10. Nambiar A, Cody JD, Jeffery ST. Single-incision sling operations for urinary incontinence in women. Cochrane Database Syst Rev. 2014;6:CD008709. Review.
11. Mostafa A, Lim CP, Hopper L, Madhuvrata P, Abdel-Fattah M. Single-incision mini-slings versus standard midurethral slings in surgical management of female stress urinary incontinence: an updated systematic review and meta-analysis of effectiveness and complications. Eur Urol. 2014;65(2):402–27.
12. Lee JK, Rosamilia A, Dwyer PL, Lim YN, Muller R. Randomized trial of a single incision versus an outside-in transobturator midurethral sling in women with stress urinary incontinence: 12 month results. Am J Obstet Gynecol. 2015;213(1):35.e1–9.
13. Tutolo M, De Ridder DJ, Montorsi F, Castagna G, Deprest J, Schellart RP, et al. A minimum of 1-year follow-up for MiniArc single incision slings compared to Monarc transobturator slings: an analysis to evaluate durability of continence and medium-term outcomes. Neurourol Urodyn. 2017;36(3):803–7.
14. Kocjancic E, Erickson T, Tu LM, Gheiler E, Van Drie D. Two-year outcomes for the Altis® adjustable single incision sling system for treatment of stress urinary incontinence. Neurourol Urodyn. 2017;36(6):1582–7.
15. Serels S, Dususo M. Long term follow up of the Solyx single incision sling in the treatment of female stress urinary incontinence (SUI). Open J Urol. 2014;4(2):13–7.
16. Fialkow MF, Newton KM, Weiss NS. Incidence of recurrent pelvic organ prolapse 10 years following primary surgical management: a retrospective cohort study. Int Urogynecol J. 2008;19(11):1483–7.
17. Whiteside JL, Weber AM, Meyn LA, Walters MD. Risk factors for prolapse recurrence after vaginal repair. Am J Obstet Gynecol. 2004;191(5):1533–8.
18. Northington GM, Hudson CO, Karp D, Huber SA. Concomitant apical suspensory procedures in women with anterior vaginal wall prolapse in the United States in 2011. Int Urogynecol J. 2016;27(4):613–9.
19. Mains LM, Magnus M, Finan M. Perioperative morbidity and mortality from major gynecologic surgery in the elderly woman. J Reprod Med. 2007;52(8):677–84.
20. Whitehead WE, Bradley CS, Brown MB, Brubaker L, Gutman RE, Varner RE, Pelvic Floor Network, et al. Gastrointestinal complications following abdominal sacrocolpopexy for advanced pelvic organ prolapse. Am J Obstet Gynecol. 2007;197(1.):78.e1-78.e7):78.e1.
21. Hiltunen R, Nieminen K, Takala T, Heiskanen E, Merikari M, Niemi K, Heinonen PK. Low-weight polypropylene mesh for anterior vaginal wall prolapse: a randomized controlled trial. Obstet Gynecol. 2007;110(2 Pt 2):455–62.

22. Nieminen K, Hiltunen R, Heiskanen E, Takala T, Niemi K, Merikari M, Heinonen PK. Symptom resolution and sexual function after anterior vaginal wall repair with or without polypropylene mesh. Int J Urogynecol. 2008;19(12):1611–6.
23. Nieminen K, Hiltunen R, Takala T, Heiskanen E, Merikari M, Niemi K, Heinonen PK. Outcomes after anterior vaginal wall repair with mesh: a randomized, controlled trial with a 3 year follow-up. Am J Obstet Gynecol. 2010;203(3):235.e1–8.
24. Glazener CM, Breeman S, Elders A, Hemming C, Cooper KG, Freeman RM, PROSPECT Study Group, et al. Mesh, graft, or standard repair for women having primary transvaginal anterior or posterior compartment prolapse surgery: two parallel-group, multicenter, randomized, controlled trials (PROSPECT). Lancet. 2017;389(10067):381–92.
25. Nguyen JN, Burchette RJ. Outcome after anterior vaginal prolapse repair: a randomized controlled trial. Obstet Gynecol. 2008;111(4):891–8.
26. Moore RD, Beyer RD, Jacoby K, Freedman SJ, McCammon KA, Gambla MT. Prospective multicenter trial assessing type I, polypropylene mesh placed via transobturator route for the treatment of anterior vaginal prolapse with 2-year follow-up. Int Urogynecol J. 2010;21(5):545–52.
27. Moore RD, Lukban JC. Comparison of vaginal mesh extrusion rates between a lightweight type I polypropylene mesh versus heavier mesh in the treatment of pelvic organ prolapse. Int Urogynecol J. 2012;23(10):1379–86.
28. Karmakar D, Hayward L, Smalldridge J, Lin S. Vaginal mesh for prolapse: a long-term prospective study of 218 mesh kits from a single Centre. Int Urogynecol J. 2015;26(8):1161–70.
29. Fatton B, Amblard J, Debodinance P, Cosson M, Jacquetin B. Transvaginal repair of genital prolapse: preliminary results of a new tension-free vaginal mesh (Prolift®™ technique) – a case series multicentric study. Int Urogynecol J Pelvic Floor Dysfunct. 2007;18(7):743–52.
30. Elmér C, Altman D, Engh ME, Axelsen S, Väyrynen T, Falconer C, Nordic Transvaginal Mesh Group. Trocar-guided transvaginal mesh repair of pelvic organ prolapse. Obstet Gynecol. 2009;113(1):117–26.
31. van Raalte HM, Lucente VR, Molden SM, Haff R, Murphy M. One-year anatomic and quality-of-life outcomes after the Prolift® procedure for treatment of posthysterectomy prolapse. Am J Obstet Gynecol. 2008;199:694.e1–6.
32. Murphy M, Sternschuss G, Haff R, van Raalte H, Saltz S, Lucente V. Quality of life and surgical satisfaction after vaginal reconstructive vs obliterative surgery for the treatment of advanced pelvic organ prolapse. Am J Obstet Gynecol. 2008;198(5):573.e1–7.
33. Withagen MI, Milani AL, den Boon J, Vervest HA, Vierhout ME. Trocar-guided mesh compared with conventional vaginal repair in recurrent prolapse: a randomized controlled trial. Obstet Gynecol. 2011;117(2, Pt 1):242–50.
34. Altman D, Väyrynen T, Engh ME, Axelsen S, Falconer C, Nordic Transvaginal Mesh Group. Anterior colporrhaphy versus transvaginal mesh for pelvic-organ prolapse. N Engl J Med. 2011;364(19):1826–36.
35. Gutman RE, Nosti PA, Sokol AI, Sokol ER, Peterson JL, Wang H, Iglesia CB. Three-year outcomes of vaginal mesh for prolapse: a randomized controlled trial. Obstet Gynecol. 2013;122(4):770–7.
36. Halaska M, Maxova K, Sottner O, Svabik K, Mlcoch M, Kolarik D, et al. A multicenter, randomized, prospective, controlled study comparing sacrospinous fixation and transvaginal mesh in the treatment of posthysterecomy vaginal vault prolapse. Am J Obstet Gynecol. 2012;207(4):301.e1–7.
37. Svabik K, Martan A, Masata J, El-Haddad R, Hubka P. Comparison of vaginal mesh repair with sacrospinous vaginal colpopexy in the management of vaginal vault prolapse after hysterectomy in patients with levator ani avulsion: a randomized controlled trial. Ultrasound Obstet Gynecol. 2014;42(4):365–71.
38. Dos Reis Brandão da Silveira S, Haddad JM, de Jármy-Di Bella ZI, Nastri F, Kawabata MG, da Silva Carramão S, et al. Multicenter, randomized trial comparing native vaginal tissue repair and synthetic mesh repair for genital prolapse surgical treatment. Int Urogynecol J. 2015;26(3):335–42.

39. Wang FM, He CN, Song YF. Prospective study of transobturator mesh kit (Prolift®™) in pelvic reconstructive surgery with vaginal hysterectomy after 3 years' follow-up. Arch Gynecol Obstet. 2013;288(2):355–9.
40. Khandwala S. Transvaginal mesh surgery for pelvic organ prolapse: one-year outcome analysis. Female Pelvic Med Reconstr Surg. 2013;19(2):84–9.
41. Alperin M, Ellison R, Meyn L, Frankman E, Zyczynski HM. Two-year outcomes after vaginal prolapse reconstruction with mesh pelvic floor repair system. Female Pelvic Med Reconstr Surg. 2013;19(2):72–8.
42. Gad N, Duvvuru A, Burchgart B. Outcome of Prolift® mesh repair in treatment of pelvic organ prolapse and its effect on lower urinary tract symptoms: 5-year retrospective case study. J Obstet Gynaecol Res. 2013;39(1):243–9.
43. Benbouzid S, Cornu JN, Benchikh A, Chanu T, Haab F, Delmas V. Pelvic organ prolapse transvaginal repair by the Prolift® system: evaluation of efficacy and complications after a 4.5 years follow up. Int J Urol. 2012;19(11):1010–6.
44. de Landsheere L, Ismail S, Lucot JP, Deken V, Foidart JM, Cosson M. Surgical intervention after transvaginal Prolift® mesh repair: retrospective single-center study including 524 patients with 3 years' median follow-up. Am J Obstet Gynecol. 2012;206(1):83.e1–7.
45. Huang WC, Lin TY, Lau HH, Chen SS, Hsieh CH, Su TH. Outcome of transvaginal pelvic reconstructive surgery with Prolift® after a median of 2 years' follow-up. Int Urogynecol J. 2011;22(2):197–203.
46. Lo TS. One-year outcome of concurrent anterior and posterior transvaginal mesh surgery for treatment of advanced urogenital prolapse: case series. J Minim Invasive Gynecol. 2010;17(4):473–9.
47. Wetta LA, Gerten KA, Wheeler TL 2nd, Holley RL, Varner RE, Richter HE. Synthetic graft use in vaginal prolapse surgery: objective and subjective outcomes. Int Urogynecol J Pelvic Floor Dysfunct. 2009;20(11):1307–12.
48. Lukban JC, Roovers JP, Vandrie DM, Erickson T, Zylstra S, Patel MP, Moore RD. Single-incision apical and posterior mesh repair: 1-year prospective outcomes. Int Urogynecol J. 2012;23(10):1413–9.
49. Stanford EJ, Moore RD, Roovers JP, Courtieu C, Lukban JC, Bataller E, et al. Elevate anterior/apical: 12-month data showing safety and efficacy in surgical treatment of pelvic organ prolapse. Female Pelvic Med Reconstr Surg. 2013;19(2):79–83.
50. Wong V, Shek KL, Rane A, Lee J, Rosamilia A, Dietz HP. A comparison of two different mesh kit systems for anterior compartment prolapse repair. Aust N Z J Obstet Gynecol. 2014;54(3):212–7.
51. Lo TS, Bt Karim N, Cortes EF, Wu PY, Lin YH, Tan YL. Comparison between elevate anterior/apical system and Perigee™ system in pelvic organ prolapse surgery: clinical and sonographic outcomes. Int Urogynecol J. 2015;26(3):391–400.
52. Long CY, Wang CL, Wu MP, Wu CH, Lin KL, Liu CM, et al. Comparison of clinical outcomes using "elevate anterior" versus "Perigee™" system devices for the treatment of pelvic organ prolapse. Biomed Res Int. 2015:479610.
53. Rogowski A, Bienkowski P, Tarwacki D, Szafarowska M, Samochowiec J, Sienkiewicz-Jarosz H, et al. Retrospective comparison between the Prolift® and elevate anterior vaginal mesh procedures: 18-month clinical outcome. Int J Urogynecol. 2015;26(12):1815–20.
54. Vu MK, Letko J, Jirschele K, Gafni-Kane A, Nguyen A, Du H, Goldberg RP. Minimal mesh repair for apical and anterior prolapse: initial anatomical and subjective outcomes. Int J Urogynecol. 2012;23(12):1753–61.
55. Jirschele K, Seitz M, Zhou Y, Rosenblatt P, Culligan P, Sand P. A multicenter, prospective trial to evaluate mesh-augmented sacrospinous hysteropexy for uterovaginal prolapse. Int J Urogynecol. 2015;26(5):743–8.
56. Letouzey V, Ulrich D, Balenbois E, Cornille A, de Tayrac R, Fatton B. Utero-vaginal suspension using bilateral vaginal anterior sacrospinous fixation with mesh: intermediate results of a cohort study. Int J Urogynecol. 2015;26(12):1803–7.

57. Altman D, Mikkola TS, Bek KM, Rahkola-Soisalo P, Gunnarsson J, Engh ME, Falconer C, Nordic TVM group. Pelvic organ prolapse repair using the Uphold™ vaginal support system: a 1-year multicenter study. Int J Urogynecol. 2016;27(9):1337–45.
58. Gutman RE, Rardin CR, Sokol ER, Matthews C, Park AJ, Iglesia CB, et al. Vaginal and laparoscopic mesh hysteropexy for uterovaginal prolapse: a parallel cohort study. Am J Obstet Gynecol. 2017;216(1):38.e1–11.
59. Ehsani N, Ghafar MA, Antosh DD, Tan-Kim J, Warner WB, Mamik MM, et al. Risk factors for mesh extrusion after prolapse surgery: a case-control study. Female Pelvic Med Reconstr Surg. 2012;18(6):357–61.
60. Sung VW, Rogers RG, Schaffer JI, Balk EM, Uhlig K, Lau J, Society of Gynecologic Surgeons Systematic Review Group, et al. Graft use in transvaginal pelvic organ prolapse repair: a systematic review. Obstet Gynecol. 2008;112(5):1131–42.
61. Abed H, Rahn DD, Lowenstein L, Balk EM, Clemons JL, Rogers RG, Systematic Review Group of the Society of Gynecologic Surgeons. Incidence and management of graft erosion, wound granulation, and dyspareunia following vaginal prolapse repair with graft materials: a systematic review. Int J Urogynecol. 2011;22(7):789–98.
62. Maher C, Feiner B, Baessler K, et al. Transvaginal mesh or grafts compared with native tissue repair for vaginal prolapse. Cochrane Database Syst Rev. 2016;2:CD012079. Review.
63. Withagen MI, Vierhout ME, Hendriks JC, Kluivers KB, Milani AL. Risk factors for exposure, pain, and dyspareunia after tensions-free vaginal mesh procedure. Obstet Gynecol. 2011;118(3):629–36.
64. Elmér C, Falconer C, Hallin A, Larsson G, Ek M, Altman D, Nordic Transvaginal Mesh Group. Risk factors for mesh complications after trocar guided transvaginal mesh kit repair of anterior vaginal wall prolapse. Neurourol Urodyn. 2012;31(7):1165–9.
65. Araco F, Gravante G, Sorge R, De Vita D, Piccione E. Risk evaluation of smoking and age on the occurrence of postoperative erosions after transvaginal mesh repair for pelvic organ prolapse. Int Urogynecol J. 2008;19(4):473–9.
66. Collinet P, Belot F, Debodinance P, Ha Duc E, Lucot JP, Cosson M. Transvaginal mesh technique for pelvic organ prolapse repair: mesh exposure management and risk factors. Int Urogyneco J. 2006;17(4):315–20.
67. Maher C, Feiner B, Baessler K, Christmann-Schmid C, Haya N, Brown J. Surgery for women with anterior compartment prolapse. Cochrane Database Syst Rev. 2016;11:CD004014. Review
68. Diez-Itza I, Aizpitarte I, Becerro A. Risk factors for the recurrence of pelvic organ prolapse after vaginal surgery. Int Urogynecol J Pelvic Floor Dysfunct. 2007;18(11):1317–24.
69. Nieminen K, Huhtala H, Heinonen PK. Anatomic and functional assessment and risk factors for recurrent prolapse after vaginal sacrospinous fixation. Acta Obstet Gynecol Scand. 2003;82(5):471–8.
70. Martin LA, Calixte R, Finamore PS. Reoperation after robotic and vaginal mesh reconstructive surgery: a retrospective cohort study. Female Pelvic Med Reconstr Surg. 2015;21(6):315–8.
71. Jambusaria LH, Murphy M, Lucente VR. One-year functional and anatomic outcomes of robotic sacrocolpopexy versus vaginal extraperitoneal colpopexy with mesh. Female Pelvic Med Reconstr Surg. 2015;21(2):87–92.
72. Juliato CR, Santos Júnior LC, Haddad JM, Castro RA, Lima M, Castro EB. Mesh surgery for anterior vaginal wall prolapse. Rev Bras Ginecol Obstet. 2016;38(7):356–64.
73. Ignjatovic I, Stojkovic I, Basic D, Medojevic N, Potic M. Optimal primary minimally invasive treatment for patients with stress urinary incontinence and symptomatic pelvic organ prolapse: tension free slings with colporrhaphy, or Prolift® with the tension free midurethral sling? Eur J Obstet Gynecol Reprod Biol. 2010;150(1):97–101.
74. Vollebregt A, Fischer K, Gietelink D, van der Vaart CH. Primary surgical repair of anterior vaginal prolapse: a randomised trial comparing anatomical and functional outcome between anterior colporrhaphy and trocar-guided transobturator anterior mesh. BJOG. 2011;118(12):1518–27.

75. El-Nazer MA, Gomaa IA, Ismail Madkour WA, Swidan KH, El-Etriby MA. Anterior colporrhaphy versus repair with mesh for anterior vaginal wall prolapse: a comparative clinical study. Arch Gynecol Obstet. 2012;286(4):965–72.
76. Turgal M, Sivaslioglu A, Yildiz A, Dolen I. Anatomical and functional assessment of anterior colporrhaphy versus polypropylene mesh surgery in cystocele treatment. Eur J Obstet Gynecol Reprod Biol. 2013;170(2):555–8.
77. de Tayrac R, Cornille A, Eglin G, Guilbaud O, Mansoor A, Alonso S, et al. Comparison between trans-obturator trans-vaginal mesh and traditional anterior colporrhaphy in the treatment of anterior vaginal wall prolapse: results of a French RCT. Int Urogynecol J. 2013;24(10):1651–61.
78. Gupta B, Vaid NB, Suneja A, Guleria K, Jain S. Anterior vaginal prolapse repair: a randomised trial of traditional anterior colporrhaphy and self-tailored mesh repair. South African J Obstet Gynaecol. 2014;20:47–50.
79. Lamblin G, Van-Nieuwenhuyse A, Chabert P, Lebail-Carval K, Moret S, Mellier G. A randomized controlled trial comparing anatomical and functional outcome between vaginal colposuspension and transvaginal mesh. Int Urogynecol J. 2014;25(7):961–70.
80. Menefee SA, Dyer KY, Lukacz ES, Simsiman AJ, Luber KM, Nguyen JN. Colporrhaphy compared with mesh or graft-reinforced vaginal paravaginal repair for anterior vaginal wall prolapse: a randomized controlled trial. Obstet Gynecol. 2011;118:1337–44.
81. Rudnicki M, Laurikainen E, Pogosean R, Kinne I, Jakobsson U, Teleman P. Anterior colporrhaphy compared with collagen-coated transvaginal mesh for anterior vaginal wall prolapse: a randomised controlled trial. BJOG. 2014;121:102–10.

Index

S. A. Shobeiri (ed.), *The Innovation and Evolution of Medical Devices*,
https://doi.org/10.1007/978-3-319-97073-8

N

O

MIX
Papier aus verantwortungsvollen Quellen
Paper from responsible sources
FSC® C105338

If you have any concerns about our products,
you can contact us on
ProductSafety@springernature.com

In case Publisher is established outside the EU,
the EU authorized representative is:
Springer Nature Customer Service Center GmbH
Europaplatz 3, 69115 Heidelberg, Germany

Printed by Libri Plureos GmbH
in Hamburg, Germany